The Hip and Pelvis in Sports Medicine and Primary Care

The Hip and Pelvis in Sports Medicine and Primary Care

Editors

Peter H. Seidenberg, MD, FAAFP
King Medical Care, Bloomsburg, PA, USA

Jimmy D. Bowen, MD, FAAPMR, CSCS, CAQ Sports Medicine
Orthopeadic Associates of Southeast Missouri,
Cape Girardeau, MO, USA

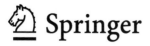

Editors
Peter H. Seidenberg
Sports Medicine and Family
 Medicine Physician
President
King Medical Care, Inc.
3151 Columbia Blvd
Suite 100
Bloomsburg, PA 17815
USA
seidenph@slu.edu

Jimmy D. Bowen
Orthopeadic Associates
 of Southeast Missouri
Cape Girardeau, MO
USA
jbowen@ortho48.com

ISBN 978-1-4419-5787-0   e-ISBN 978-1-4419-5788-7
DOI 10.1007/978-1-4419-5788-7
Springer New York Dordrecht Heidelberg London

Library of Congress Control Number: 2010924819

© Springer Science+Business Media, LLC 2010
All rights reserved. This work may not be translated or copied in whole or in part without the written permission of the publisher (Springer Science+Business Media, LLC, 233 Spring Street, New York, NY 10013, USA), except for brief excerpts in connection with reviews or scholarly analysis. Use in connection with any form of information storage and retrieval, electronic adaptation, computer software, or by similar or dissimilar methodology now known or hereafter developed is forbidden.
The use in this publication of trade names, trademarks, service marks, and similar terms, even if they are not identified as such, is not to be taken as an expression of opinion as to whether or not they are subject to proprietary rights.
While the advice and information in this book are believed to be true and accurate at the date of going to press, neither the authors nor the editors nor the publisher can accept any legal responsibil-ity for any errors or omissions that may be made. The publisher makes no warranty, express or im-plied, with respect to the material contained herein.

Printed on acid-free paper

Springer is part of Springer Science+Business Media (www.springer.com)

Preface

What a great opportunity it is to participate in the body of information advancing the study of musculoskeletal medicine. As the physician, the readers can attest that didactic presentations of musculoskeletal complaints are at a minimum during undergraduate training. The advancement of individual clinical understanding of this field many times is left to the practitioner. Out of imagination, passion, or frustration, we the musculoskeletal practitioners seek to improve our abilities to provide better clinical diagnostic endeavors. The hip and pelvis is an area in musculoskeletal and sports medicine that provides continued mystery. It is the last great bastion of the unknown. Our hope in bringing together many excellent clinician authors is to provide the basis for improved approach to the patient and athlete who have complaints involving the hip and pelvis. Each chapter begins with a clinical case which is probably similar to the patients you see in your practices. Each chapter provides an approach to the diagnosis of hip and pelvis pain and dysfunction that hopefully is easily applicable to your daily activities as a practitioner. Most importantly, we hope that the material contained within this book helps you provide improved care, satisfaction, and function for your patient athletes.

Jimmy D. Bowen

Contents

1 Epidemiology of Hip and Pelvis Injury 1
  BRANDON LARKIN

2 Physical Examination of the Hip and Pelvis 9
  DEVIN P. MCFADDEN AND PETER H. SEIDENBERG

3 Functional and Kinetic Chain Evaluation
  of the Hip and Pelvis 37
  PER GUNNAR BROLINSON AND MARK ROGERS

4 Gait Assessment 71
  JIMMY D. BOWEN AND GERRY SALTER

5 Imaging of Hip and Pelvis Injuries 87
  DONALD J. FLEMMING AND ERIC A. WALKER

6 Adult Hip and Pelvis Disorders 115
  PETER H. SEIDENBERG

7 Hip and Pelvis Injuries in Childhood
  and Adolescence 149
  CHRISTOPHER S. NASIN AND MARJORIE C. NASIN

8 Specific Considerations in Geriatric Athletes 171
  ROCHELLE M. NOLTE

9 Hip and Pelvis Injuries in Special Populations 187
  DORIANNE R. FELDMAN,
  MARLÍS GONZÁLEZ-FERNÁNDEZ, AARTI A. SINGLA,
  BRIAN J. KRABAK, AND SANDEEP SINGH

10 Functional Therapeutic and Core Strengthening 207
   GERARD A. MALANGA AND STEVE M. AYDIN

11 Manual Medicine of the Hip and Pelvis 233
   CHARLES W. WEBB AND JAYSON CANNON

12 Taping and Bracing for Pelvic and Hip Injuries 263
   SCOTT A. MAGNES, LANCE RINGHAUSEN,
   PETER H. SEIDENBERG

13	Nonsurgical Interventions.	271
	MICHAEL D. OSBORNE AND TARIQ M. AWAN	
14	Treatment Options for Osteoarthritis of the Hip.	297
	HEATHER M. GILLESPIE AND WILLIAM W. DEXTER	
15	Surgical Interventions in Hip and Pelvis Injuries	317
	CARL WIERKS AND JOHN H. WILCKENS	
Appendix		337
Index		349

Contributors

Tariq M. Awan, DO, Department of Sports Medicine, Detroit Medical Center, Warren, MI, USA

Steve M. Aydin, DO, Department of Physical Medicine and Rehabilitation, UMDNJ–NJMS, Kessler Institute for Rehabilitation, Mahwah, NJ, USA

Jimmy D. Bowen, MD, FAAPMR, CSCS, CAQ Sports Medicine, Orthopeadic Associates of Southeast Missouri, Medical Director for Sports Medicine, Saint Francis Medical Center, Cape Girardeau, MO, USA

Per Gunnar Brolinson, DO, FAOASM, FAAFP, Associate Professor, Department of Family Medicine, Blacksburg, VA, USA; Team Physician, Virginia Tech and US Freestyle Ski Team, Blacksburg, VA, USA; Edward Via Virginia College of Osteopathic Medicine, Blacksburg, VA, USA; Virginia Tech, Blacksburg, VA, USA; Discipline Chair, Department of Sports Medicine, Blacksburg, VA, USA

Jayson Cannon, DC, Cannon Chiropractic, Atoka, TN, USA

William W. Dexter, MD, FACSM, Director, Sports Medicine Program, Maine Medical Center, Portland, ME, USA

Dorianne R. Feldman, MD, MSPT, Chief Resident, Department of Physical Medicine and Rehabilitation, Johns Hopkins University School of Medicine, Baltimore, MD, USA

Donald J. Flemming, MD, Associate Professor, Department of Radiology, Penn State Hershey Medical Center, Hershey, PA, USA

Heather M. Gillespie, MD, MPH, Sports Medicine Fellow, Sports Medicine Program, Maine Medical Center, Portland, ME, USA

Marlís González-Fernández, MD, PhD, Assistant Professor,
Department of Physical Medicine and Rehabilitation,
School of Medicine, Johns Hopkins University,
Baltimore, MD, USA

Brian J. Krabak, MD, MBS, Clinical Associate Professor,
Department of Rehabilitation, Orthopaedics and Sports
Medicine, Seattle Children's Hospital, University of Washington,
Seattle, WA, USA

Brandon Larkin, MD, Primary Care Sports Medicine,
St. Peters Bone and Joint Surgery, St. Peters, MO, USA

Scott A. Magnes, MD, ACT, FAAOS, FAAFP, FACSM,
Chairman, Department of Orthopaedic Surgery, Naval Hospital,
Jacksonville, FL, USA

Gerard A. Malanga, MD, Director, New Jersey Sports Institute,
NJ, USA; Associate Professor, Department of Physical Medicine
and Rehabilitation, Verona, NJ, USA

Devin P. McFadden, MD, Family Medicine Resident,
Department of Family Medicine, DeWitt Army Community
Hospital, Ft. Belvoir, VA, USA

Christopher S. Nasin, MD, Gaithersburg, MD, USA

Marjorie C. Nasin, MD, Gaithersburg, Virginia

Rochelle M. Nolte, MD, FAAFP, Family Physician, Primary Care
Sports Medicine, US Coast Guard, San Diego, CA, USA

Michael D. Osborne, MD, Assistant Professor of Physical Medicine
and Rehabilitation, and Assistant Professor of Anesthesiology,
Mayo Clinic College of Medicine, Jacksonville, FL, USA;
Mayo Clinic Jacksonville, Jacksonville, FL, USA;
Department of Physical Medicine and Rehabilitation,
Jacksonville, FL, USA; Department of Pain Medicine,
Jacksonville, FL, USA

Lance Ringhausen, ATC, Head Athletic Trainer, McKendree
College, Lebanon, IL, USA

Mark Rogers, DO, MA, Primary Care Sports Medicine Fellow, Edward Via Virginia College of Osteopathic Medicine, Blacksburg, VA, USA; Department of Sports Medicine, Virginia Tech, Blacksburg, VA, USA

Gerry Salter, MBA, PT, ATC, CSCS, Director, Orthopaedic Service Line, Saint Francis Medical Center, Cape Girardeau, MI, USA

Peter H. Seidenberg, MD, FAAFP, President and Co-founder, King Medical Care Inc., Bloomsburg, PA, USA

Sandeep Singh, MD, Clinical Associate, Department of Physical Medicine and Rehabilitation, Johns Hopkins University, Baltimore, MD, USA

Aarti A. Singla, MD, Resident, Department of Physical Medicine and Rehabilitation, Johns Hopkins University, Baltimore, MD, USA

Eric A. Walker, MD, Assistant Professor, Department of Radiology, Penn State Milton S. Hershey Medical Center, Hershey, PA, USA

Charles W. Webb, DO, Director, Department of Family Medicine, Sports Medicine, Oregon Health and Science University, Portland, OR, USA

Carl Wierks, MD, Resident, Department of Orthopaedic Surgery, Johns Hopkins Bayview Medical Center, Baltimore, MD, USA

John H. Wilckens, MD, Chairman, Department of Orthopaedic Surgery, Johns Hopkins University, Johns Hopkins Bayview Medical Center, Baltimore, MD, USA

Chapter 1
Epidemiology of Hip and Pelvis Injury

Brandon Larkin

CLINICAL PEARLS

- Injuries to the hip and pelvis are common among both athletes and the general population.
- The incidence and etiology of hip and pelvis injury vary depending on patients' age, gender, and the sport in which they participate.
- Hip and pelvis injury and pain are most common in adolescents and older adults.
- Explosive and contact sports carry the highest risk of hip and pelvis injury.
- Women are twice as likely to suffer from hip pain as men.

CASE REPORT: PRESENTATION

Chief Complaint and History
A 17-year-old female high school basketball player presents with pain in the lateral aspect of the right hip that radiates down the lateral thigh. She reports a painful "snapping" sensation as she runs down the court. Initially, she noted this pain only while running during practices and games, but it has recently begun to bother her during normal ambulation.

Physical Examination
Examination of the right hip reveals no obvious deformity. There is tenderness to palpation of the greater trochanter. Range of motion of the hip is full in flexion, extension, abduction, adduction,

internal rotation, and external rotation. While lying on the left side, passive internal and external rotation of the right hip reproduces symptoms. There is a positive Trendelenberg test bilaterally.

INTRODUCTION

Hip and pelvis injuries are typically not the most common etiology for pain in lower extremity in athletes or in the general population. However, many of these conditions carry significant associated morbidity that makes them important in the scope of musculoskeletal care. Diagnosis is often challenging, as hip and pelvis pain is often secondary to numerous pathologic processes. Twenty-seven to ninety percent of patients presenting with groin pain are eventually found to have more than one associated injury.[1] In children and adolescents, those with hip pain have a higher prevalence of pain in the lower back and lower extremity joints, further clouding the diagnosis.[2] Additionally, in patients presenting with hip pathology, the hip is not initially recognized as the source of pain in 60% of all cases.[3] An individual's predisposition to injury and the type of injury sustained vary greatly on the basis of age and type of recreational activity.

Hip pain is often caused by sports-related injury. Ten to twenty-four percent of injuries sustained during athletics or recreational activities in children are hip related,[4] and 5–6% of adult sports injuries originate in the hip and pelvis.[3,5] Pain may result from either acute injury or chronic pathology due to excessive or repetitive activity that places significant demand on the hip and pelvis. The hip bears a tremendous burden during typical weight-bearing activities of daily living. Hip loading is further increased by up to 5–8% during exercise, leading to elevated risk of injury.[6] As a significant element of the body's core musculature, the pelvis also provides an important biomechanical foundation for the lower extremities and is often a hidden contributor to pain in more distal joints.

This chapter will consider the incidence of hip and pelvis pain and injury in the general population as well as in selected subsets. It will also discuss factors that have been shown to increase the risk of injury to this region, including both anatomic features and characteristics of specific sport participation.

AGE

The age of the patient is the single most important factor in determining the etiology of hip and pelvis pain. In very young children, there is rarely a significant acute injury, but several common orthopedic entities involving this region may initially present with exercise-associated pain. As a child grows, skeletal development occurs in a predictable pattern with the appearance of apophyses and epiphyses and their eventual fusion. During growth, these are areas of relative weakness, and avulsion injuries to the developing apophyses are more common than those involving the musculotendinous unit. During adolescence, ossification continues, but the immature skeleton remains more prone to injury as the high physical demands of sports participation exceed the capacity of the musculoskeletal system. Additionally, rapid increases in muscular power related to hormonal changes accentuate the mismatch between muscular and physeal strength.

In children and adolescents, the most common disorder that causes hip pain is transient synovitis. In addition, Legg–Calve–Perthes disease has been shown to have an incidence of 1.5–5 per 10,000 children of ages 2–12 years. Slipped capital femoral epiphysis, with an incidence of 0.8–2.2 per 10,000, is also an oft-encountered etiology for hip pain that usually presents in the early adolescent period. Developmental hip dysplasia, noted in 1.5–20 cases per 1,000 births in developed countries depending on the diagnostic modality used and timing of the evaluation, may lead to hip pain later in life.[2] Each entity should be considered not only in the investigation of hip pain in the limping child, but also in complaints of knee pain in this population. Each is discussed further in this text. (Please see Chap. 7 – Hip and Pelvis Injuries in Pediatrics and Adolescence).

The epidemiologic data regarding incidence of hip and pelvis injury in children have been studied at length, often in association with investigation of injury incidence at other anatomical sites. Data have been further divided into acute and chronic injury, with acute injury occurring much more commonly in this population. In retrospective studies, injuries to hip and thigh in children encompassed 17–25% of all acute, but only 2.2–4.8% of chronic injuries.[7] Sports injuries to the hip and groin have been noted in 5–9% of high school athletes.[1,5]

Investigation involving primary school through high school-aged individuals in the general population has found an incidence of hip pain in 6.4%.[2] This can be further divided into 4% in the primary school-aged population, compared with 7.8% in the high school group. These data portend a higher risk in the older child of suffering from hip pain. Interestingly, in the same study, 2.5% of the subjects were found to have clinical evidence of hip pathology on examination, the most commonly noted findings being pelvic obliquity, limb length discrepancy, and snapping hip. In only 0.6% of those who reported hip pain was any pathology noted by a physician on physical examination. This may suggest that objectively dysfunctional hips are relatively common in the school-aged and adolescent population, but that these pathologic features do not typically result in pain. One may further conclude that most hip pain in this population is functional, as examination findings are typically lacking in those who do report pain.

Among adults, the spectrum of hip and pelvis injury evolves. As these patients age, the risk of pain from hip osteoarthritis increases substantially. The prevalence of hip and pelvis pain in adults from all etiologies ranges from 2.8% to 22.4%, and reports of pain tend to increase with age.[2] Over the age of 60, fully 14.3% of adults report significant activity limiting hip pain.[8]

SPORT

Participation in athletic activity of any kind has been shown to increase the risk of hip and pelvis injury, as well as the eventual development of hip osteoarthritis.[9] Men with high long term exposure to sports had a relative risk of developing hip osteoarthritis of 4.5 when compared to those with lower exposure.[9] In those with exposure to high physical loads from both sports and occupation, the relative risk increased to 8.5 for the development of hip osteoarthritis when compared to those with low physical loads in both activities.[9]

Overall, hip and groin injuries are more prevalent in athletes participating in explosive or contact sports.[7] Such injuries are seen in a wide variety of sports, including those that feature cutting activities and quick accelerations and decelerations, such as football and soccer, those with repetitive rotational activities, such as golf and martial arts, as well as dancing, running, and skating.[1,6]

By far, dancers possess the highest incidence of hip and pelvis injury among athletes. Ballet dancers are at particularly high risk, as most studies note that the hip is implicated in between 7% and 14.2% of all injuries in this population.[10] Often, these athletes substitute proper technique with exaggerated external rotation of the lower extremity, placing further stress on the hip joint and pelvis.

Runners and soccer players are also at higher risk than other athletes. The incidence of hip and groin injury in these participants has been found to be 2–11% and 5.4–13%, respectively of all reported injuries.[4] The most common injuries that involve these sites in runners are adductor strains and iliac apophysitis.[11] The injuries to the groin in soccer athletes fall on a spectrum, and may range from mild adductor and hip flexor strains to the often debilitating "sports hernia." A common etiology for groin injury is the adductor strain, where the leg is overstretched at the groin while the hip is abducted and externally rotated, sometimes against an opposing force, such as the ground or an opponent.

Seven percent of all injuries to participants in high school football involve the hip and thigh, compared to 20% involving the knee and 18% involving the ankle.[12] Injuries such as hip pointers and thigh contusions are common in this population. Track and field, rugby, martial arts, and racket sports have been implicated as being hazardous to the hip joint itself, specifically for the later development of hip osteoarthritis.[3,9]

GENDER

Injuries of the hip and pelvis are more commonly suffered by women in direct comparisons with men, regardless of age or sport. Most studies note incidences of hip pain in women that are twice that in men. In a study of primary and high school-aged children, 8.2% of all girls reported hip pain, compared with 4.4% of the boys.[2] In the adult population, the risk of hip pain in women is more than double that in men.[8,13]

In a comparison of injuries in high school basketball athletes, injuries to the hip and thigh ranked third in female students compared with fourth in male students. Incidences of ankle and knee injuries were much more common in both groups, with facial injuries also more common than hip and thigh injuries in boys.[14] Isolated injuries of the pelvis were noted in less than 1% of both genders.

The etiology of the increased incidence of hip pain in women is likely because of both anatomic and functional factors. The anatomic differences of the lower extremities in women are well described in the literature. Regarding the hip, larger femoral anteversion may predispose women to hip pain. Furthermore, during running, female subjects have a higher degree of hip abduction, hip internal rotation, and knee abduction compared to men.[2,15] This increased motion is likely to at least partly contribute to higher injury statistics in this region. In addition, acquired anatomic laxity secondary to hormonal changes in pregnancy may contribute to increased incidence of hip and pelvis complaints in women.

CASE REPORT: CONCLUSION

Assessment and Plan

The athlete is diagnosed with external snapping hip syndrome, characterized by subluxation of the iliotibial band over the greater trochanter of the femur. Additionally, she exhibits signs of core weakness, which partly contributes to her symptoms. A physical therapy regimen addressing core strengthening and stabilization and iliotibial band flexibility is instituted. Corticosteroid injection into the greater trochanteric bursa can be considered if relief is not obtained through therapy alone.

SUMMARY

As this chapter has discussed, injury to the hip and pelvis is prevalent in all populations, from the very young to the elderly, among athletes in numerous sports, and in men and women. In the chapters that follow, specific entities affecting this often diagnostically challenging anatomic location will be further explored, including appropriate workup and management strategies that are useful to not only the sports medicine physician but the primary care physician as well.

References

1. Morelli V, Weaver V. Groin injuries and groin pain in athletes: part 1. Prim Care 2005; 32(1):163–183.
2. Spahn G, Schiele R, Langlotz A, et al. Hip pain in adolescents: results of a cross-sectional study in German pupils and a review of the literature. Acta Paediatr 2005; 94(5):568–573.
3. Braly BA, Beall DP, Martin HD. Clinical examination of the athletic hip. 2006; 25(2):199–210, vii.
4. Boyd KT, Peirce NS, Batt ME. Common hip injuries in sport. Sports Med 1997; 24(4):273–288.
5. DeAngelis NA, Busconi BD. Assessment and differential diagnosis of the painful hip. Clin Orthop Relat Res 2003; (406):11–18.
6. Bharam S, Philippon MJ. Hip injuries. Clin Sports Med 2006; 25(2):xv–xvi.
7. Watkins J, Peabody P. Sports injuries in children and adolescents treated at a sports injury clinic. J Sports Med Phys Fitness 1996; 36(1):43–48.
8. Christmas C, Crespo CJ, Franckowiak SC, et al. How common is hip pain among older adults? Results from the Third National Health and Nutrition Examination Survey. J Fam Pract 2002; 51(4):345–348.
9. Vingard E, Alfredsson L, Goldie I, et al. Sports and osteoarthrosis of the hip. An epidemiologic study. 1993; 21(2):195–200.
10. Reid DC. Prevention of hip and knee injuries in ballet dancers. Sports Med 1988; 6(5):295–307.
11. Ballas M, Tytko J, Cookson D. Common overuse running injuries: Diagnosis and management. Am Fam Physician 1997; 55(7):2473–2484.
12. DeLee JC, Farney WC. Incidence of injury in Texas high school football. Am J Sports Med 1992; 20(5):575–580.
13. Tuchsen F, Hannerz H, Burr H, et al. Risk factors predicting hip pain in a 5-year prospective cohort study. Scand J Work Environ Health 2003; 29(1):35–39.

14. Messina DF, Farney WC, DeLee JC. The incidence of injury in Texas high school basketball. A prospective study among male and female athletes. 1999; 27(3):294–299.
15. Ferber R, Davis IM, Williams DS 3rd. Gender differences in lower extremity mechanics during running. Clin Biomech 2003; 18(4):350–357.

Chapter 2
Physical Examination of the Hip and Pelvis

Devin P. McFadden and Peter H. Seidenberg

CLINICAL PEARLS

- Hip and pelvis injuries are common in both sports medicine and primary care practices.
- The hip and pelvis are often viewed as a "black box" because of the complex anatomy and overlapping pain referral patterns.
- Use of a systemic physical examination will assist the clinician in demystifying this region of the body and narrowing the differential diagnosis.
- A thorough lower extremity neurologic examination should be included in the evaluation of the hip and pelvis.
- Special tests are used in concert to gather a more complete picture of the patient's biomechanical deficits.

CASE REPORT: PRESENTATION

Chief Complaint and History

T.R. is a 20-year-old male NCAA Division I cross-country runner who presents to the sports medicine clinic complaining of "right hip dislocation." He has noticed lateral hip pain over the past 2 months which has been gradually increasing in severity. He states that it feels as though his hip is "going out of place." Initially, the patient noticed the pain only at the end of a run. Now, he complains of a constant dull ache that sharpens during runs. He has no radiation of the pain and no complaints of paresthesias. His running shoes are only 2 months old, and he used his prior pair for only 4 months. A change to his training regimen – the addition of hill workouts – corresponded to the onset of his pain. His first scheduled meet of the season is in 4 weeks.

He denies fevers, chills, night sweats, anorexia, and weight loss. He has no gastrointestinal symptoms or genitourinary symptoms. He denies a history of back pain.

He has no personal history of cancer. He had a left distal tibial stress fracture, and 2 years ago that healed without complication. There is no family history of cancer or rheumatologic disorders other than osteoarthritis in his grandparents.

T.R. takes ibuprofen prn. He is a non-smoker, uses alcohol socially, and does not use recreational drugs or dietary supplements.

Physical Examination Results

T.R.'s vital signs are within normal limits. He is a well developed, well nourished, Caucasian man. He is in no acute distress, alert, and oriented to person, place, and time with normal affect.

The abdomen is non-distended and non-tender, with normal active bowel sounds. There is no abdominal mass.

A back examination reveals no tenderness to palpation of the lumbar spinous or transverse processes. There is no sacroiliac (SI) joint tenderness and no tenderness of the lumbar musculature. The back demonstrates full range of motion in all planes and the Stork test is negative. No pelvic obliquity is present.

On neurological examination, T.R. demonstrates normal gait, mildly positive Trendelenburg on left and grossly positive Trendelenburg on right. The straight leg raise is negative, and hip abduction strength is 4+/5 right and 5/5 left. The remainder of lower extremity strength testing is 5/5 bilaterally, sensation is intact, and lower extremity reflexes are +2 and symmetrical.

Right hip examination reveals no obvious deformity. T.R. is able to reproduce an audible, palpable pop by flexing and abducting the hip. Log roll is negative. Hip range of motion tests' results are as follows:

Extension: 20° bilaterally
Flexion: full bilaterally
Abduction and adduction: equal and full bilaterally
Internal rotation and external rotation full and equal bilaterally.

There is no tenderness at the anterior superior iliac spine (ASIS), anterior inferior iliac spine (AIIS), ischial spine, iliac crest, or lesser trochanter. There is tenderness just posterior to the greater trochanter. Ober's test is positive; Stinchfield, piriformis, and Gaenslen's tests are negative. Leg lengths are equal.

The FABER (Flexion, ABduction, External Rotation), modified Thomas, and Ely's tests are all negative. The popliteal angles are equal at 30° bilaterally.

INTRODUCTION

Hip and pelvis injuries are seen commonly in sports medicine and primary care clinics. In fact, certain groups of athletes such as runners, dancers, and soccer players have been identified as being at particularly high risk of injuring these regions,[1] likely secondary to the extremes of motion and high-level forces exerted on the hip during participation in these sports. Studies suggest that up to 10–24% of all pediatric patients as well as 5–6% of all adult patients presenting with musculoskeletal complaints have involvement of the hip.[1] Yet despite the commonplace nature of hip and pelvis injuries, many still view the evaluation of this area as a proverbial "black box." Such a view may result from the combination of complex anatomy and overlapping pain referral patterns that often present as hip complaints. As such, the clinician is required to maintain a broad differential diagnosis of both musculoskeletal and non-musculoskeletal etiologies. The following chapter strives to arm the reader with a systematic method for evaluation of this potentially intimidating area.

ANATOMY

The hip derives its stability from the fact that, unlike the shoulder, it is a true ball-and-socket joint, with the femoral head held snugly in place by the pelvic acetabulum. Yet despite its stable construction, the hip maintains a considerable deal of flexibility in the frontal, sagittal, and transverse planes of motion. Because of its unique design, the partially spherical articulation of the femoral head with the acetabulum is ideally designed to receive and distribute the forces of daily activity, which studies have shown can range from three to five times the patient's bodyweight with simple tasks such as walking or running.[2]

The bony joint of the hip is derived from the articulation of the head of the femur and the convergence of the ilium, ischium, and pubis bones of the pelvis to form the acetabulum. These bones, which are commonly referred to as innominate bones, collectively comprise the "hip bone." Like the shoulder, the articular surface of the acetabular cartilage possesses a thickened rim, or labrum, at its periphery which serves to deepen the acetabulum and lend additional support without significantly sacrificing flexibility. When one considers the extra support provided by the three ligaments which surround and enmesh the joint capsule as well as the small ligamentum teres which connects directly to the femoral head, it is easy to see why the hip is one of the most stable joints in the body.[3] The innominate bones also articulate anteriorly at the symphysis pubis, while the posterior articulation of the pelvic girdle is completed by the sacrum and coccyx, providing the connection of the distal appendicular skeleton to the axial skeleton and torso.

The muscular anatomy of the hip is typically divided for simplicity into the medial adductor region, the anterior flexor region, the lateral abductor region, and the posterior extensor region. This breakdown oversimplifies the muscular anatomy insofar as such a strict classification does not take into account the ability of the hip to internally and externally rotate. However, it serves as a convenient way to conceptualize the cooperative muscle groups that mobilize the hip joint. When evaluating the individual muscles, it is important to remember that the musculature of the "hip" includes origins as proximal as the lumbar spine and insertions as far distal as the tibia. The major muscles from each of the cardinal groupings and their respective functions will be discussed in greater detail later in this chapter.

HISTORY

One of the primary difficulties in definitively diagnosing a patient who presents with hip pain is the sheer number of possible sources of this seemingly simple complaint. Aside from the articulation of the femur and acetabulum (i.e., hip joint proper), potential causes of pain include a variety of local bony and soft tissue sources, several potential peripheral nerve palsies, and radiculopathies referring pain from the lumbar spine. In light of the many potential etiologies of hip pain, it is important to consider a broad differential diagnosis before devising a treatment strategy.

Further complicating matters is the significant effect of age on the differential diagnosis of hip pain. Developmental dysplasia of the hip, Legg–Calve–Perthes disease, and slipped capital femoral epiphyses all have their own classical age ranges for presentation in the pediatric population (see Chap. 7).[4] In addition, a mechanism of injury which likely would cause tendinopathy at the musculotendinous junction in a skeletally mature individual is far more likely to cause an apophysitis or apophyseal avulsion fracture in children or adolescents with open growth plates as their tendons are frequently stronger than the apophyses to which they attach. Fortunately, the incidence of all the previously cited pediatric hip disorders decreases as a patient reaches skeletal maturity.[5] Because of these variables, accurate assessment of both the patient's chronologic and physiologic age is an elementary yet essential part of any evaluation of the hip.

Systemic causes of intra-articular hip pathology, such as transient synovitis and septic arthritis, are also more common in pediatric populations. Such examples illustrate the importance of assessing constitutional symptoms as well as musculoskeletal complaints.[6,7] Non-musculoskeletal diseases, particularly those involving the genitourinary and gastrointestinal systems (e.g., pelvic inflammatory disease, appendicitis), have also been known to masquerade as vague hip discomfort. A final yet critical point entails the possible diagnosis of cancer, as hematopoietic and metastatic tumors frequently invade the hip region,[8] making the presence of a long-standing limp or recent weight loss an integral part of the patient history.

Despite the complex interplay of biomechanical, developmental, and systemic contributions to "hip pain," the responsible healthcare practitioner should find that a detailed, thorough, and systematic history and physical examination can efficiently narrow an initially broad differential diagnosis.

As with any musculoskeletal complaint, the patient presenting with hip pathology should always be questioned regarding the onset, provoking and alleviating factors, quality, radiation, severity, and timing (duration) of symptoms (OPQRST). Characterization of the pain as sharp or dull, constant or intermittent, severe or mild can also be helpful. Other historical points of emphasis should include the presence or absence of neurological signs and symptoms and a clear description of any clicking or snapping of the joint.

One of the primary objectives of the history with any joint complaint should be to determine whether the injury is acute, chronic, or acute-on-chronic in nature. Detailed questions regarding athletic involvement, exercise habits, training regimen and modifications, equipment use, and nutritional practices often yield useful information to help elucidate the mechanism of injury. One must also inquire about any previous or concurrent injuries sustained to the back or lower extremities, as injury to either the ipsilateral or contralateral leg, knee, ankle, or foot can cause a compensatory alteration to gait pattern and potentially contribute to sustained hip pain (see Chap. 3).[9] Once one determines the nature of the injury, considering the progression or regression of symptoms along with behavioral modifications preceding those changes may help unmask the precise biomechanical "culprit" of the disease process, which is an imperative step in healing the "victim" and preventing recurrence.

The presence of radiating symptoms can be helpful in accurately diagnosing hip pain as well. The hip serves as a conduit through which all the nerves innervating the lower extremity must pass;

as such, it is a frequent location of nerve injury. The surface area and skin distribution affected can vary widely with these complaints and should be definitively delineated to ensure an accurate diagnosis. Sciatica presents with its classic nerve impingement syndrome, but smaller nerves such as the ilioinguinal nerve may also be damaged and should also be included in the differential diagnosis. If neurological symptoms are present, the healthcare professional must differentiate between functionally-predominant and sensory-predominant symptomatology and pursue an immediate diagnosis more aggressively when functional decline is apparent (SOR-C).

Finally, the value of an accurate past medical history and medication list must never be underestimated, as a history of osteoporosis or recent steroid treatment, for example, can alter the differential diagnosis and treatment plan significantly.

PHYSICAL EXAMINATION

The evaluation of hip complaints should begin before the physician has even entered the room. An astute physician can gather vital information simply by observing the patient's affect, posture, and gait pattern as he or she is escorted to an exam room. In doing so, the physician should be able to identify obvious muscular atrophy or weakness, pelvic obliquity, and abnormal scoliotic or lordotic curves resulting in gross postural abnormalities.[10] Knowledge of normal gait biomechanics and frequently encountered compensatory reactions to traditional disturbances is essential for integrating this information into the clinical picture (see Chap. 4). For example, a patient with a Trendelenburg gait most likely has hip abductor weakness, but the cause may also be related to a tight iliotibial band or coxa externa saltans (snapping hip).[9] Likewise, a hyperlordotic lumbar curve may indicate a compensatory reaction employed to preserve balance in a patient with flexion contractures of one or both hips.

Range of Motion

Range-of-motion testing can be very informative and, therefore, should constitute a distinct part of the standard hip exam. Normal parameters for range of motion have been well defined, giving the practitioner a reliable standard against which to compare collected data (Table 2.1). When performing this portion of the exam, it is important to pay special attention to abduction and internal rotation, as these are the most commonly compromised motions in many pathological conditions involving the hip (SOR-C).

2. PHYSICAL EXAMINATION OF THE HIP AND PELVIS

TABLE 2.1. Normal parameters for hip range of motion[17]

Motion	Flexion	Extension	Abduction	Adduction	Internal Rotation	External Rotation
Range in degrees	110–120	0–15	30–50	30	30–40	40–60

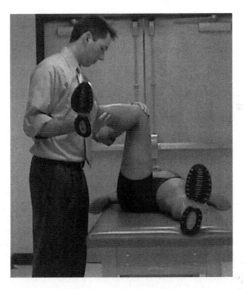

FIGURE 2.1. Internal rotation.

The majority of the range-of-motion testing can easily be performed with the patient supine. One can assess internal and external rotation by having the patient lying with his or her legs slightly separated and passively rolling the entire lower extremity as if performing a log roll. An alternate method involves flexing the patient at the knee and rotating the leg around the vertical axis of the femur (Fig. 2.1 and Fig. 2.2). This method may make measurements easier, but it is important to remember that pivoting the ankle in one direction causes the hip to rotate in the opposite plane. For example, moving the ankle laterally, while using this method, causes internal rotation at the hip. Abduction (Fig. 2.3) and adduction (Fig. 2.4) are performed by anchoring the patient's pelvis with one hand while moving one leg at a time through the transverse plane with the other. When the hip begins to rotate (despite the

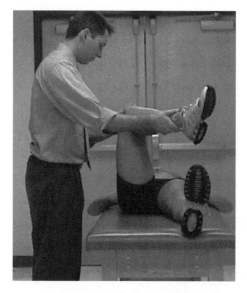

FIGURE 2.2. External rotation.

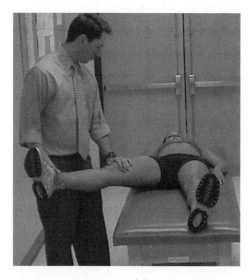

FIGURE 2.3. Abduction.

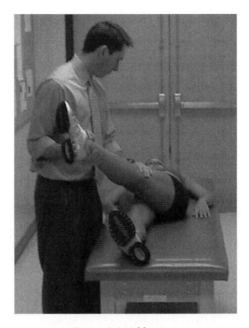

FIGURE 2.4. Adduction.

added support provided by the examiner) the full range of motion in that plane has been reached. Hip flexion should be tested in the supine position by having the patient draw both knees to his or her chest, as flexion at the knee eliminates hamstring tightness as a potential limiting factor for this exam. Extension, on the other hand, is best performed with the patient in the prone position by raising the selected thigh from the exam table (Fig. 2.5).

Palpation

Palpation constitutes another significant portion of the exam. The musculature, tendinous origins and insertions, bony prominences (e.g., the greater trochanter), bony articulations (including the SI joint (Fig. 2.6) and pubic symphysis), bursae, and apophyses all must be palpated to the extent possible. The examiner must be attentive to any snapping or popping throughout the range of motion. While this usually indicates benign tendinous friction over a bony prominence, it can at times indicate an intra-articular lesion or free-floating loose body.[11] This information may be obtained by palpating the portion of the joint being assessed with the free hand while performing the range of motion testing as detailed above.

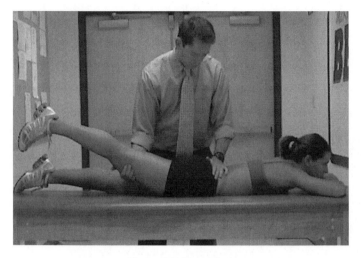

FIGURE 2.5. Extension.

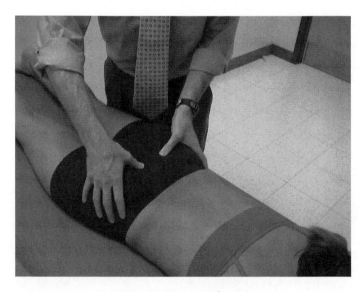

FIGURE 2.6. SI joint palpation.

Neurologic Testing

The hip and pelvis channel numerous nerves from the back to the groin and lower extremity. Accordingly, a thorough neurologic exam is essential even when neurological involvement is not suspected. Strength testing of the lower extremity must include each of the major muscle complexes that mobilize the hip and knee. As described previously, these muscle complexes can be divided into four cardinal muscle groups: the flexors (e.g., iliopsoas and rectus femoris), the extensors (e.g., gluteus maximus and hamstrings), the abductors (e.g., gluteus medius and gluteus minimus), and the adductors (e.g., adductor longus, adductor brevis, adductor magnus, pectineus, and gracilis.) Strength should then be graded on a scale from 1 to 5 (Table 2.2).

After palpating the muscle bellies and tendinous junctions of the individual muscles, the examiner may proceed to test the strength of each muscle grouping. In order to test the flexor group, the examiner places his or her hand over the seated patient's thigh and asks the patient to push upward against his or her hand while offering resistance. Similarly, to test the hip extensors, the patient is placed in a prone position and instructed to raise his or her thigh from the exam table as resistance is applied from behind the knee. Abduction and adduction may be assessed from the supine position with knees extended. The patient is instructed to separate the legs as the examiner offers resistance from the lateral malleoli and then to squeeze the legs together as resistance is applied to the medial malleoli. These latter tests may also be performed with the patient in the lateral decubitus position with the hips neutral. In this scenario, the patient is instructed to abduct the upper thigh to 30° and strength testing proceeds as above for the elevated leg (Fig. 2.7). The authors suggest that this technique may offer a greater degree of sensitivity to subtle deficits of strength (SOR-C).

TABLE 2.2. Strength testing values

Strength test value	Meaning of the value
1/5	No signs of muscle firing
2/5	Visible twitching or fibrillations of the contracted muscle group without any movement
3/5	Active movement when gravity is eliminated
4/5	Active muscle activity against resistance with decreased strength
5/5	Indicating normal strength

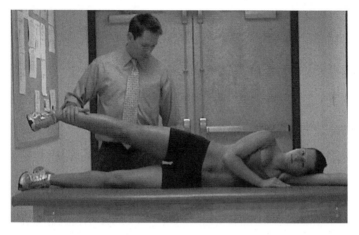

Figure 2.7. Abduction strength testing.

Special Tests

One may employ a number of special tests to narrow the differential diagnosis after history, range-of-motion testing, neurologic testing, and palpation have been completed. Despite variability in sensitivity and specificity, as well as significant crossover, such tests can be helpful when employed within the context of the previously obtained information.

Trendelenburg's sign is a test used to determine whether the patient has adequate hip abductor strength, particularly of the gluteus medius. To perform this test the patient is instructed to stand on both feet and slowly raise one foot off of the ground without additional support. If the patient has adequate abductor strength, then the iliac crest of the raised leg should remain parallel with or elevated slightly in relation to the contralateral side (Fig. 2.8). In addition, the patient should maintain an upright posture without significant tilt of the upper trunk, which would indicate a compensatory mechanism to help the patient maintain his or her balance (Fig. 2.9). A positive Trendelenburg sign is defined as either a compensatory tilt of the torso (vide supra) or a drop of the contralateral iliac crest (Fig. 2.10), indicating that the ipsilateral hip abductors are unable to contract with adequate force to maintain a level pelvis. Instability of the pelvis from other etiologies may also create a positive Trendelenburg's sign resulting from increased tensile forces on the bony structures of

2. PHYSICAL EXAMINATION OF THE HIP AND PELVIS 21

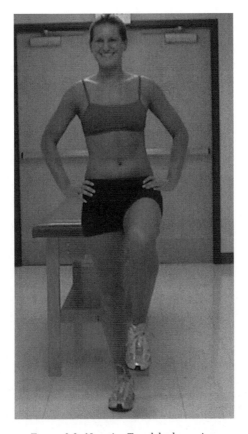

FIGURE 2.8. Negative Trendelenburg sign.

the hip. Therefore, diagnoses causing pelvic instability, such as Legg–Calve–Perthes disease or acetabular fractures of any etiology, may be considered as alternate causes of a positive test.[12]

The *FABER test*, sometimes referred to as *Jansen's test* or *Patrick's test*, was designed to isolate hip joint, SI joint, or iliopsoas pathology. The most commonly used name of this test is an acronym for the positioning of the hip during the test (i.e. FABER). The patient lies supine and one leg is placed in a *f*lexed, *ab*ducted, *e*xternally *r*otated position, as if creating the number 4, with the foot of the leg being tested resting on the contralateral knee (Fig. 2.11). From this position, the examiner places gentle downward traction on the ipsilateral knee. Pain or a decreased range of

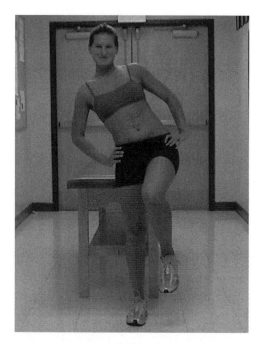

Figure 2.9. Compensated Trendelenburg sign.

motion indicates a positive test. A study by Broadhurt and Bond published in 1998 demonstrated a sensitivity of 0.77 and specificity of 1.0 when using the symptom of SI pain during the FABER test to indicate SI dysfunction.[11] The examiner should note, however, that a restricted range of any of the individual planes of motion being tested in the FABER results in decreased specificity of the test, as any individual restriction would be expected to decrease range of motion in this composite motion exam as well, thereby leading to false positive results.[13,14]

Ober's test is useful for evaluating the iliotibial band, tensor fascia lata, and greater trochanteric bursa. The patient is placed in a lateral decubitus position with hips and knees each flexed to 90°. Initially, the examiner passively abducts and extends the upper leg until the thigh is in line with the torso, followed by passive adduction until the extremity returns to a natural position (Fig. 2.12). A positive test is indicated by a leg maintained in relative abduction, in contrast to a negative test in which the leg may rest on the table without causing significant discomfort.[15] Inflexibility indicated by

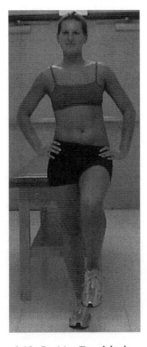

FIGURE 2.10. Positive Trendelenburg sign.

a positive test suggests excessive tightness of the iliotibial band, whereas focal pain overlying the trochanter points towards a possible trochanteric bursitis.

The *Thomas test*[10] and *modified Thomas test* are used to assess hip flexor flexibility, particularly of the iliopsoas muscle. To perform the Thomas test, the patient is placed in a supine position and instructed to flex one leg and pull it to the chest. A flexion contracture would be indicated by passive flexion of the contralateral straight leg lifting off of the exam table (Figs. 2.13 and 2.14). A more informative version, the modified Thomas test, is performed by having the patient sit on the end of the exam table and pull a single leg to his or her chest. The patient is then instructed to lie back on the exam table while maintaining the knee against the chest wall, as the examiner watches carefully to insure that the patient does not fall. Once again, a flexion contracture of the iliopsoas is indicated by the contralateral thigh rising off of the table. In the modified Thomas, however, the patient may

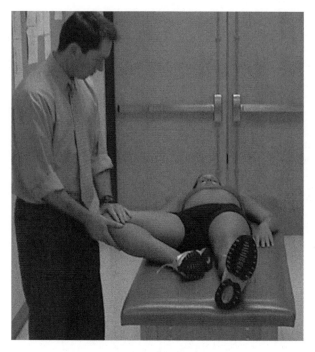

Figure 2.11. FABER test.

also demonstrate a rectus femoris contracture via extension of the contralateral knee from its passively flexed position, making this a higher-yield test.[10]

The *piriformis* or *FAIR (flexion, adduction, internal rotation) test* is performed with the patient in the lateral decubitus position, with the upper leg flexed to 60° and the lower leg maintained in full extension. The examiner places one hand on the patient's shoulder and, with the other hand, exerts mild pressure on the flexed leg at the knee. A positive test is defined as classical "shooting" pain elicited by direct impingement of the sciatic nerve by the tight piriformis muscle. In 1992, Fishman and Zybert showed that when used to demonstrate sciatic nerve impingement, these symptoms have a sensitivity of 0.88 and a specificity of 0.83 in comparison to electrodiagnostic studies as a gold standard.[16] It is important to distinguish this classical description, however, from other sources of pain which may result from the added pressure placed on the hip joint during the exam.

2. PHYSICAL EXAMINATION OF THE HIP AND PELVIS   **25**

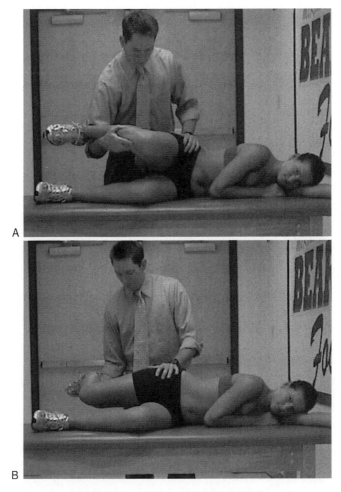

FIGURE 2.12. Ober test. (**A**) Start (**B**) End.

The *Log Roll test*[17] is a simple but useful test for demonstrating acetabular or femoral neck pathology. To perform the test, the practitioner passively internally and externally rotates both fully extended legs of the supine patient. Pain in the anterior hip or groin is considered positive. When significant bony injury is suspected, this test can be used to offer a preliminary assessment of

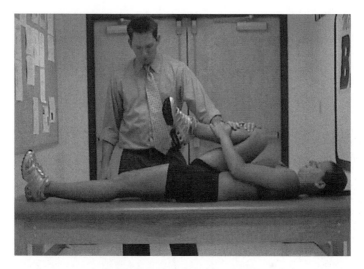

FIGURE 2.13. Negative Thomas test.

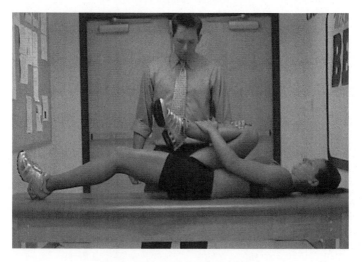

FIGURE 2.14. Positive Thomas test.

bony integrity in order to guide subsequent exam maneuvers and minimize risk of further injury (**SOR-C**).

The *Stinchfield test* is performed with the patient in the supine position with the symptomatic hip flexed to 20° and the knee maintained in full extension. A gentle downward pressure is then exerted

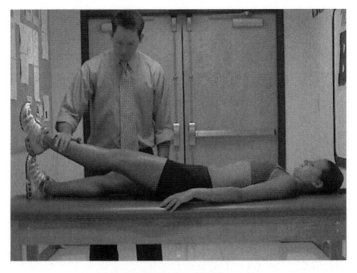

FIGURE 2.15. Stinchfield test.

on the distal end of the elevated leg (Fig. 2.15). Pain in the anterior hip or groin indicates a positive test and may suggest femoral fracture, acetabular injury, or osteoarthritis of the affected hip.[18]

Ely's test is used to assess the flexibility of the rectus femoris. To perform this test, the patient is instructed to lie in the prone position with legs fully extended. The examiner then passively hyperflexes the knee to the extreme of its range of motion taking care to avoid rotation or extension of the hip joint, and observes the ipsilateral hip for vertical separation from the exam table (Fig. 2.16). If the hip is forced to lift off of the table, then the test is considered positive, suggesting a rectus femoris contracture. Again, the examiner must cautiously avoid any extension or rotation of the hip which can cause false positive results by eliciting pain from other areas.[8]

The *straight leg raise* test classically has been used in descriptions of patients suffering from lumbar herniated disk disease, but it can also be used to differentiate various types of hip pathology from those of gluteal etiology. To perform the exam, the patient is placed in a supine position, and the examiner passively flexes (raises) one leg at a time while maintaining full extension at the knee. If the patient experiences pain or is too inflexible to perform an adequate exam, then the knee may be slightly flexed and continued flexion of the hip attempted. If the examiner is unable to further flex the hip despite this modification, then a pathology of the buttock such as

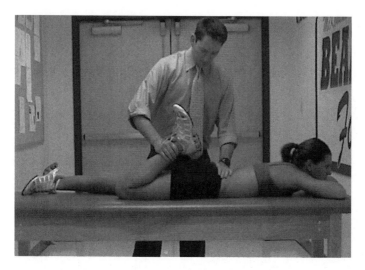

Figure 2.16. Ely's test.

ischial bursitis or an abscess, rather than intra-articular hip pathology, is likely. Pain radiating distally in either leg represents a positive test and suggests some form of sciatic nerve irritability, either at the level of the piriformis or possibly at the site of a more proximal lumbar disk herniation. A meta-analysis by Vroomen and Knottnerus in 1999 suggested that the ipsilateral straight leg raise was the most sensitive physical exam maneuver used to rule out a herniated disk, with a pooled sensitivity of 0.85 compared to a specificity of just 0.52.[19] The contralateral straight leg raise, on the other hand, was the most specific exam technique for identification of a herniated disk, with a specificity of 0.84 in contrast to its poor sensitivity of 0.30.[19] For this reason, when used, the straight leg raise should always be evaluated bilaterally (SOR-B).

An accurate *leg length assessment* is critical in the evaluation of hip pain, as a significant discrepancy sometimes may represent a masked "culprit" masquerading as secondary pathology. These secondary problems, or "victims," are destined to recur unless the primary etiology is addressed appropriately. While it may be difficult for the practitioner to definitively diagnose an anatomic leg length discrepancy,[20] it is equally important to make the diagnosis of a functional leg length discrepancy due to its effects on the athlete's kinetic chain. One proposed method for determining anatomical leg length requires the patient to stand fully erect with his or her feet 6–8 in. apart as the examiner measures the distance from the ASIS to the medial malleolus of each lower extremity.[20] Confounding factors such as the patient shifting weight to alleviate pain and the potential for asymmetrical soft tissue distribution, however, sometimes decrease the reliability of the obtained measurements. In addition, even in cases in which the measurements are reliable, this method offers no information as to where the discrepancy arises, thus limiting its clinical utility.

The *Weber–Barstow maneuver* was subsequently designed to address these limitations. In this technique, the patient is asked to lie supine with both knees and hips flexed to approximately 45°. The patient is then instructed to reset the pelvis by pushing off of the table and gently lowering himself or herself back down (Fig. 2.17). The examiner can then assess the length of the femur and tibia individually by aligning the medial malleoli and examining the profile of the knees from both the front and side. A vertical discrepancy between the level of the knee joints most visible from the front would indicate a discrepancy of the structures distal to the knee (i.e., tibia), while an anterior–posterior discrepancy more apparent from the lateral view indicates that the discrepancy lies proximally (i.e., femur). After making these observations, the examiner then passively extends the knees and uses the medial

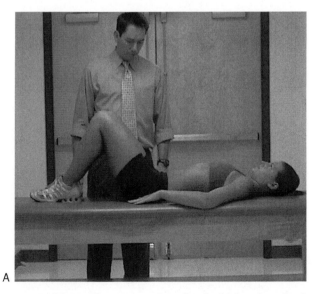

FIGURE 2.17. (**A**) Start for resetting the pelvis for leg length evaluation.

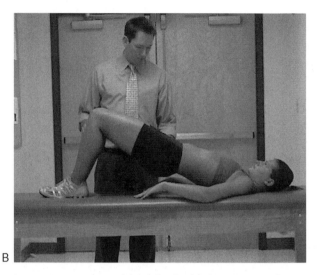

FIGURE 2.17. *Continued* (**B**) Pelvic bridge for resetting pelvis.

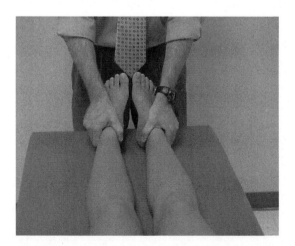

FIGURE 2.18. Measuring position for Weber–Barstow maneuver.

malleoli as landmarks to indicate whether a discrepancy appears to be present (Fig. 2.18). Similarly, the examiner can compare the position of the patellas and ASISs to evaluate for proper and symmetrical body alignment.

The *prone knee flexion test* can be used as a confirmatory examination when the Weber–Barstow suggests that a discrepancy may exist. It is performed with the knees flexed to 90° and the patient in a prone position. The clinician's thumbs are placed transversely across the soles of the feet distal to the calcaneus bilaterally, and the heights of the thumbs are compared. A discrepancy in thumb position would suggest a tibial length discrepancy. Unfortunately, the inter-examiner reliability of the prone knee flexion test has only been found to be 0.21–0.26.[21,22]

The *supine to sit test* or *long sitting test* is employed to differentiate functional versus anatomical leg length discrepancy. To perform this test, the patient is placed in the supine position with legs fully extended and the medial malleoli aligned. The patient is then instructed to rise to a sitting position without moving his or her legs. The examiner observes this motion, paying particular attention to the medial malleoli. If the patient is unable to rise without one leg shifting proximally to the other, then there is likely some degree of pelvic dysfunction or malrotation contributing to any discrepancy present (Fig. 2.19). Bemis and Caniel evaluated 51 asymptomatic individuals and found the test to have a sensitivity of 0.17 and specificity of 0.38.[23] However, a limitation of this study was that all of the subjects were asymptomatic.

The *standing flexion test* is also used to assess for pelvic dysfunction. The posterior superior iliac spines are palpated while the patient stands vertically and then maximally flexes at the waist. A positive test is marked by migration of one side cephalad (cranially) and suggests SI joint hypomobility. Cohort studies have found inter-examiner reliability of the standing flexion test to range from 0.08 to 0.68.[21,24–28]

The *Gillet test* is another assessment of the SI joint. The patient stands with feet separated by about a foot, and the examiner's thumbs are again placed on the posterior superior iliac spines. The patient is then instructed to balance himself or herself on a single leg while pulling the opposite leg toward his or her chest wall. The maneuver is performed bilaterally, and a positive finding is noted if the posterior superior iliac spine on the flexed side migrates vertically or remains still, indicating inadequate SI flexibility or hypomobility. Dreyfuss et al. determined the sensitivity and specificity of this particular test to be 0.43 and 0.68 respectively making it a poor screening tool if SI dysfunction is suspected.[29]

The *Gaenslen sign* is also used to elicit symptoms of SI disorders. This test is performed by positioning a supine patient on the edge of the table with both legs flexed to his or her chest. The patient is then instructed to allow the outside leg to hang off of

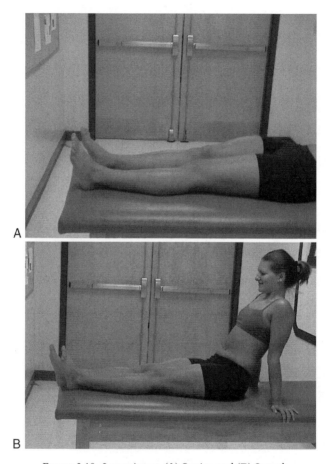

FIGURE 2.19. Long-sit test. (**A**) Supine and (**B**) Seated.

the side of the table as the examiner stabilizes the patient's torso. Pain in the SI region with this maneuver indicates a positive test. Sensitivity and specificity of this test have varied widely in multiple studies, with ranges from 0.21 to 0.71 and 0.26 to 0.72 respectively.[29,30]

Craig's test[10] is used to test for femoral torsion. The normal range of femoral anteversion, or forward projection of the femoral neck, changes throughout life from an average range of 30–40° in infants to 8–15° in adults. Excessive anteversion, or less commonly femoral retroversion, can be problematic and presents most frequently in the pediatric population. To perform the exam, the patient is instructed to lie prone on the exam table with the knee of the side being tested flexed to 90°. From this position the examiner palpates the greater trochanter of the flexed knee and internally and externally rotates the hip to find the position in which the greater trochanter is most lateral. The degree of femoral anteversion can then be estimated using a goniometer with the stationary arm perpendicular to the floor and the moving arm at the angle of the leg.

Passive abduction and *resisted adduction* are useful maneuvers for differentiating pubic symphysis pathology from other midline pelvic symptoms.[31] The exam is performed with the patient in the lateral decubitus position and 90° flexion of the knees and hips. Pain at the pubic symphysis with either maneuver from this position is considered a positive test and may be indicative of osteitis pubis.

The *lateral pelvic compression test* is also performed from the lateral decubitus position with knees and hips flexed. To perform this test, the examiner places direct downward pressure to the greater trochanter. Once again, midline pain overlying the pubic symphysis is consistent with bony injury or osteitis pubis.[17]

The *Scour test* or *Quadrant test* is used for investigation of possible labral pathology. To perform this test the examiner axial loads, adducts, and flexes the hip to its end range of motion with the patient in a supine position. If performed correctly, the ipsilateral knee should point to the patient's contralateral shoulder. From this position the leg is taken in an arc-like motion to the point of full abduction. Any positive exam, defined as pain, apprehension, or catching of the hip during the maneuver, is presumably caused by either labral pathology or a loose body within the hip joint.[10] The authors suggest that this maneuver is analogous in technique to the McMurray test for the knee, lending a useful method for conceptualizing the exam.

The *fulcrum test* is performed with the patient seated on the exam table with legs hanging from the edge. The examiner's forearm is positioned under the patient's thigh for use as a fulcrum as pressure is applied to the ipsilateral knee by the examiner's spare hand. In this manner, the examiner moves up and down the entire shaft of the femur attempting to elicit any point tenderness which may indicate a stress fracture of the overlying bone.[10] Either sharp pain or apprehension indicates a positive test.

CASE REPORT: CONCLUSION

Assessment
- External snapping of the right hip secondary to inflexibility of the iliotibial band and tensor fascia lata which is secondary to core instability, specifically gluteus medius weakness.
- Poor hamstring flexibility bilaterally.

Plan
Physical therapy to address the above biomechanical deficits with specific attention to the core instability. Cross train to maintain cardiovascular fitness. Decrease weekly running mileage in half and decrease running pace by 1 min/mile.

Follow-up
After 4 weeks of physical therapy, the patient's pain had resolved. Once the patient became completely pain free, his running mileage and pace were gradually increased. When he was able to run on level ground at his previous pace, hills were slowly re-introduced. He was back competing at pre-injury levels by his second competition, which was 6 weeks after presentation.

References
1. Scopp, M. The assessment of athletic hip injury. Clin Sports Med 2001; 20(4):647–659.
2. Hurwitz DE, Foucher KC, Andriacchi TP. A new parametric approach for modeling hip forces during gait. J Biomechanics 2003; 36(1):113–119.
3. Jenkins DB. The bony pelvis, femur, and hip joint. In: Hollinshead's Functional Anatomy of the Limbs and Back, Jenkins DB, ed. Philadelphia PA: W.B. Saunders; 1998:239–248.
4. Adkins SB III, Figler RA. Hip pain in athletes. Am Fam Physician 2000; 61(7):2109–2118.
5. Metzmaker JN, Pappas AM. Avulsion fractures in the pelvis. Am J Sports Med 1985;13(5):349–358.
6. Vijlbrief AS, Bruijnzeels MA, vand der Wouden JC, van Suijelkom-Smit LW. Incidence and management of transient synovitis of the hip: a study in Dutch general practice. Br J Gen Pract 1992; 42(363): 426–428.
7. Tolat V, Carty H, Klenerman L, Hart CA. Evidence for a viral aetiology of transient synovitis of the hip. J Bone Joint Surg (Br) 1993; 75(6):973–974.
8. Hage WD, Aboulafia AJ, Aboulafia DM. Orthopedic management of metastatic disease: incidence, location, and diagnostic evaluation of metastatic bone disease. Orthop Clin North Am 2000; 31(4):515–528.
9. Geraci MC Jr, Brown W. Evidence-based treatment of hip and pelvic injuries in runners. Phys Med Clin Rehabil Clin North Am 2005; 16(3):711–747.

10. Magee DJ. Pelvis. In: Magee DJ, ed. Orthopedic Physical Assessment, 3rd ed. Philadelphia PA: WB Saunders; 1997.
11. Allen WC, Cope R. Coxa Saltans: The snapping hip syndrome. J Am Acad Orthop Surg 1995; 3:303.
12. Hardcastle P, Nade S. The significance of the Trendelenburg test. J Bone Joint Surg (Br) 1985; 67(5):741–746.
13. Broadhurst N, Bond M. Pain provocation tests for the assessment of sacroiliac dysfunction. J Spinal Disord 1998; 11:341–345.
14. Ross MD, Nordeen MH, Barido M. Test–retest reliability of Patrick's hip range of motion test in healthy college-aged men. J Strength Condition Res 2003; 17(1):156–161.
15. Gajdosik RL, Sandler MM, Marr HL. Influence of knee positions and gender on the Ober test for length of the iliotibial band. Clin Biomech 2003;18(1):77–79.
16. Fishman L, Zybert P. Electrophysiologic evidence of piriformis syndrome. Arch Phys Med Rehabil 1992;73:359–364.
17. Seidenberg PH, Childress MA. Evaluating hip pain in athletes. J Muscoloskel Med 2005 May; 22(5):246–254.
18. McGrory BJ. Stinchfield resisted hip flexion test. Hosp Phys 1999; 35(9):41–42.
19. Vroomen PC, de Krom MC, Knotterus JA. Diagnostic value of history and physical examination in patients with sciatica due to disc herniation; a systematic review. J Neurol 1999;246(10):899–906.
20. Rhodes DW, Mansfield ER, Bishop PA, Smith JF. The validity of the prone leg check as an estimate of standing leg length inequality measured by X-ray. J Manipulative Physiol Ther 1995;18(6):343–346.
21. Riddle D, Freburger J. Evaluation of the presence of sacroiliac joint dysfunction using a combination of tests: a multicenter intertester reliability study. Phys Ther 2002; 82:772–781.
22. O'Haire C, Gibbons P. Inter-examiner and intraexaminer agreement for assessing sacroiliac anatomical landmarks using palpation and observation: pilot study. Manual Ther 2000; 5:13–20.
23. Bemis T, Caniel M. Validation of the long sitting test on subjects with iliosacral dysfunction. J Orthop Sports Phys Ther 1987; 8:336–345.
24. Touissaint R, Gawlik C, Rehder U, Ruther W. Sacroiliac dysfunction in construction workers. J Manipulative Physiol Ther 1999; 22:134–139.
25. Touissaint R, Gawlik C, Rehder U, Ruther W. Sacroiliac joint diagnosis in the Hamburg Construction Workers study. J Manipulative Physiol Ther 1999; 22:139–143.
26. Vincent-Smith B, Gibbons P. Inter-examiner and intra-examiner reliability of the standing flexion test. Manual Ther 1999;4:87–93.
27. Potter N, Rothstein J. Intertester reliability for selected clinical tests of the sacroiliac joint. Phys Ther 1985; 65:1671–1675.
28. Flynn T, Fritz J, Whitman J, et al. A clinical prediction rule for classifying patients with low back pain who demonstrate short-term improvement with spinal manipulation. Spine 2002; 27:2835–2843.
29. Dreyfuss P, Michaelen M, Pauza K, et al. The value of the medical history and physical examination in diagnosing sacroiliac joint pain. Spine 1996; 21:2594–2602.

30. van der Wuff P, Hagmeijer R, Meyne W. Clinical tests of the sacroiliac joint. Manual Ther 2000;5:30–36.
31. Nuccion S, Hunter D, Finerman G. Hip and pelvis. In: DeLee J, Drez D, Miller MD, (eds). DeLee and Drez's Orthopaedic Sports Medicine, 2nd ed. Philadelphia PA: Saunders; 2003.

Chapter 3
Functional and Kinetic Chain Evaluation of the Hip and Pelvis

Per Gunnar Brolinson and Mark Rogers

> *Dedicated to the memory of Kevin Granata, PhD, Virginia Tech, 4-16-07, husband, father, and pre-eminent biomechanical researcher.*

CLINICAL PEARLS
Some common signs of kinetic chain dysfunction:
- Abnormal muscle firing sequences on muscle testing
- Poor proprioception
- Need for frequent manual medicine or manipulation
- "Weak" phasic muscles on exam
- Easy fatigability of phasic muscles
- Chronic musculoskeletal pain

CASE PRESENTATION

Chief Complaint and History
B.L. is an 18-year-old varsity college third baseman at a Division I university with the complaint of right hip and right low back pain (LBP). He noted waxing and waning discomfort for the past 2 years, and for the past 6 months, his pain has been progressively worsening resulting in altered batting mechanics and reduction in hitting power and efficiency. His initial injury occurred, while playing high school baseball, when he was sliding into second base and collided with another player. That player's knee struck the posterior aspect of B.L.'s right hip. He was unable to finish playing the game and took 3 weeks off from competitive baseball secondary to the right hip pain. He gradually resumed activities

and returned to baseball, but was never completely free from pain. He sustained a second injury about 1 year later consisting of an axial load through the right femur after falling down on his right knee and ultimately landed again on the right posterior hip. He was diagnosed with "right hip spasm" and placed on muscle relaxers and given a course of physical therapy. He improved but never really felt 100% healthy. Prior to coming to college, he had had no diagnostic workup.

When initially seen in our sports medicine clinic, he complained of his "typical" right low back and right posterior hip discomfort. He had some radiation of pain into the low back and posterior hip regions but denied true radicular symptoms.

Physical Examination

Nerve root tension signs were negative, but straight leg raise did produce some mild upper hamstring and posterior hip discomfort. Neurovascular and motor exams were normal. The right hamstring was tight. He had reduced motion in internal and external hip rotation with some reproduction of hip and low back discomfort at extremes of motion. Functional structural evaluation revealed a positive standing forward flexion test (Fig. 3.1) with an

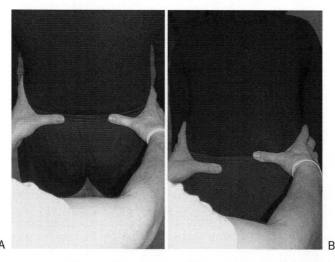

FIGURE 3.1. Standing flexion test in neutral (*left*) and forward (*right*) flexion. Note elevated right thumb with forward flexion, signifying a positive standing flexion test on the right.

associated sacral torsion as well as restricted motion and tissue texture changes noted at the lumbosacral and thoracolumbar regions. He had multiple tender points noted in the right quadratus lumborum. His gait was normal. Anteroposterior pelvis with a frog leg view of the right hip was obtained and was normal. Films of the sacrum and coccyx were normal. He was initially treated with anti-inflammatory medicine, manipulation to correct the dysfunctions noted on exam, and was seen in the training room for functional therapeutic exercise and modalities as indicated.

He had a partial response to this treatment but continued to experience episodic discomfort. A lumbar spine magnetic resonance image (MRI) was obtained to evaluate him for potential disk pathology and revealed signal change and mild bulging of the L4 disk centrally which was not felt to be clinically significant. Despite aggressive conservative management and transient improvement in symptoms following manipulation, he continued to demonstrate a recurrent dysfunctional pattern in the hip, pelvis, and low back area. Ultimately, a magnetic resonance (MR) arthrogram of the right hip was obtained demonstrating a right hip labral tear anteriorly and inferiorly with an associated paralabral cyst.

INTRODUCTION

A *kinetic chain* can be described as the sequencing of individual body segments and joints to accomplish a task. It generally functions from a base of support proximally and then proceeds distally, but this is entirely dependent on the task at hand. Because of the unique nature of sport and the tremendous demands that most sporting activities place on the spine, pelvis, and hip, the ability to recognize kinetic chain disorders related to these specific structures and their interactions with related components of the musculoskeletal system is important for athletic medical practitioners. Because of the complexity of the anatomic and biomechanical interactions as well as neuromuscular control issues, evaluation and accurate diagnosis are problematic.

The hip and pelvis serve as a force transfer link between the lower extremities and torso, and as such, is an at-risk region for athletic injury. The evaluation and treatment of hip and pelvis dysfunction is controversial. One issue is the broad categorization and terminology utilized for the anatomic etiologies of the pain by various health care practitioners. There is no specific or salient historical issue or single clinical examination technique that is both sensitive and specific for the diagnosis of hip and/or pelvis dysfunction. To date, imaging studies do not always distinguish the asymptomatic from symptomatic patient population, nor is there a gold standard for the treatment of the symptom complex associated with these problems in the active patient population.[1]

As noted in Chap. 1, sports injuries to the hip and groin region have been noted in 5–9% of high school athletes[2,3] and 1.4–15.8% of collegiate athletes, according to the NCAA Injury Surveillance System from 2004 to 2005 seasons.[4] These injuries occur most commonly in athletes participating in sports involving side-to-side cutting, quick accelerations and decelerations, and sudden directional changes. The sports medicine practitioner must diligently evaluate hip and pelvis pain and carefully monitor the athlete's response to initial conservative management. This is paramount not only because of the difficulty in making an accurate diagnosis, but also because 27–90% of patients presenting with groin pain have more than one coexisting injury.[5–7] This emphasizes the need for a thorough and comprehensive functional biomechanical evaluation of the region.

NATURAL HISTORY

The clinical evidence suggests that hip and pelvis dysfunction may not simply be an acute process that resolves with time alone. Typically, hip and pelvis pain and dysfunction are often a recurrent problem similar to other chronic musculoskeletal conditions that may have symptom-free periods interspersed with exacerbations. Therefore, physicians must approach hip and pelvis dysfunction with this mindset and be aware of its potential episodic, recurrent, and chronic nature. They should initially seek treatment methods that are active and physical in nature to help restore the body's normal balance of regional and segmental joint motion, posture, and neuromuscular control, with appropriate functional strength and flexibility (SOR = B).

There are emerging studies indicating that physical activity is a risk factor for the development of osteoarthritis of the hip and pelvis. Unfortunately, osteoarthritis of the hip is relatively common in athletes, second only to osteoarthritis of the knee. It may be the result of chronic overuse or secondary to specific traumatic events, such as transient subluxation or chondral injury.[8,9] Kujala et al. performed a retrospective review on former elite male athletes.[10] Using a registry of Finnish male athletes who competed at an Olympic or other international level between 1920 and 1965, the study looked at relative risks of development of chronic disease. Although the participants had significant improvement in health with respect to coronary artery disease, diabetes, and hypertension, an increase in the development of osteoarthritis was noted in these athletes. The cohort was divided into endurance sports (runners and cross country skiers), mixed sports (soccer, basketball, and ice hockey), and power sports (boxing, wrestling, and weight lifting). The relative risks for osteoarthritis were 2.42, 2.37, and 2.68, respectively.[10] In another retrospective study, Spector et al. evaluated 81 female ex-elite middle long-distance runners and tennis players.[11] In comparison to 997 age-matched controls, the athletes demonstrated a relative risk of 2.5 for hip arthritis, and 3.5 for knee arthritis. A cross-sectional study performed by Lindberg et al. demonstrated a 5.8% incidence of hip osteoarthritis in 286 ex-soccer players compared with a 2.8% incidence in controls.[12]

Contradicting this information are studies in long-distance runners, which fail to demonstrate an increased risk for osteoarthritis. Lane et al retrospectively studied 41 long-distance runners averaging 5 h\week of running over 9 years, concluding that there was no increased risk of osteoarthritis in runners.[13] Konradsen et al evaluated 58 ex-long-distance runners who averaged more than 20 km\week of running over 40 years and compared them to age, weight, and occupation-matched controls. Radiographically, the athletic cohort had no significant changes suggestive of osteoarthritis when compared with controls.[14]

Multiple studies have demonstrated a risk of hip osteoarthritis for professional soccer players that may be as high as 13.2%, or 10.2 times that of the general population, even in the absence of identifiable injury to the joint.[15-17] Other studies have shown other significant increases in risk in rugby players,[18] javelin throwers,[19] high jumpers, track, and field sports.[20] Hip arthritis is also common among former National Football League (NFL) players, with 55.6% reporting some arthritic problem in a 2001 NFL Player's Association Survey.[21,22] This association of hip osteoarthritis with significant athletic activity has been demonstrated in female as well as male athletes.[23-25]

Although it is not a consensus opinion of these articles, excessive microtrauma from exercise and cumulative overuse can potentially increase the risk of developing joint injury and osteoarthritis. This risk is dependent on the amount, type, and intensity of the exercise, as well as the genetics, joint structure, fitness, and body habitus of the individual.[26,27] Other specific risk factors include high loads, sudden or irregular impact,[28] and preexisting abnormalities such as dysplasia.[18,29] Recently, labral tears of the hip have been implicated in early osteoarthritis.[30]

In summary, the clinician should view athletic hip and pelvis pain and dysfunction as a common injury with a potentially episodic nature that can affect the athlete's ability to function in both sports and personal life. Treatment must be focused on complete functional recovery and prevention, not just elimination of acute pain, as there appears to be significant risk for the development of hip arthritis if the pain and resultant kinetic chain dysfunction is left untreated (SOR = B).

FUNCTIONAL ANATOMIC CONCEPTS AND NEUROMUSCULAR CONTROL

Arthrokinetic responses are transmitted through the neuromuscular system as proprioceptive data processed by the central nervous system (CNS). These responses are separate from stretch reflexes, though some of the same pathways are utilized. The four nerve types responsible for transmitting afferent information from the joint are globular (static and dynamic mechanoreceptors), conical (dynamic mechanoreceptors), fusiform (mechanoreceptor), and plexus (nociceptor)[31] (see Chap. 2).

The gamma loop mechanism functions in the following fashion. A dynamic load applied to the tendon stretches the spindle muscle fibers. This activates the afferent nerve fibers which synapse in the anterior horn (we are skipping the numerous interneurons for simplicity) on the alpha motor neurons in the same and adjacent spinal segments, simultaneously inhibiting the antagonist muscle groups. If the capsule or ligament becomes stretched beyond what its programming allows for as a normal range of motion (or if too rapid a stretch occurs), inhibitory signals are sent to the agonist muscle responsible for loading the joint in the plane in question and stimulatory signals to the antagonist musculature.[31]

An *engram* is a memorized series of muscle activation patterns (MAPs), for example, tying your shoes, or changing lanes when driving a car. They free up your conscious mind from the task at hand, allowing you to focus on other tasks simultaneously. The development and "burning in" of successful engrams as well as kinetic chain movement patterns (a specific sequence of engrams resulting in a motion) result in successful athletic performance. Injuries and overload can happen when there is compensation for dysfunction (motion loss) in the earlier (temporally speaking) components of the kinetic chain and can lead to injury in the later components, as the tissues either cannot handle the load or the neuromuscular system fires inappropriately.[31]

Neuromuscular imbalance in the postural musculature, either due to hypertonicity or inhibition, allows microtrauma to begin to insidiously accumulate. With repetitions of these dysfunctional MAPs, dysfunctional kinetic chains and engrams develop that "burn in" the dysfunctional, although usually asymptomatic, pathways even more. Pain and/or pathology usually will begin in the local stability system, which cannot maintain its functioning, thus perpetuating the loop.[31] Tendons and ligaments lose their tensile properties over time. Proprioceptive inputs become less reliable and actually can become harmful as MAPs and their kinetic chains are thereby altered, leading to abnormal loading of bone and the supporting soft tissues.

CLINICAL BIOMECHANICS

Much of our understanding of the biomechanics of the hip joint has been obtained through simple static diagrams, gait analysis, and through the insertion of force-measuring implants. The muscles about the hip joint are generally at a mechanical disadvantage because of a relatively short lever arm and must produce forces across the joint that are several times body weight. It has been calculated that level walking can produce forces of up to six times body weight and that jogging with a stumble increases these forces to up to eight times body weight.[32] Although forces, when measured in vivo, tend to be less than the calculated values, one can anticipate potentially greater loads during vigorous sports athletic competition.[33] The structures about the hip are uniquely adapted to transfer such forces. The body's center of gravity is located within the pelvis, anterior to the second sacral vertebra; thus, the loads that are generated or transferred through this area are important in virtually every athletic endeavor.[34]

The normal hip joint is capable of a flexion and extension arc of approximately 140°, but one study has shown that slow-paced jogging used only about 40° of this arc.[35] This increases somewhat as pace increases. Analysis of electromyelographic (EMG) activity shows that the rectus femorus and iliac muscles are very active with swing-phase hip flexion, while the hamstring muscles act eccentrically to control hip flexion and decelerate knee extension.[36] It is of note that, when running, the body is propelled forward primarily through hip flexion and knee extension rather than by push-off with ankle plantar flexion.

Sahrmann has described a hip lateral rotation (HLR) movement impairment that she has observed in people with LBP.[37] The impairment is described as early coupling[38,39] of the primary hip rotation motion with lumbopelvic rotation during a clinical test of active HLR in prone position.[40] The HLR test was performed with the patient in the prone position, the knee flexed to 90°, and the hip in neutral rotation and neutral abduction/adduction. At a self-selected movement speed, patients laterally rotate the hip as far as possible toward the opposite leg, and then return it to the starting position. This is done both actively and passively and the amount and quality of the motion is noted by the clinician.[37] The relationship between LBP and repeated early coupling of hip and lumbopelvic rotation may be of particular importance in people who put rotational demands on both the hip and lumbopelvic region.[37] Passive tissue stiffness about the hips has the potential to contribute to early motion of the lumbopelvic region during HLR.[39]

Patients may, therefore, demonstrate lumbopelvic-coupled movement early during HLR because they have a greater amount of passive stiffness in the hip musculature. The difference in the pattern of movement during the HLR test may be the result of an interaction of biomechanical factors, such as passive tissue stiffness, and motor control factors, such as timing and magnitude of muscle activity. Identifying how movement patterns differ during this clinical test is important because it provides information that can assist the clinician in treatment of a person with hip and pelvis pain and dysfunction.

Atraumatic instability can occur because of overuse or repetitive motion. This is a common complaint in athletes who participate in sports involving repetitive hip rotation with axial loading (i.e., figure skating, golf, football, baseball, martial arts, ballet, gymnastics, etc.). The history provides the greatest clues to the diagnosis because patients can usually describe the motion that causes the pain, such as swinging a golf club during a drive or throwing a football toward the sideline. These repetitive stresses may directly injure the iliofemoral ligament or labrum and alter the balance of forces in the hip. These abnormal forces cause increased tension in the joint capsule, which can lead to capsular redundancy, painful labral injury, and subsequent microinstability. On physical examination, patients will usually experience anterior hip pain while in the prone position with passive hip extension and external rotation.[41,42]

Once the static stabilizers of the hip, including the iliofemoral ligament and labrum, are injured, the hip must rely more on the dynamic stabilizers to maintain stability during activity. It is hypothesized that when capsular laxity is present, the psoas major, a dynamic stabilizer of the hip, contracts to provide hip stability. Over time, this condition can lead to stiffness, coxa saltans, or flexion contractures of the hip.[43,44] In addition, because of the origin of this muscle from the lumbar spine, a chronically contracted or tightened psoas major may be a major contributor to LBP. Thus, hip instability or capsular laxity can trigger a whole spectrum of disorders that the physician must take into consideration when considering various treatment options.[39]

The relationship between hip rotation motion, hip stability, and LBP is important because external forces must be sequentially transmitted from distal body segments to more proximal ones during movement. Movement at the hip could, therefore, influence movement and loading at the lumbar spine. When performed repeatedly, such hip movement could result in excessive loading on tissues in the low back region, and eventually LBP.[37]

In 2001, Vleeming et al.[45] described their integrated model of joint dysfunction. This functional description comes from extensive study of the sacroiliac joint (SIJ) over the past 10–15 years, and is the most studied and supported model for sacroiliac joint dysfunction (SIJD). It integrates structure (form and anatomy), function (forces and motor control), and the mind (emotions and awareness) on human performance. Integral to the biomechanics of SIJ stability is the concept of a self-locking mechanism. The SIJ is the only joint in the body that has a flat joint surface that lies almost parallel to the plane of maximal load. Its ability to self-lock occurs through two types of closure – form and force.

Form closure describes how specifically shaped, closely fit contacts provide inherent stability independent of external load. Force closure describes how external compression forces add additional stability (Fig. 3.2). It had long been thought that only the ligaments in this region provided that additional support. However, it is the fascia and muscles within the region that provide significant self-bracing or self-locking to the SIJ and its ligaments through their cross-like anatomic configuration. Ventrally, this is formed by the external abdominal obliques, linea alba, internal abdominal obliques, and transverse abdominals, whereas dorsally the latissimus dorsi, thoracolumbar fascia, gluteus maximus, and iliotibial tract contribute significantly. In addition, there appears to be an arthrokinetic reflex mechanism by which the nervous system actively controls this added support system. These supports are critical in asymmetric loading, when the SIJ is most prone to subluxation. The important concept to gain from this understanding of integrated function with regard to treatment and prevention of LBP is that SIJD is a *neuromyofascialmusculoligamentous* injury.[1]

The relationship of the abdominal musculature and the erector muscles of the spine, along with their role in stabilization of the lumbosacral spine, is being studied extensively because of the high incidence of LBP in our society. Decreased spinal mobility and trunk muscle strength have been identified in patients with recurrent LBP.[46] These muscles must also be considered for their role in conditions that affect pelvic tilt and the hip joint. The transversus abdominis has been shown to be the key muscle to functional stability of the lumbosacral pelvic region to generate stability and retraining of the core, because of its observed patterns

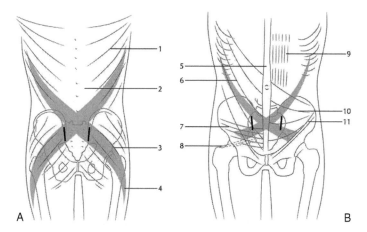

FIGURE 3.2. The cross-like configuration demonstrating the force closure of the sacroiliac joint. The SIJ becomes stable on the basis of dynamic force closure via the trunk, arm, and leg muscles that can compress it, as well as its structural orientation. The cross-like configuration indicates treatment and prevention of low back pain with strengthening and coordination of trunk, arm, and leg muscles in torsion and extension rather than flexion. The crossing musculature is noted. (**A**) (1) Latissimus dorsi; (2) thoracolumbar fascia; (3) gluteus maximus; (4) iliotibeal tract. (**B**) (5) Linea alba; (6) external abdominal obliques; (7) transverse abdominals; (8) piriformis; (9) rectus abdominis; (10) internal abdominal obliques; (11) ilioinguinal ligament[1].

of firing before and independent of the other abdominal muscles. Most recently, a study by Richardson et al.[47] appears to show that these clinical benefits focusing on the transversus abdominis occur as a result of significantly reduced laxity in the SIJ. The balance of the muscles of the upper thigh, particularly the adductor muscles, with those of the lower abdomen requires further study. Conditioning programs have traditionally focused on strengthening of the extremities. Only recently have there been rehabilitation programs designed to address the power and endurance of the trunk and postural muscles.[48,49]

Vleeming et al.[50] defined the posterior layer of the thoracolumbar fascia as a mechanism of load transfer from the ipsilateral latissimus dorsi and the contralateral gluteus maximus. This load transfer is critical during rotation of the trunk, helping to stabilize the lower lumbar spine and pelvis. This was demonstrated through cadaveric and EMG studies.[51] The stretched tissue of the posterior thoracolumbar fascia assists the muscles by generating an extensor influence and by storing elastic energy during lifting to improve muscular efficiency.[1]

In recent years, intramuscular EMG studies of the hip flexor muscles during human locomotion have revealed a separate role of the psoas and iliacus muscles for stability and movement of the lumbar spine, pelvis, and hip.[51-53] In 1995, Vleeming et al. presented evidence that the iliacus muscle was selectively recruited in the standing position with extension of the contralateral leg and in standing, maximal ipsilateral abduction, significantly higher levels of activation in the iliacus muscle, when compared with the psoas muscle, were found.[50] This suggested preferential action of involved single-joint muscles when possible to achieve local pelvic control. In another study, Anderson et al studied walking and running and found that the iliacus muscle was the main "switch muscle" during low-speed walking.[51] Therefore, it is the key to reversing lower extremity motion from extension to flexion. In a later study, they reported that the iliacus and sartorius muscles performed a static function needed to prevent a backward tilting of the pelvis during trunk flexion sit-ups.[53] Also, with static supine leg lifts, there was progressively more activation of these muscles with increasing elevation of the extremity; they recognized that a change in pelvic tilt influenced activation of the iliacus and sartorius muscles. A backward pelvic tilt combined with a hyperlordotic back decreased activation of these muscles, whereas forward pelvic tilt combined with a hyperlordotic back increased activation of the these muscles. This suggests an important and separate role of the iliacus from the psoas in function and dysfunction of the low back and pelvis region.[52]

Recent studies show there is both a functional and anatomic connection between the biceps femoris muscle and the sacrotuberous ligament.[54-56] This relationship allows the hamstring to play an integral role in the intrinsic stability of the pelvis and SIJ. It appears that the biceps femoris, often found to be short on the pathologic side in LBP, may actually be a compensatory mechanism via the previously described arthrokinetic reflexes to help stabilize the SIJ. In healthy individuals, a normal lumbopelvic rhythm exists, during which the first 65° of forward bending is via the lumbar spine, followed by the next 30° via the hip joints. Increased hamstring tension prevents the pelvis from tilting forward, which diminishes the forward bent position of the spine, which results in reducing the spinal load.[56] Normalization of the lumbopelvic rhythm is an essential component to treatment of LBP, hip, pelvis, and SIJD.[1]

In the normal gait cycle, (see Chap. 4: Gait Analysis) there are combined activities that occur conversely in the right and

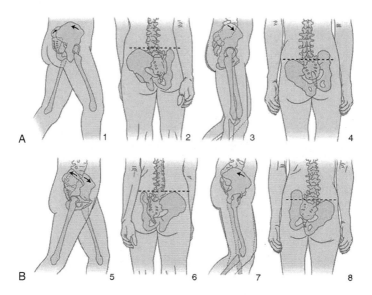

FIGURE 3.3. Sacroiliac joint motion during walking. (**A**) (1) and (2): At right heel strike. (1) Right innominate has rotated in a posterior and left innominate in an anterior direction. (2) Anterior surface of sacrum is rotated to left and superior surface is level, while spine is straight but rotated to the left. (3) and (4): At right mid-stance. (3) Right leg is straight and innominate is rotating anterior. (4) Sacrum has rotated right and sidebent left, while lumbar spine has side-bent right and rotated left. (**B**) (5) and (6): At left heel strike. (5) Left innominate begins anterior rotation; after toe-off, right innominate begins posterior rotation. (6) Sacrum is level but with anterior surface rotated to the right. The spine, although straight, is also rotated to the right, as is the lower trunk. (7) and (8): At left leg stance. (7) Left innominate is high and left leg straight. (8) Sacrum has rotated to the left and sidebent right, while lumbar spine has side-bent left and rotated right[1].

left innominates and function in connection with the sacrum and spine (Fig. 3.3).[57] As one steps forward with the right foot, at heel strike the right innominate rotates posterior and the left innominate rotates anterior. During this motion, the anterior surface of the sacrum is rotated to the left and the superior surface is level, while the spine is straight but rotated to the left. Toward mid-stance, the right leg is straight and the innominate is rotated anterior. The sacrum is rotated right and side-bent left, while the lumbar spine is side-bent right and rotated left. At left heel strike, the opposite sequence will occur and the cycle is repeated.

Throughout this cycle, there is a rotatory motion at the pubic symphysis, which is essential to allow normal motion through the SIJ. Several authors[58,59] have suggested that pubic symphysis dysfunction in walking is one of the essential or leading causes of the development of hip and pelvic dysfunction. In static stance, when one bends forward and the lumbar spine regionally extends, the sacrum regionally flexes, with the base moving forward and the apex moving posterior. During this motion, both innominates go into a motion of external rotation and out-flaring. This combination of motion during forward bending is called nutation of the pelvis. The opposite occurs in extension, which is called counternutation. As the sacrum goes into extension with the base moving posterior and the apex anterior, the innominate components internally rotate and in-flare. This motion is clearly demonstrated and illustrated by Kapandji.[60]

The model of suboptimal posture, though incomplete, has shown to be effective when used as a model to guide treatment.[61-63] Posture can be defined as the size, shape, and attitude of the musculoskeletal system with respect to gravitational force.[64] Subtle departure from ideal posture has been implicated as an important biomechanical factor in athletes with regard to injury because it results in increased mechanical stress throughout the body. Posture must always be evaluated as part of the biomechanical evaluation. The size, shape, and attitude of three cardinal bases of support should always be included – standing surface, the feet, and the base of the sacrum.[1]

Muscles respond to dysfunctional joints in a predictable, characteristic pattern. This pattern is not random and occurs irrespective of the clinical diagnosis or specific regional injury. Tonic or postural muscles are facilitated and hypertonic, which maintain a low level of tone nearly all the time. These muscles tend to utilize more fibers of an oxidative nature to avoid fatigue. Phasic or dynamic muscles are inhibited, hypotonic, or "weak" (pseudoparesis). They exhibit quicker, shorter bursts of activity with phases of rest in between and more often utilize the glycolytic pathway fibers.[35] The specific response pattern of the muscles in the lower half of the body is seen in Fig. 3.4.

Tonic muscles will increase their resting tone and become less pliable. Phasic musculature will become less responsive and weak. Both responses will carry negative impact for the kinetic chain resulting in compensatory phenomenon. This muscle dysfunction, referred to as neuromuscular imbalance, is characterized by a change in the sequence of MAPs. This has been described both as an upper crossed syndrome and a lower (pelvic) crossed syndrome

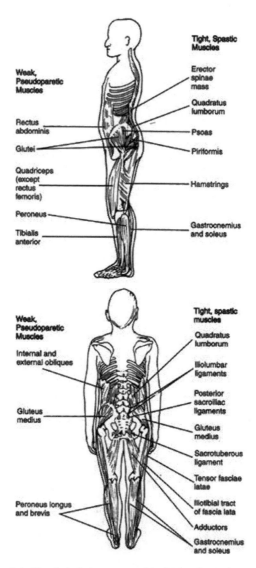

FIGURE 3.4. Muscle imbalance caused by biomechanical stressors.[58]

that when combined produce a layered syndrome that can be appreciated throughout the body (Fig. 3.2). Superficial and deep EMG analysis reveals that there are delays in the activation of phasic muscles, a decrease in amplitude, and recruitment of phasic muscles, and that normal input can have an inhibitory effect.[65]

Triggers of muscle imbalance patterns include muscle disuse, repetitive movements, development of inflexibility, and pain. Of these, pain seems to be the single dominant factor in the maintenance of these patterns. Muscle imbalance should be suspected any time there are abnormal firing sequences on range-of-motion testing, poor balance, recurrent somatic dysfunction, "weak" or easily fatigable phasic muscles on clinical exam, history of recurrent injury or other overuse injury in the same region, chronic pain, and postural imbalance. It is critical to understand these muscle imbalances because they may be a dominant factor in the cause of musculoskeletal pain and/or a major factor in the continuance of the pain. Failure to rehabilitate these patterns is sure to be a significant factor in recurrent injury.[65]

Initially the pseudoparesis, as described above, may be seen as a CNS inhibition, not a true weakness. Over a prolonged time period of inhibition, the muscles actually may become weak. Attempts at strengthening the "weak" muscles only increase inhibition. Physiologically, a decrease in recruitment is seen with added resistance. These muscles actually may not appear grossly weak on initial testing but they are seen to fatigue quickly and demonstrate poor endurance. This can lead to poor motor control or neuromuscular instability, in which there is marked irregularity in sensory-motor balance. It is important to remember that treatments and rehabilitation must be directed at the cause of inhibition, the neural reflex, first as most likely this will be a major factor in recurrent injury.

COMMON HIP AND PELVIS DYSFUNCTIONS

Strains of the adductor group (adductor longus, magnus, and brevis; gracilis; pectineus; and obturators) are the most common causes of acute groin pain in athletes. Their primary function is stabilization of the lower extremity and pelvis in the closed kinetic chain, as well as adduction of the thigh in the open kinetic chain and assisting in femoral flexion and rotation.[66] Strains are more common with eccentric loading. The adductor longus is most frequently affected, at the musculotendinous junction, likely because of its lack of mechanical advantage.[67]

Among soccer players, incidence rates ranging between 10% and 18% have been reported.[57,68,69] Risk factors associated with increased incidence of strains include decreased hip range of motion, decreased adductor strength, and prior injury with 32–44% of injuries classified as recurrent.[70–73] In addition, biomechanical abnormalities of the lower limb such as, leg-length discrepancy, imbalance of the surrounding hip musculature, and muscular fatigue, have also been postulated to increase the risk of adductor strain.[72] Although there have been no controlled clinical studies proving these latter elements to be causative, prevention programs focused on ameliorating some of these abnormalities have been shown to be effective in professional hockey players.[74]

In 2002, National Hockey League (NHL) statistics demonstrated that adductor strains occurred 20 times more frequently during training camp as opposed to the regular season, implying that deconditioning might contribute to these injuries, and therefore, strengthening programs may be preventative. Such strengthening of the musculature of the hip, pelvis, and lower extremities has long been thought to be an important part of adductor injury prevention programs[75]; recently these programs have been documented to be effective in preventing groin injuries in soccer and hockey players.[73,76] In one study, Tyler et al.[73] presented their strengthening and injury prevention programs focused on decreasing adductor weakness (with a goal of keeping at least 80% of abductor strength). They found that adductor strengthening significantly reduced injury in NHL players.

Strains and tendonitis of the iliopsoas muscle usually occur at the musculotendinous junction during resisted hip flexion or hyperextension. Iliopsoas bursitis can occur alone or in conjunction with strain. The two conditions commonly occur concomitantly and are essentially identical in their clinical presentations.[77] The iliopsoas bursa is the largest bursa in the body. It communicates with the hip joint in 15% of people and can be a source of significant groin pain. Bursitis results from overuse and friction as the tendon rides over the iliopectineal eminence of the pubis (Fig. 3.5). This condition occurs in activities requiring extensive use of the hip flexors including soccer, ballet, uphill running, hurdling, and jumping. Iliopsoas bursitis is characterized by deep groin pain that sometimes radiates to the anterior hip or thigh and is often accompanied by a snapping sensation. If this is severe enough, the athlete may exhibit a limp.[78] Because of poor localization and reproducibility of the pain, the average time from the onset of symptoms to diagnosis has been reported from 32 to 41 months.[77]

Pain may also be reproduced when the flexed, abducted, externally rotated hip is extended and brought back into a neutral

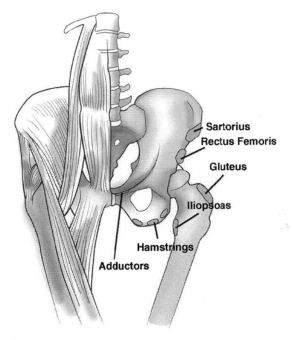

FIGURE 3.5. Attachment of the muscles in the groin region.[5]

position (extension test). During this maneuver, the iliopsoas is stretched as the hip is extended and symptoms are reproduced. Another diagnostic test is to have the supine athlete raise his or her heels off the table to about 15°; in this position, the only active hip flexor is the iliopsoas, and provocative testing as such will elicit pain.[79] Tenderness may be felt during this maneuver by palpating the psoas muscle below the lateral inguinal ligament at the femoral triangle.[80] The biomechanical abnormalities that may contribute to the injury must be sought and corrected as previously described.

High hamstring strains occur most commonly in dancers, hurdlers, runners, water skiers, and other athletes who place excessive stress on the stretched hamstrings.[81] Muscle fatigue may increase risk of injury.[67] It must be remembered that the ischial tuberosity may not fused until the third decade[82] and that some of these injuries may actually represent an apophysitis rather than a true strain.[82] Patients usually present with posterior thigh pain and can have radiation to the groin as well. The diagnosis may be easily made with pain on palpation directly over the muscle insertion on the ischial tuberosity; however, it must be remembered that the adductor magnus also originates from the ischial tuberosity and that injuries to this muscle must also be considered in the differential diagnosis. These injuries occur usually with the hip extended and knee flexed when the sartorius undergoes a sudden contraction. Because the anterior superior iliac spine (ASIS) ossification center fuses relatively late, commonly at 21–25 years of age, a diagnosis of both strain and apophysitis must be entertained in these age groups.[5]

Because rectus femoris is the only member of the quadriceps muscle group that spans two joints, it is subject to more stress and subsequently more injuries. Muscular injuries often result from the explosive hip flexion experienced in kicking or sprinting. Clinically, there is swelling and tenderness over the anterior thigh or at the anterior inferior iliac spine (AIIS) if the injury occurs at the tendon–bone interface. Conservative treatment is effective for most acute partial ruptures; however, small subsets of these patients go on to have chronic pain and disability.[5]

Osteitis pubis, or inflammation of the symphysis pubis, is seen commonly in runners,[83] hockey players,[80] and soccer players. Shearing forces across the pubic symphysis may result in symphysis inflammation or even joint disruption.[84] Repetitive adductor traction on the symphysis has also been proposed as a possible mechanism.[85] Cutting and twisting forces may transmit even greater forces to the pubic symphysis in athletes lacking ideal ranges of hip flexibility.[86,87] Although no published studies have addressed the role biomechanical abnormalities of the lower limb (e.g., leg-length discrepancies or excessive pronation play), in the genesis of osteitis pubis, it is intuitive that such abnormalities might increase forces acting across the os pubis and thus increase susceptibility to the condition.

The symptoms may be initially indistinguishable from an adductor strain and may be aggravated by kicking and running. Symptoms may increase in severity if athletic activity is not reduced. A clinical review[80] noted that in athletes who have documented osteitis pubis, adductor pain occurred in 80%, pain around the pubic symphysis in 40%, lower abdominal pain in 30%, and hip pain in 12%, while scrotal pain, previously described as a classic complaint, was found in only 8%. Physical examination usually reveals tenderness over the pubic symphysis.[88] Pain can often be provoked by active adduction if the distal symphysis is involved or by partial sit-ups if the proximal portion is involved.

The two most common stress fractures of the groin region are femoral neck stress fractures and pubic ramus fractures. These are often seen in distance runners, endurance athletes, or military recruits and are caused by repetitive overuse and overload. Additional risk factors include relative osteoporosis in young female athletes who have nutritional or hormonal imbalances, changes in shoes or training surface, sudden increases in intensity or duration of training regimens, and muscle fatigue, which may reduce shock-absorbing abilities of the hip and pelvis region.[89,90]

An estimated 1% of stress fractures occur at the femoral neck. Although most femoral neck fractures are nondisplaced at presentation, diagnostic delay is common, especially as initial radiographs are often normal. There has been a reported average diagnostic delay of up to 14 weeks.[91] A decreased range of motion at the hip has also been detected in athletes diagnosed with pubic bone stress injury.[92]

During walking or running, the loads on the femoral head can exceed three to five times body weight. These loads occur because of gravity and the torque on the medial side of the hip joint, and are counteracted by contraction of the gluteus medius and minimus muscles. The force on the femoral head is transmitted through the neck to the femoral shaft, creating stresses and strains in the femoral neck secondary to compression and bending. If the abductor muscles fatigue and are unable to provide the normal compensatory tension, the tensile stress in the femoral neck will increase. Muscle fatigue also returns in gait alterations that affect the position of the body's center of mass and alter the stress and strain patterns within the femoral neck.[93]

Pelvic biomechanical studies lend support to this view of increased stress to the central pubic bone area. These studies consider that during weight-bearing loads the superior pubic rami and the pubic symphysis act as a compression strut linking the femur to the posterior pelvic structures and spine,[94] with the centers of rotation being near the pubic symphysis. Therefore, the pubic symphysis area is the region of the anterior pelvis most vulnerable to the stressors of athletic activity. Having a hip joint range-of-motion restriction will contribute to dysfunction, resulting in a greater stress across the superior pubic ramus and pubic symphysis. This, in turn, may lead to increased stress through this vulnerable area and increased likelihood of the athlete having chronic groin injury consistent with a pubic bone stress injury.[95]

Although first reported by Patterson in 1957,[96] it is only in the last 10 years that acetabular labrum tears have become more widely recognized as a cause of hip and groin pain. In one prospective study of patients presenting to a sports medicine center with chronic groin pain, 22% were found to have labral tears.[97]

Awareness and clinical suspicion of this condition among healthcare providers are important, especially in those athletes who have not responded to the prescribed treatment for the more familiar causes of hip and groin pain; early diagnosis and appropriate management lend themselves to improved outcomes.[98]

The labrum is a fibrocartilaginous rim which encompasses the acetabulum, effectively deepening the socket, much like the glenoid labrum of the glenohumeral joint.[98] It can vary in form and thickness. It has three main surfaces: an internal articular surface, an external surface which is in contact with the joint capsule, and a basal surface which is attached to the acetabular bone and transverse ligaments. Its distal edge is free, forming the lateral limit of the acetabulum. Anteriorly, the labrum is equilaterally triangular in shape; posteriorly, it is square with a rounded distal surface, making it more bulbous.

In contrast to the glenoid labrum, the acetabulum in the hip is much deeper and, therefore, provides substantially more stability to the hip joint. Thus, the deepening of the acetabulum that is provided by the labrum is thought to play less of a role in hip joint stability. The acetabular labrum, however, may enhance stability by providing negative intra-articular pressures within the hip joint with joint distraction, thereby adding a "sealing" function to the joint.[99] The sealing function of the labrum also may enhance the lubrication mechanism of the joint by preventing direct contact of the joint surfaces and more evenly distribute the applied forces across the cartilaginous surface.[100] The role of the acetabular labrum in load transmission was further examined in a cadaveric biomechanical study by Konrath et al.,[101] in which they found no significant changes with regard to contact area, load, and mean pressure after removal of the labrum. From these findings they concluded that removal of the acetabular labrum does not predispose to premature hip osteoarthritis.

Femoroacetabular impingement is a more recently described entity as a cause of hip and pelvis pain as well as early development of osteoarthritis in young athletes.[102–104] There have been two mechanisms described which cause impingement between the femoral head and the acetabulum. The cam-type involves an abnormally shaped, non-spherical femoral head with decreased offset at the anterolateral head–neck junction, leading to impingement on the normal acetabulum and medial displacement of the labrum with flexion and internal rotation. The pincer type, causes impingement of the normally shaped femoral head on a retroverted or abnormally deep acetabulum. Both types occur on a spectrum and can coexist.[66]

3. FUNCTIONAL AND KINETIC CHAIN EVALUATION

Most tears are caused by relatively atraumatic mechanisms such as twisting or pivoting during athletic activity, by chronic degenerative disease, or associated with developmental dysplasia,[30,105] as only about one-third of athletes recall a specific traumatic event as the cause of symptom onset.[106]

Athletes commonly present with diffuse, poorly localized groin pain, night pain, pain with pivoting or walking, and mechanical symptoms in the hip and pelvis area; some may present with a painful snapping hip syndrome.

On examination, passive and/or active range of motion may not be limited but pain may be present at the extremes. There are a number of clinical tests that have been reported to reproduce pain, clicking, or locking sensations in the hip and pelvis, specifically they are as follows:

- The impingement test – performed by inducing hip flexion, adduction, and internal rotation, especially in anterior–superior tears.[66,106,107]
- Passive hyperextension, abduction, and external rotation, particularly with posterior tears.[106,107]
- Acute flexion of the hip with external rotation and full abduction, followed by extension, abduction, and internal rotation (anterior tears).[108]
- Extension, abduction, and external rotation brought to a flexed, adducted, and internally rotated position (posterior tears).[108]

In one study, a clicking sensation of the hip was both sensitive (100%) and specific (85%) in predicting labral tears.[66] On physical examination, the internal rotation/flexion/axial compression maneuver was 75% sensitive but only 43% specific,[95] and the flexion/abduction/external rotation (FABER) test was found to be 88% sensitive.[109]

In 2006, Burnett et al.[110] reported an average time from the initial onset of symptoms to the definitive diagnosis of 21 months (range, 2–156 months; median, 12 months). In addition, an average of 3.3 health-care providers (range, 0–11 health-care providers) had been seen prior to the establishment of a definitive diagnosis. Therefore, clinicians must keep in mind that these physical maneuvers are imperfect and must maintain a high index of suspicion for such injuries.

Although plain radiographs and computed tomography may show hip dysplasia, arthritis, and acetabular cysts in patients with acetabular labrum tears, they cannot be counted as reliable tools for diagnosing the condition itself.[106,107,111–113] Even when arthrograms are obtained as well, there does not seem to be an appreciable improvement in the ability of these investigations to detect labral tears.[112] They are, however, useful for excluding other types of hip pathology. MRI, by virtue of its superior soft tissue contrast and ability to directly depict the labrum, has begun to show promise in detecting labral tears over the last two decades.[98]

The use of MR arthrography (MRA) to evaluate labral tears in patients yielded a sensitivity of 79%.[110] However, in 27% of the patients who had an arthroscopically verified tear, preoperative MRA failed to detect the lesion. Despite this limitation in sensitivity, this test frequently confirms the diagnosis and reliably rules out other uncommon conditions (e.g., osteonecrosis, stress fracture, neoplasm) that could present with hip symptoms suggestive of labral disease.[110]

Conservative treatment is usually tried for at least 6 weeks before definitive surgical intervention. This is done to insure that mechanical symptoms are not due to snapping hip syndrome or other functional pathologies as identified above and that any associated soft tissue injuries are given a chance to heal.[66]

EVALUATION

In the clinical evaluation of the patient with suspected kinetic chain dysfunction resulting in hip and pelvis pain with associated altered biomechanics, we have found the following schema to be helpful (Fig. 3.6).

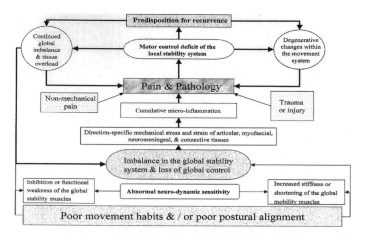

FIGURE 3.6. Kinetic chain dysfunction.[31]

The physical examination begins with observation of the athlete both statically and dynamically. One should evaluate the patient in standing, supine, and prone positions, and assess symmetry of the heights of the iliac crests, ASISs, posterior superior iliac spines, ischial tuberosities, gluteal folds, and greater trochanters, as well as symmetry of the pubic tubercles, sacral sulci, and inferior lateral angles. Next, determine if there is any leg-length discrepancy. One should realize that true leg-length discrepancies will generally cause asymmetry and pain, whereas a functional leg-length discrepancy is usually the result of SIJ, hip, or pelvic dysfunction.[1]

Leg-length discrepancies allow for an unequal transmission of forces across the spine and pelvis during weight-bearing activities. These forces can be amplified in sport because of the rapid acceleration of body mass or repetitive stress transmitted. Although traditional orthopedic teaching is that a minimum of 1–2 cm difference is essential to cause dysfunction, many in the sports medicine community feel that a short leg is clinically relevant and consider differences of as little as 4 mm to be significant.[114]

Assess posture for increased lumbar lordosis, which can result from sacrum, pelvis, and/or hip dysfunction. Dynamic observation assesses for any asymmetry during both gait and specific motions characteristic of the patient's sport. SIJ pain, pathology, and restriction may cause a decrease in stride length, leading to a limp or cause reflex inhibition of the gluteus medius, leading to a Trendelenburg gait.[1]

The examiner should then look for decreases in both passive and active range of motion of the entire spine, hips, pelvis, knees, and feet. Perform the HLR test as previously described. If pain with motion testing occurs, the patient should specifically identify the area of pain and the clinician should then perform a thorough examination of the relevant structures. A neurologic examination for radiculopathy should also be conducted, in addition to evaluating core strength and overall flexibility.[1]

There have been numerous functional (motion) and provocative (pain-producing) tests reported in the literature; however, none has consistently been shown to reliably diagnose hip and pelvic joint dysfunction.[115–119] We feel that there are two major flaws in how these studies and others like them have been carried out. Dreyfuss et al.[120] assumed that pain production is an essential prerequisite to dysfunction. We would suggest that hip and pelvic dysfunction can be diagnosed on the basis of motion restriction and tissue texture changes, especially in chronic pain syndromes when pain location can vary greatly because of muscle imbalance and other factors. Also hip and pelvis screening tests should always be followed up with segmental motion testing and tissue palpation.

When these tests are used together with a thorough history to create a clinical picture, they become significantly more reliable.[119] A detailed discussion of the numerous tests described for dysfunction is beyond the scope of this review, but the reader is referred to several excellent sources.[65,121–123] In osteopathic medicine, hip and sacrum joint somatic dysfunction is diagnosed primarily by the standing and seated flexion tests and asymmetry of pelvic and sacral bony landmarks.[65]

Functional Diagnostic Imaging

There is no specific gold standard imaging test to diagnose hip and pelvis dysfunction, largely because of the location and complexity of the joint and the associated structures that may make visualization difficult. However, a variety of normal radiographic indices have been described to differentiate normal from abnormal bony anatomy and these play an important role in understanding why some patients develop instability (see Chap. 5: Imaging of the Hip and Pelvis).

PRINCIPLES OF TREATMENT

Recurrent hip and pelvis dysfunction and altered postural alignment should provide clue to the physician for the diagnosis of chronic neuromuscular dysfunction or postural imbalance related to kinetic chain dysfunction. Gravitational strain results in a systemic neuromuscular response of postural musculature and muscle firing patterns related to chronic gravitational stress. Other findings may include chronic or recurrent sprains/strains, pseudoparesis, articular dysfunction, myofascial trigger points, muscle imbalance, and ligamentous laxity. Gravitational stress, an obligatory consequence of bipedal posture, is a constant and a greatly underestimated systemic stressor.[124,125] It is most important that one understands that postural imbalance is a systemic neuromuscular dysfunction.

Initial treatment in hip and pelvis dysfunction must focus on the re-education of the neuromuscular system. This is partially accomplished by seeking optimization of posture and can be achieved through the use of one or more of the following modes of physical manipulation[126]:

- Contoured orthotics worn in the shoes to optimize foot and lower extremity biomechanics
- A flat orthotic of sufficient thickness to level the sacral base
- Joint manipulation and/or mobilization directed to restore resilience to soft tissues and motion of restricted joint segments
- Daily practice of a therapeutic posture for 20 min to counter the bias of soft tissues reflective of the initial posture

During the implementation of the above, a principle-centered, functional rehabilitation program[126] that focuses first on the stretching of tight, hypertonic postural muscles, strengthening of weak phasic muscles, and proprioceptive retraining must be carried out.[127-130] It is critical to remember that muscle imbalances must be eliminated and coordinated movement patterns returned to normal before strengthening of the core can begin effectively.

Principles of Sequencing the Exercise Prescription

1. Normalization of segmental function through manual medicine and bodywork as clinically indicated
2. Sensorimotor balance retraining
3. Comprehensive, symmetric, flexibility
   a. Stretch to symmetry
   b. Go for overall increase in length
4. Re-educate movement patterns – PRECISION
   a. Normalize firing patterns – slow, precise, minimalist movements
   b. Quality of movement (neuromotor control) over quantity
   c. Start unloaded, progressive load, sports specific movements
5. Strengthening
6. Sport-specific conditioning

CASE REPORT, CONCLUSION

B.L., our 18-year-old college third baseman, subsequently underwent arthroscopic debridement of the labrum, and his hip and LBPs dramatically improved with no subsequent evidence of the previously noted dysfunctional movement patterns.

This case illustrates the important contribution of hip labral pathology and the resultant transverse plane motion loss in the hip causing recurrent hip, low back, and pelvis pain. The patient's motion loss on functional examination, as well as recurrent biomechanical abnormalities partially responsive to conservative management, is an excellent demonstration of a dysfunctional kinetic chain pattern which resolved once the primary pathology was identified and treated.

SUMMARY

So, as sports medicine clinicians, when should we suspect kinetic chain dysfunction? Some common signs are as follows:

- Abnormal muscle firing sequences on muscle testing
- Poor proprioception
- Need for frequent manual medicine or manipulation

- "Weak" phasic muscles on exam
- Easy fatigability of phasic muscles
- Chronic musculoskeletal pain
- Progressive postural decline
- Symptoms of tendonopathy
- Poor "core" strength

While each one of these elements may not be considered relevant on its own, when you see several of these findings together you should consider a thorough functional biomechanical examination with emphasis on identifying kinetic chain issues and treating them in an integrated manner.

References

1. Brolinson PG, Kozar AJ, Cibo G. Sacroiliac joint dysfunction in athletes. Curr Sports Med Rep 2003; 2: 47–56.
2. DeLee JC, Farney WC. Incidence of injury in Texas high school football. Am J Sports Med 1992; 20 (5):575–580.
3. Gomez E, DeLee JC, Farney WC. Incidence of injury in Texas girls' high school basketball. Am J Sports Med 1996; 24 (5):684–687.
4. NCAA Injury Surveillance System (ISS). At: http://www1.ncaa.org/membership/ed_outreach/health-safety/iss/index.html. Accessed 27 September 2008.
5. Morelli V, Espinoza L. Groin injuries and groin pain in athletes: part 1. Prim Care Clin Office Pract 2005, 32:163–183.
6. Lovell G. The diagnosis of chronic groin pain in athletes: a review of 189 cases. Aust J Sci Med Sport 1995; 27 (3):76–79.
7. Westlin N. Groin pain in athletes from Southern Sweden. Sports Med Arthros Rev 1997; 5:280–284.
8. Koh J, Dietz J. Osteoarthritis in other joints (hip, elbow, foot, ankle, toes, wrist) after sports. Clin Sports Med 2005, 24:57–70.
9. Olsen O, Vingard E, Koster M, Alfredsson L. Etiologic fractions for physical work load, sports and overweight in the occurrence of coxarthrosis. Scand J Work Environ Health 1994; 20 (3):184–188.
10. Kujala UM, Marti P, Kaprio J, et al. Occurrence of chronic disease in former top-level athletes. Predominance of benefits, risks or selection effects? Sports Med 2003; 33 (8):553–561.
11. Spector TD, Harris PA, Hart DJ, et al. Risk of osteoarthritis associated with long-term weight-bearing sports: a radiologic survey of the hips and knees in female ex-athletes and population controls. Arthritis Rheum 1996; 39 (6):988–995.
12. Lindberg H, Roos H, Gardsell P. Prevalence of coxarthrosis in former soccer players. 286 players compared with matched controls. Acta Orthop Scand 1993; 64 (2):165–167.
13. Lane NE, Bloch DA, Jones HH, et al. Long-distance running, bone density, and osteoarthritis. JAMA 1986; 255 (9):1147–1151.
14. Konradsen L, Hansen EM, Sondergaard L. Long distance running and osteoarthrosis. Am J Sports Med 1990; 18 (4):379–381.

15. Shepard GJ, Banks AJ, Ryan WG. Ex-professional association footballers have an increased prevalence of osteoarthritis of the hip compared with age matched controls despite not having sustained notable hip injuries. Br J Sports Med 2003; 37 (1):80–81.
16. Drawer S, Fuller C. Propensity for osteoarthritis and lower limb joint pain in retired professional soccer players. Br J Sports Med 2001; 35:402–408.
17. Lindberg H, Roos H, Gardsell P. Prevalence of coxarthrosis in former soccer players. 286 players compared with matched controls. Acta Orthop Scand 1993; 64 (2):165–167.
18. Lequesne MG, Dang N, Lane NE. Sport practice and osteoarthritis of the limbs. Osteoarthritis Cartilage 1997; 5 (2):75–86.
19. Schmitt H, Brocai DR, Lukoschek M. High prevalence of hip arthrosis in former elite javelin throwers and high jumpers: 41 athletes examined more than 10 years after retirement from competitive sports. Acta Orthop Scand 2004; 75 (1):34–39.
20. Vingard E, Sandmark H, Alfredsson L. Musculoskeletal disorders in former athletes. A cohort study in 114 track and field champions. Acta Orthop Scand 1995; 66 (3):289–291.
21. Callahan L. Osteoarthritis in retired National Football League (NFL) players: The role of injuries and playing position. Abstract presentation: American College of Rheumatology Annual Meeting New Orleans (LA); October, 2002.
22. <http://www.medicalpost.com/mpcontent/article.jsp?content=/content/extract/rawart/3811/19a.html>. Accessed March 3, 2007.
23. Vingard E, Alfredsson L, Malchau H. Osteoarthrosis of the hip in women and its relation to physical load at work and in the home. Ann Rheum Dis 1997; 56 (5):293–298.
24. Spector TD, Harris PA, Hart DJ, et al. Risk of osteoarthritis associated with long-term weight-bearing sports: a radiologic survey of the hips and knees in female ex-athletes and population controls. Arthritis Rheum 1996; 39(6):988–995.
25. Lane NE, Hochberg MC, Pressman A, et al. Recreational physical activity and the risk of osteoarthritis of the hip in elderly women. J Rheumatol 1999; 26 (4):849–854.
26. Buckwalter JA, Lane NE. Athletics and osteoarthritis. Am J Sports Med 1997; 25 (6):873–881.
27. Gorsline RT, Kaeding CC. The use of NSAIDs and nutritional supplements in athletes with osteoarthritis. Clin Sports Med 2005, 24:71–82.
28. Kujala UM, Kaprio J, Sarna S. Osteoarthritis of weight bearing joints of lower limbs in former elite male athletes. BMJ 1994; 308 (6923): 231–234.
29. Leunig M, Casillas MM, Hamlet M, et al. Slipped capital femoral epiphysis: early mechanical damage to the acetabular cartilage by a prominent femoral metaphysis. Acta Orthop Scand 2000; 71 (4): 370–375.
30. McCarthy JC, Noble PC, Schuck MR, et al. The Otto E. Aufranc award: the role of labral lesions to development of early degenerative hip disease. Clin Orthop 2001; 393:25–37.

31. Kerger S. Exercise principles. In: Steven J, Karageanes J, (eds). Principles of Manual Sports Medicine. Philadelphia: Lippincott, Williams & Wilkins. 65–76, 2005.
32. Wertheimer LG, Lopes SD. Arterial supply of the femoral head: A combined angiographic and histological study. J Bone Joint Surg 1971; 53A:545–556.
33. Brand RA, Pedersen DR, Davy DT, et al. Comparison of hip force calculations and measurements in the same patient. J Arthroplasty 1994; 9:45–51.
34. Anderson K, et al. Hip and groin injuries in athletes. AJSM. 2001; 29 (4):521–533.
35. Pink M, Perry J, Houglum PA, et al. Lower extremity range of motion in the recreational sport runner. Am J Sports Med 1994; 22:541–549.
36. Montgomery WH III, Pink M, Perry J. Electromyographic analysis of hip and knee musculature during running. Am J Sports Med 1994; 22:272–278.
37. Sahrmann SA. Diagnosis and Treatment of Movement Impairment Syndromes. St. Louis: Mosby, 2002.
38. Panjabi MM, White AA. Biomechanics in the Musculoskeletal System, first ed. Philadelphia: Churchill Livingstone, 2001.
39. Gajdosik RL. Passive extensibility of skeletal muscle: review of the literature with clinical implications. Clin Biomech 2001; 16(2), 87–101.
40. Gombatto SP, Collins DR, Sahrmann S, et al. Gender differences in pattern of hip and lumbopelvic rotation in people with low back pain. Clin Biomech 2006, 21:263–271.
41. Philippon MJ. The role of arthroscopic thermal capsulorrhaphy in the hip. Clin Sports Med 2001; 20(4):817–829
42. Bellabarba C, Sheinkop MB, Kuo KN. Idiopathic hip instability. An unrecognized cause of coxa saltans in the adult. Clin Orthop 1998; 355:261–271.
43. Shindle MK, Ranawat AS, Kelly BT. Diagnosis and management of traumatic and atraumatic hip instability in the athletic patient. Clin Sports Med 2006; 25:309–326.
44. Crowninshield RD, Johnston RC, Andrews JG, et al. A biomechanical investigation of the human hip. J Biomech 1978; 11:75–85.
45. Vleeming A, Lee D, Ostgaard HC, et al. An integrated model of "joint" function and its clinical application. Presented at the 4th Interdisciplinary World Congress on Low Back and Pelvic Pain. Montreal, Canada; November 8–10, 2001.
46. Hodges PW, Richardson CA. Feedforward contraction of transverses abdominis is not influenced by the direction of arm movement. Exp Brain Res 1997; 114:362–370.
47. Richardson CA, Snijders CJ, Hides JA, et al. The relation between the transversus abdominis muscles, sacroiliac joint mechanics, and low back pain. Spine 2002; 27:399–405.
48. Leinonen V, Kankaanpaa M, Airaksinen O, et al. Back and hip extensor activities during trunk flexion/extension: effects of low back pain and rehabilitation. Arch Phys Med Rehabil 2000; 81:32–37.

49. Sparto PJ, Parnianpour M, Reinsel TE, et al. The effect of fatigue on multi-joint kinematics, coordination, and postural stability during a repetitive lifting test. J Orthop Sports Phys Ther 1997; 25:3–12.
50. Vleeming A, Pool-Goudzwaard AL, Stoeckart R, et al. The posterior layer of the thoracoabdominal fascia: its function in load transfer from spine to legs. Spine 1995; 20:753–758.
51. Anderson E, Nilsson J, Thorstensson A. Intramuscular EMG from the hip flexor muscles during human locomotion. Acta Physiol Scand 1997; 161:361–370.
52. Anderson E, Oddsson L, Grundstrom H, et al. The role of the psoas and iliacus muscles for stability and movement of the lumbar spine, pelvis and hip. Scand J Med Sci Sports 1995; 5:10–16.
53. Anderson E, Nilsson J, Zhijia M, et al. Abdominal and hip flexor muscle activation during various training exercises. Eur J Appl Physiol 1997; 75:115–123.
54. Vleeming A, Stoeckart R, Snijders CJ. The sacrotuberous ligament: a conceptual approach to its dynamic role in stabilizing the sacroiliac joint. Clin Biomech 1989, 4:201–203.
55. Vleeming A, van Wingerden JP, Snijders CJ, Stoeckart R. Load application to the sacrotuberous ligament: influences on sacroiliac joint mechanics. Clin Biomech 1989; 4:204–209.
56. van Wingerden JP, Vleeming A, Stam HJ, Stoeckart R. Interaction of the spine and legs: influence of the hamstring tension on lumbopelvic rhythm. Second Interdisciplinary World Congress on Low Back Pain. San Diego, CA; November 9–11, 1993.
57. Renstrom P, Peterson L. Groin injuries in athletes. Br J Sports Med 1980; 14 (1):30–36.
58. Kuchera ML. Treatment of gravitational strain pathophysiology. In Vleeming A, Mooney V, Dorman T, et al, eds. Movement, Stability, and Low Back Pain: The Essential Role of The Pelvis. New York: Churchill Livingstone, 1997; 477–499.
59. Greenman PE. Clinical aspects of the sacroiliac joint in walking. In Vleeming A, Mooney V, Dorman T, et al, eds. Movement, Stability, and Low Back Pain: The Essential Role of The Pelvis. New York: Churchill Livingstone, 1997.
60. Kapandji IA. The physiology of the joints. In Vol 3: the trunk and the vertebral column, 2nd ed. New York: Churchill Livingstone; 1994.
61. Irvin RE. Reduction of lumbar scoliosis by use of a heal lift to level the sacral base. J Am Osteopath Assoc 1991; 1:33–44.
62. Hoffman K, Hoffman L. Effects of adding sacral base leveling to osteopathic manipulative treatment of low back pain: a pilot study. J Am Osteopath Assoc 1994; 3:217–226.
63. Kuchera ML, Jungman M. Inclusion of a Levitor orthotic device in management of refractory low back pain patients. J Am Osteopath Assoc 1986; 10:673.
64. Irvin RE. Suboptimal posture: the origin of the majority of idiopathic pain of the musculoskeletal system. In Vleeming A, Mooney V, Dorman T, et al, eds. Movement, Stability, and Low Back Pain: The Essential Role of the Pelvis. New York: Churchill Livingstone; 1997:133–155.

65. Greenman PE. Principles of Manual Medicine, 2nd ed. Baltimore: Williams & Wilkins; 1996.
66. Macintyre J, Johson C, Schroeder EL. Groin pain in athletes. Curr Sports Med Rep 2006, 5:293–299.
67. Verrall GM, Slavotinek JP, Barnes PG, et al. Diagnostic and prognostic value of clinical findings in 83 athletes with posterior thigh injury: comparison of clinical findings with magnetic resonance imaging documentation of hamstring muscle strain. Am J Sports Med 2003; 31 (6):969–973.
68. Ekstrand J, Gillquist J. Soccer injuries and their mechanisms: a prospective study. Med Sci Sports Exerc 1983; 15 (3):267–270.
69. Nielsen AB, Yde J. Epidemiology and traumatology of injuries in soccer. Am J Sports Med 1989; 17 (6):803–807.
70. Ekstrand J, Gillquist J. The avoidability of soccer injuries. Int J Sports Med 1983; 4 (2):124–128.
71. Tyler TF, Nicholas SJ, Campbell RJ, et al. The association of hip strength and flexibility with the incidence of adductor muscle strains in professional ice hockey players. Am J Sports Med 2001; 29 (2):124–128.
72. Holmich P, Uhrskou P, Ulnits L, et al. Effectiveness of active physical training as treatment for long-standing adductor-related groin pain in athletes: randomised trial. Lancet 1999; 353 (9151):439–443.
73. Tyler TF, Nicholas SJ, Campbell RJ, et al. The effectiveness of a preseason exercise program to prevent adductor muscle strains in professional ice hockey players. Am J Sports Med 2002; 30 (5):680–683.
74. Broadhurt N. Iliopsoas tendinitis and bursitis. Aust Fam Physician 1995; 24 (7):1303.
75. Emery CA, Meeuwisse WH. Risk factors for groin injuries in hockey. Med Sci Sports Exerc 2001; 33:1423–1433.
76. Nicholas SJ, Tyler TF. Adductor muscle strains in sport. Sports Med 2002; 32:339–344.
77. Hoelmich P. Adductor-related groin pain in athletes. Sports Med Arthroscop Rev 1997; 5:285–291.
78. Fricker PA. Management of groin pain in athletes. Br J Sports Med 1997; 31:97–101.
79. Johnston CA, Wiley JP, Lindsay DM, et al. Iliopsoas bursitis and tendinitis. A review. Sports Med 1998; 25 (4):271–283.
80. Fricker PA, Taunton JE, Ammann W. Osteitis pubis in athletes. Infection, inflammation or injury? Sports Med 1991; 12 (4):266–279.
81. Orava S, Kujala UM. Rupture of the ischial origin of the hamstring muscles. Am J Sports Med 1995; 23 (6):702–705.
82. Anderson K, Strickland S, Warren R. Hip and groin injuries in athletes. Am J Sports Med 2001; 29 (4):521–533.
83. Kujala UM, Orava S, Karpakka J, et al. Ischial tuberosity apophysitis and avulsion among athletes. Int J Sports Med 1997; 18 (2):149–155.
84. Renstroem AF. Groin injuries: a true challenge in orthopaedic sports medicine. Sports Med Arthroscop Rev 1997; 5:247–251.
85. Koch RA, Jackson DW. Pubic symphysitis in runners. A report of two cases. Am J Sports Med 1981; 9 (1):62–63.

86. Williams JG. Limitation of hip joint movement as a factor in traumatic osteitis pubis. Br J Sports Med 1978; 12(3):129–133.
87. Paletta GA Jr, Andrish JT. Injuries about the hip and pelvis in the young athlete. Clin Sports Med 1995; 14 (3):591–628.
88. Westlin N. Groin pain in athletes from Southern Sweden. Sports Med Arthroscop Rev 1997; 5:280–284.
89. Roos HP. Hip pain in sport. Sports Med Arthrosc 1997; 5:292–300.
90. Rolf C. Pelvis and groin stress fractures: a cause of groin pain in athletes. Sports Med Arthrosc 1997; 5:301–304.
91. Clough TM. Femoral neck stress fracture: the importance of clinical suspicion and early review. BJSM, 2002; 36:308–309.
92. Egol KA, Koval KJ, Kummer F, Frankel VH. Stress fractures of the femoral neck. Clin Ortho Relat Res 1998; 348:72–78.
93. Canale ST, Beaty JH. Pelvic and hip fractures. In: Rockwood CA Jr, Wilkins KE, Beaty JE, et al, editors. Rockwood and Green's fractures in adults, 4th ed. Philadelphia: Lippincott-Raven; 1996:1109–1147.
94. Beaty JH. Pelvis, hip and thigh. In: Sullivan JA, Anderson SJ, eds. Care of the young athlete. Rosemont (IL): American Academy of Orthopaedic Surgeons and American Academy of Pediatrics; 2000:365–376.
95. Boyd KT, Peirce NS, Batt ME. Common hip injuries in sport. Sports Med 1997; 24 (4):273–288.
96. Patterson I. The torn acetabular labrum. J Bone Joint Surg [Br] 1957; 39:306–309.
97. Narvani AA, Tsiridis E, Kendall S, et al. A preliminary report on prevalence of acetabular labrum tears in sports patients with groin pain. Knee Surg Sports Traumatol Arthrosc 2003; 11(6):403–408.
98. Narvani, AA, Tsiridis E, Tai, CC, et al. Acetabular labrum and its tears. BJSM 2003, 37:207–211.
99. Takechi H, Nagashima H, Ito S. Intra-articular pressure of the hip joint outside and inside the limbus. J Jpn Orthop Assoc 1982; 56:529–536.
100. Ferguson SJ, Bryant JT, Ganz R, et al. The acetabular labrum seal: a poroelastic finite element model. Clin Biomech 2000; 15:463–468.
101. Konrath GA, Hamel AJ, Olsen SA, et al. The role of the acetabular labrum and the transverse acetabular ligament in load transmission in hip. J Bone Joint Surg [Am] 1998; 80:1781–1787.
102. Ganz R, Parvizi, J, Beck, M, et al. Femoroacetabular impingement: a cause for osteoarthritis of the hip. Clin Orthop Relat Res 2003; 412:112–120.
103. Crawford, JR, Villar RN. Current concepts in the management of femoroacetabular impingement. J Bone Joint Surg [Br] 2005; 87-B:1459–1462.
104. Philippon, MJ. Arthroscopy for the treatment of femoroacetabular impingement in the athlete. Clin Sports Med 2006; 25:299–308.
105. Ikeda T, Awaya G, Suzuki S, et al. Torn acetabular labrum in young patients. Arthroscopic diagnosis and management. J Bone Joint Surg Br 1988; 70 (1):13–16.
106. Klaue K, Durni CW, Ganz R. The acetabular rim syndrome: a clinical presentation of dysplasia of the hip. J Bone Joint Surg [Br] 1991; 73:423–429.

107. Leunig M, Werlen S, Ungersbock A, et al. Evaluation of the acetabulum labrum by MR arthrography. J Bone Joint Surg [Br] 1997; 79:230–234.
108. Fitzgerald RH. Acetabular labrum tears. Diagnosis and treatment. Clin Orthop 1995; 311:60–68.
109. Laorr A, Greenspan A, Anderson MW, et al. Traumatic hip dislocation: early MRI findings. Skeletal Radiol 1995; 24 (4):239–245.
110. Burnett RSJ, Della Roca GJ, Prather H, et al. Clinical presentation of patients with tears of the acetabular labrum. J Bone Joint Surg 2006; 88:1448–1457.
111. Hase T, Ueo T. Acetabular labral tear: arthroscopic diagnosis and treatment. Arthroscopy 1999; 15:138–141.
112. Hofmann S, Tschauner C, Urban M, et al. Clinical and radiological diagnosis of lesions of the labrum of the hip. Orthopade 1998; 27:681–689.
113. Czerny C, Hofmann S, Neuhold A, et al. Lesions of the acetabular labrum: accuracy of MR arthrography in detection and staging. Radiology 1996; 200:225–230.
114. Waters PM, Millis MB. Hip and pelvic injuries in the young athlete. Clin Sports Med 1988; 7 (3):513–526.
115. Hochschuler SH. The Spine and Sports. Philadelphia: Hanley and Belfus; 1990.
116. Slipman CW, Sterenfeld EB, Chou LH, et al. The predictive value of provocative sacroiliac joint stress maneuvers in the diagnosis of sacroiliac joint syndrome. Arch Phys Med Rehabil 1998; 79:288–292.
117. Van der Wurff P, Hagmeijer RHM, Meyne W. Clinical tests of the sacroiliac joint: A systematic methodological review. Part I: reliability. Man Ther 2000; 5:30–36.
118. Van der Wurff P, Hagmeijer RHM, Meyne W. Clinical tests of the sacroiliac joint: a systematic methodological review. Part II: validity. Man Ther 2000; 5:89–96.
119. Cibulka MT, Koldehoff R. Clinical usefulness of a cluster of sacroiliac joint tests in patients with and without low back pain. J Orthop Sports Phys Ther 1999; 29:83–92.
120. Dreyfuss P, Dreyer S, Griffin J, et al. Positive sacroiliac screening tests in asymptomatic adults. Spine 1994; 19:1138–1143.
121. Ward RC, Jerome JA, Jones JM III. Foundations for Osteopathic Medicine, 2nd ed. Baltimore: Lippincott Williams & Wilkins; 2002.
122. Magee DJ. Orthopedic Physical Assessment, 3rd ed. Philadelphia: WB Saunders; 1997.
123. Morelli V, Espinoza L. Groin injuries and groin pain in athletes: part 2. Prim Care Clin Office Pract 2005; 32:185–200.
124. Reynolds D, Lucas J, Klaue K. Retroversion of the acetabulum. A cause of hip pain. J Bone Joint Surg Br 1999; 81(2):281–288.
125. Kuchera ML. Treatment of gravitational strain pathophysiology. In: Vleeming A, Mooney V, Dorman T, et al, eds. Movement, Stability, and Low Back Pain: The Essential Role of The Pelvis. New York: Churchill Livingstone; 1997:477–499.
126. Kuchera ML. Gravitational stress, musculoligamentous strain, and postural alignment. Spine: State of the Art Reviews 1995; 9:463–490.

127. Brolinson PG, Gray G. Principle-centered rehabilitation. In: Garrett WE, Kirkendall DT, Squire DH, eds. Principles and Practice of Primary Care Sports Medicine. Philadelphia: Lippincott Williams and Wilkins; 2001:645–652.
128. Jones PS, Tomski MA. Exercise and osteopathic manipulative medicine: the Janda approach. PM&R: State of the Art Reviews 2000; 14:163–179.
129. Comerford MJ, Mottram SL. Functional stability re-training: principles and strategies for managing mechanical dysfunction. Man Ther 2001; 6:3–14.
130. Schlink MB. Muscle imbalance patterns associated with low back problems. In: The Spine in Sports. Los Angeles: Robert & Watkins; 1996.

Chapter 4
Gait Assessment

Jimmy D. Bowen and Gerry Salter

CLINICAL PEARLS

- The understanding of gait is paramount in understanding an athlete's impairment and the diagnosis, treatment, and rehabilitation of that impairment.
- Walking and running are universal endeavors while efficient athletic walking and running are not. Know the difference.
- The examination of a lower limb injury begins at the feet and extends to the spine and must pass through the hip and pelvis, regardless of the joint or segment injured.
- Understanding the differences that occur in gait as we age will help you promote the continued athletic performance of your "baby boomer" patients.
- Differences in gait between genders exist, it is important to know the variability in order to design your differential diagnoses and treatments.

CASE PRESENTATION

Chief Complaint
A 42-year-old female long distance runner presents with right anterior knee pain and complaint of right foot placement changes during running.

History of Present Illness
She has been a competitive runner for 15 years, at times running up to 60 miles a week. During the last 15 years, she has had a number of bilateral lower extremity injuries including

patellofemoral knee pain, iliotibial band friction syndrome, plantar fasciitis, peroneal tendonitis, right groin pain, and sacroiliac malalignment. These ailments normally abated with relative rest, nonsteroidal anti-inflammatory agents (NSAIDS), manual physical therapy, and rare corticosteroid injections. About 2 years ago, she began insidiously catching her right foot while running, occasionally falling to the ground. After relative rest and treatment, she had been able to return to pain-free running but has continued to have problems regarding right foot placement. She has no symptoms with other activities, such as activities of daily living or athletic activities, including elliptical trainers and road biking. The persistent right foot catching and inability now to push off correctly have affected her to the point that she has not run in the last 3 months.

Review of Systems
She denies any neurological symptoms, neck or back problems, and is currently on no medications except for occasional use of NSAIDS. She has had serial examinations and multiple diagnostic testing that have yet to reveal the etiology of her problem.

Physical Examination
Her physical examination reveals normal spinal alignment and range of motion without pain. Her pelvic and spinal static alignment demonstrates no imbalances. She demonstrates frontal plane (Table 4.1 and Fig. 4.1) genu valgus of less than 10° bilaterally that are symmetric. During relaxed double stance, she has 9° more frontal plane rear foot eversion (calcaneal valgus) on the right versus the left. While walking, she demonstrates more right hip transverse plane internal rotation and more right foot pronation than on the left. During running, there was an increase of hip internal rotation and adduction with increased genu valgus. Interestingly, the right foot supinated during plantar flexion of stance phase with internal rotation and forefoot transverse plane adduction during push off, causing her foot to catch. She compensated for this by circumduction of her right lower extremity so that she could clear her foot during swing phase. This caused her to be off balanced during running and she consistently lunged to the right. Her hip, knee, and ankle ranges of motion were normal and symmetric. She was noted to have adductor tightness on the right compared to the left. She was also noted to have decreased strength on manual muscle testing of the right hip abductors and external rotators. The remainder of her neurological and vascular examination was normal.

TABLE 4.1. Anatomic plane classification

Region	Sagittal	Frontal/coronal	Transverse/rotational
Foot	Toe flex/ext	Pronation/supination	Adduction/abduction
Ankle	Plantar flexion Dorsiflexion	Varus/valgus	
Tibia			Internal/external torsion
Knee	Flex/extension	Varum/valgum	
Femur			Internal/external rotation
Hip	Flex/extension	Adduction/abduction	
Pelvis	Ant/post tilt	Elevated/depressed	Rotation
Spine	Lordosis/kyphosis	Lateral scoliosis	Rotational scoliosis

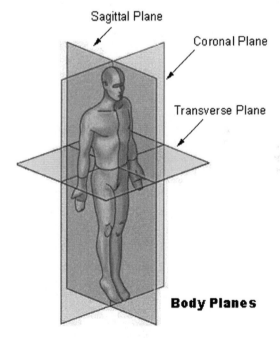

FIGURE 4.1. Anatomic planes. Sagittal plane divides body into left and right. Coronal/frontal plane divides it into front and back or anterior and posterior. Transverse/axial plane divides body into cranial and caudal portions. This picture is in the *public domain* in the United States.

Testing

Radiographic images of her lumbar spine, hips and pelvis, and knees were all normal except for minimal degenerative changes of her knees. Scanogram of her pelvis to ankles demonstrated no anatomic leg length discrepancy. An electrodiagnostic study (EDX) of her right lower extremity and back was normal.

GAIT ASSESSMENT

I spent this last weekend at a local track meet and for the countless time noted that no two people seem to run the same way. Anthropometric differences, turn over speeds, stride lengths, arm swing, endurance, and the will to succeed all seem to dictate how a runner performs. Great, now how do I take this observation of idiosyncratic differences and translate it into a clinically relevant enterprise when I see a runner with a problem? Well to begin with, walking and running are two of the most obvious and fundamental actions of life. Being able to visualize and discern gait patterns is the beginning of understanding the complexities of gait.[1] Ultimately, it is important for the sports medicine provider to appreciate the complexities of gait: what makes for an efficient gait; are there differences in gait relative to age or gender; what is the importance of symmetry for an individual; and do identified impairments have a functional impact or cause limitations?[2] We all have an idea of what an optimal gait should look like. Consider the sprinting power of a Michael Johnson in the 200 M or 400 M run, or the graceful efficiency of no wasted motion of the great Kenyan long distance runners, and you have an observational *gestalt* of what the optimal gait pattern is for running.

THE ELEMENTS OF GAIT

"Walking is the simple act of falling forward and catching oneself."[3] The tasks of walking and running involve forward propulsion, alternately balancing the body on one limb and then the other by repeated adjustments of limb length, and supporting the body in an upright position. The assessment of these activities takes time, practice, and technical skill.[3] It begins with an understanding of the definitions, phases, and determinants of gait.

Walking involves always having one foot in contact with a surface for support, in fact it involves periods of single limb and double limb support. Running involves periods in which neither foot is in contact with a surface, in effect a "double float" (Fig. 4.2). The basic unit of walking and running is the gait cycle; also known as "stride." During the gait cycle, Perry et al.[4] describe temporal and functional variables. The functional aspects of the

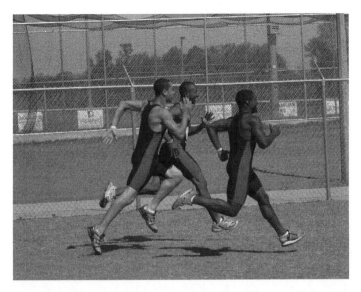

FIGURE 4.2. Two of three runners in *running double float* phase. Picture by Kevin Lewter.

gait cycle are weight acceptance and support during stance and limb advancement during swing. Classically there are eight phases of the gait cycle beginning with the initial contact of the loading response and progressing to terminal swing before the next initial contact (Table 4.2 and Fig. 4.3). Temporal–spatial gait parameters also must be understood including the *stride time*, initial contact on right to initial contact on right, and *step time*, initial contact on right to initial contact on the left. The stride length is the distance covered during a stride with the gait velocity being the stride distance divided by the time taken.[1-3]

Walking and running demonstrate a reversal of the percentage of stance and swing phase. During walking stance phase represents 60% of the time during the gait cycle while swing represents 40%. The slower the walking speed, the more is the time spent in double limb support and the faster the walking speed, the less is the time in double limb support, until a time is reached when no interval exists which would be considered double limb support. At this time, you are running.

The *kinematics of gait* of the individual during walking or running is evaluated by observing the body as composed of body

Table 4.2. Normal gait cycle

Loading response	Initial double support stance phase beginning with initial contact. Some literature may include initial contact as separate phase of cycle.
Mid-stance	First half of single support representing the time the opposite limb leaves the floor until body weight is aligned over the forefoot.
Terminal stance	Second half of single support representing the time the opposite limb makes contact with the floor and the body weight moves ahead of the forefoot.
Push off	Late stance when there is an ankle plantar flexion moment advancing the limb into swing phase. Some literature references include this as part of pre-swing phase.
Pre-swing	Final double support representing the time of initial contact of the contralateral limb to ipsilateral toe-off.
Initial swing	Initial third of the swing phase representing the time from toe-off to when the swing limb foot is opposite the stance limb.
Mid swing	Middle third of swing, time the swing foot is opposite the stance limb to when the tibia is vertical.
Terminal swing	Final third of the swing phase, time from tibia being vertical until initial contact.

segments (links) and connections (joints) between segments.[1] The kinematics of the individual or system is known when the orientation and position of the segments are recognized. Each link has a center of mass (COM) or center of gravity (COG). The whole system, the body, also has a COM or COG. As segments move, their positions in time and space affect the balance and energy use of the system as the whole body COM distribution changes.[5] Kinematics is best evaluated through quantitative and not qualitative means (SOR = A). Three-dimensional (3D) gait analysis provides information relative to degrees of movement of the joint and relationships to the links in terms of frontal, sagittal, and transverse arrangements. The flexion–extension, abduction–adduction, and internal rotation–external rotation relationship of the segments and joints are evaluated and compared to "norms" as well as the side to side, front to back symmetry within an individual. The COM for the segments and the COM of the body are expressed in terms of vertical, anterior to posterior, and medial to lateral relationships.[6,7] The body COM reaches its highest point in stance when

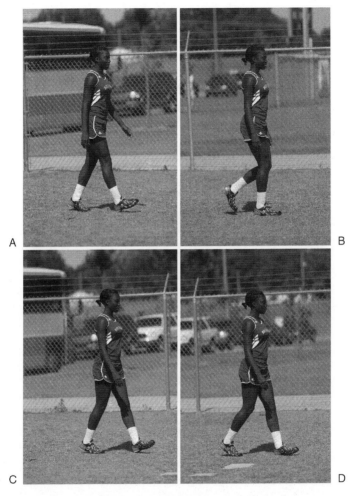

FIGURE 4.3. (**A**) Initial contact, the beginning of the *loading response*. (**B**) Mid stance. (**C**) Terminal stance. (**D**) Push off, beginning of pre-swing. (**E**) Pre-swing. (**F**) Initial swing. (**G**) Mid swing. (**H**) Terminal swing. Pictures by Kevin Lewter.

the speed is minimal (i.e., double stance phase during walking).[8] This is illustrated in a classic oral board examination question. A person stands at the entrance of a 100 yard tunnel. Standing erect weight bearing on both feet, the top of the tunnel is 1 cm above

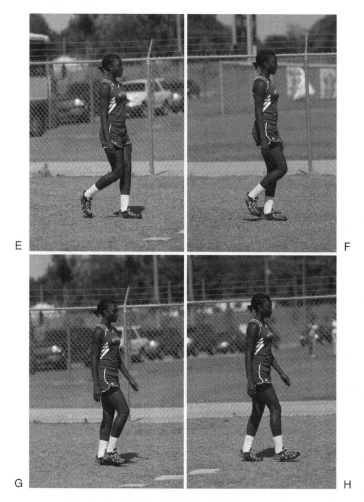

FIGURE 4.3. *Continued.*

the person's head. If the person begins to walk in the tunnel, will the person hit his or her head on the tunnel ceiling? The answer of course is NO. For walking, the maximums of COM and height are during double stance phase. But, if the individual is running, the maximums of COM and height are during "double float" at maximum velocity. Always a good idea not to run in a low tunnel!

The muscles play an important role in what occurs at the joints. The function at the hip during gait is simplistically to extend the thigh during stance and flex the thigh during swing. The ligaments of the hip stabilize the joint during extension. The extensors and flexors of the hip work phasically and cooperatively. The iliopsoas will contract eccentrically to slow extension while the hamstrings will contract eccentrically to control hip flexion. The abductors and adductors of the hip provide static and phasic co-contraction stability of the stance leg during single leg support. If the mobility of the hip is reduced, there will be an increased moment of the ipsilateral knee, contralateral hip, and the lumbar spine to compensate. The knee acts as a shock absorber during weight bearing, a stride length extender, and a pendulum for leg and foot swing. The knee flexes during the first three levels of stance phase, and then extends during stance to push-off. If the knee has a flexion deformity, it will decrease extension at the hip during stance and reduce hip extension power. The gastrosoleus complex provides restraint for the individual's forward momentum during forward movement. Using 85% maximum voluntary contraction during normal walking,[9] it stabilizes the knee and ankle providing restraint of forward rotation of the tibia on the talus. During stance, it will minimize the vertical displacement of the COM. The foot and ankle work independently during normal walking. Movements and stresses are absorbed by the structures of the leg and foot during initial heel contact through push-off during terminal stance phase.

The *kinetics of gait* represents the study of forces and moments that cause movement.[1] An example in gait research would be the expression of the forces exerted on the foot during contact called the ground reactive force (GRF). The center of the distribution of these forces is called the center of pressure.

The kinetics of gait during the phases of the gait cycle are best realized during the clinical qualitative evaluation by observation of the parameters, parametrics, or "determinants" of gait (SOR = B). Normal determinants of gait are seen between 8 and 45 years of age, but, may be seen as young as 3 years old and well into the eighth decade in some individuals. Gait differences are seen between different ages and different genders. The determinants of gait change within an individual depending on age, segment and joint maintenance, health, strength, and flexibility. Non-impaired walking is almost effortless. This efficiency is made possible by minimizing the displacement of the body's COM during ambulation. Vertical displacement is far more relevant than lateral displacement when considering optimization of this efficiency.[10] During walking, the

COM normally travels along an inverted pendulum with a sinusoidal, up and down, side to side path with each step. A series of maneuvers described by Saunders and colleagues, are the mechanism by which the body minimizes the COM displacement during walking; they are known as "the determinants of gait."[11] The COM is normally 5 cm anterior to the second sacral vertebrae, slightly higher in males on average. The vertical and horizontal displacements of the COM describe a figure of eight within a relatively small 5 cm square during walking. Vertical displacement is seen as head height decreasing during weight acceptance and unloading, and increasing during stance. During normal gait cadence of 90–120 steps/min,[12,13] if factors increase the vertical displacement, greater energy is needed, cardiovascular responses are elevated, and a self-selected slower walking speed will be entertained for compensation. If not for the combined action of the determinants of gait, the average total vertical displacement of the COM would be two times the value it actually is in normal gait.

THE DETERMINANTS OF GAIT
1. *Pelvic rotation in the transverse/axial plane:* Decreases the drop in COM during double limb support. The pelvis rotates anterior 4° during swing and posterior 4° during stance phase. This decreases the amplitude of displacement along the COM's path. To maintain balance, the thorax and pelvis rotate in opposite directions. Weakness or inflexibility in these *core* areas will increase the amplitude of displacement of the COM and cause less efficient progression. During pelvic rotation, the other joints of the lower limb are involved in rotation as well. In fact, the greater the joint's distance from the trunk, the greater is the rotation (i.e., the tibial rotation is three times the rotation of the pelvis).[8]
2. *Pelvic obliquity in the frontal/coronal plane*: Slight pelvic obliquity reduces the peak COM during single limb support. During swing phase the hip of the swing limb is lowered, the knee is flexed, and the ankle dorsiflexed to clear the toe of the swing leg. Flexion of the lower limb joints and lowering of the hip keeps the COM from moving up and down less than 5 cm (2 in.) during normal gait.
3. *Lateral pelvic shift in the frontal/coronal plane*: Necessary for balancing over the stance leg. The pelvis lists to the side, causing relative adduction of the stance weight bearing lower limb. There is a side to side movement of the pelvis during walking that is normally 2½–5 cm (1–2 in.). The natural valgus between the femur and the tibia brings the feet closer together during

forward progression. The amount of lateral displacement can be altered because of changes in foot placement width and relative weakness of the hip abductors.

4. *The interchange of knee, ankle, and foot motions*: This interchange reduces the displacement of the COM and gives a smooth sinusoidal movement pattern. The ankle controls plantar flexion from initial contact to loading, the knee flexes slightly to reduce the peak of COM during single stance, the ankle progresses to dorsiflexion during single support also reducing the peak of COM displacement, and the foot progresses from a supinated to a pronated position during weight acceptance to push off. Inability to flex or lower the hip or flex the knee or ankle will be seen during the qualitative evaluation as *circumduction* of the relatively longer limb during swing phase or *vaulting* during stance phase, with a noticeable increased vertical displacement of the head (bobbing). This is more energy consuming and less efficient.

AGE AND DIFFERENCES IN GAIT

The inverted pendulum model accurately predicts the general pattern of mechanical energy fluctuations of the body during walking and an optimal walking speed.[14]

For adults the hip vaults over the stance leg like an inverted pendulum. Two times during each gait cycle both hips simultaneously lift during midstance. The recovery of mechanical energy of the COM in each gait cycle is similar for older children and adults.[15] Toddlers are more variable from step to step than older children and adults. The sinusoidal hip oscillations seen in adults are lacking in toddlers. Also the forward energy of the displacement of the COM is very irregular. Newly locomotive toddlers do not implement the classic inverted pendulum mechanism, but they do develop this over the first few months of ambulation.

As adults age, it is not unusual to observe decreased walking speed and step length. This and the increased double support time are well established by epidemiological and clinical literature.[16] Winter et al.[17] noted that the reasons for these changes were not well understood, questioning whether it was a "voluntary" self selection for safety or physiologic decline and neuromuscular adaptation. Studies done recently[18–22] suggest that the changes in gait in the aged have a physiologic basis. These changes may include decreased range of motion, muscular strength, vestibular function, vision, proprioception, and cardiopulmonary vitality. Studies have pointed to a neuromuscular basis, but they have been inconsistent.

A literature review by McGibbon[16] gives strong evidence that neuromuscular adaptations seen are responses to a primary impairment and exist to provide a compensatory role.

A dramatic decrease in ankle power output during terminal stance phase represents a consistent finding in age and impaired related gait. This limits gait speed, length of steps, and may cause variable stride characteristics that may be linked to falls in adults.[23] Inconsistent results from studies do point to compensation of this reduced ankle power through increased hip concentric and eccentric power. This may possibly provide trunk stabilization with hip extensors and in assisting with leg swing initiated by the use of the hip flexors. Hip flexor contractures seen commonly with sedentary adults may present additional limiting impairment in combination with weak ankle push-off power.

MALE AND FEMALE GAIT

Relative weakness and reduced ability to stabilize the hip, pelvis, and trunk are documented in women and female athletes.[24–28] This has been demonstrated as reduced endurance of side bridging activity and decreased hip abduction and external rotation isometric strength relative to men. But what are the consequences, if any, of these findings? Women may be more vulnerable to large external forces experienced by these proximal segments during athletics, especially in the transverse and frontal planes. They may be predisposed to excessive motion in the hip and trunk compared to men, potentially permitting their entire lower extremity to move into positions frequently associated with non-contact injuries. Many studies[29–31] observe that women display greater hip internal rotation and adduction during athletic tasks (Fig. 4.4). This functional positioning has been demonstrated to be associated with increased injury in retrospective and cross sectional studies.[32]

Leetun et al.[24] provided the first prospective study that demonstrated this relationship and that the strength rather than the endurance of core stability is the key to maximizing the capacity of the lumbo–pelvic–hip complex during weight bearing athletic activity.

CASE ASSESSMENT AND TREATMENT

This female runner demonstrated weakness of the proximal stabilizers of the pelvis resulting in an abnormal running pattern. Relative weakness of the external rotators and abductors of the right hip placed the right hip in a more internally rotated and adducted position during running. Initially, she was given a routine of open and closed chain exercises designed to improve

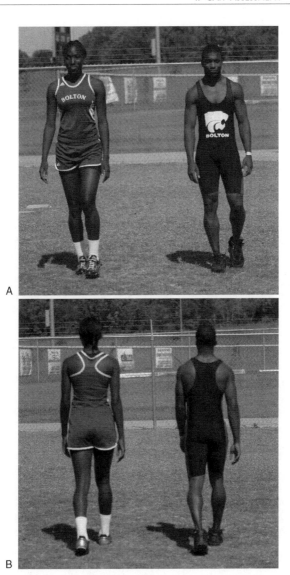

FIGURE 4.4. (**A**) Female and male walking (front). Note the relative hip internal rotation and adduction in our female athlete. (**B**) Female and male walking (back). Note the relatively lower COM and the relative increase of hip internal rotation and adduction in our female athlete. Pictures by Kevin Lewter.

the functional motion and stability of her spine, pelvis, and hips through all plans of movement. Then she was placed on a series of exercises that emphasized concentric, isometric, and eccentric progressive strengthening in a functional fashion needed to reduce this proximal muscle weakness. After 8 weeks of three times a week conditioning, she was released to a progressive return to running program. Her impaired movement pattern did not return and she is currently running without difficulty.

SUMMARY

Gait evaluation is an essential part of the assessment of hip and pelvic integrity in an athlete. The evaluators' implementation of the examination takes time and patience to develop a clinically efficient and effective evaluation, and a functional and anatomic gestalt for identification of impairments which may be relatively subtle. Through systematic understanding of the anatomy, neuromuscular interaction, kinematics, and kinetics involved in the enterprise of locomotion, a more comprehensive clinical evaluation can be achieved. An understanding of differences of age and gender of athletes and patients can help the evaluator develop a more definitive recommendation for resolution of pain and impairment, and optimization of activities.

References

1. Kerrigan D, Croce U. Gait analysis. In: O'Connor F, Sallis R, Wilder R, et al, eds. Sports Medicine: Just the Facts. New York: McGraw-Hill Medical Publishing Division; 2005:126–130.
2. Malanga G, Delisa J. Clinical observation. In: Delisa J, ed. Gait Analysis in the Science of Rehabilitation. Department of Veterans Affairs. Darby: Diane Publishing; 2000:1–10.
3. Magee D. Gait assessment In: Magee D, ed. Orthopedic Physical Assessment, 3rd ed. Philadelphia: WB Saunders Company; 1997: 673–696
4. Perry J. Gait Analysis, Normal and Pathological Function. Thorofare, NJ: SLACK; 1992.
5. Birrer R, Buzermanis S, DellaCorte M, et al. Bio-mechanics of running. In: O'Connor F, Wilder R, eds. The Textbook of Running Medicine. New York: McGraw Hill; 2001:11–19.
6. Novacheck T. The Biomechanics of Running. Gait Posture 1998; 7:77–95.
7. Adams J, Perry J. Gait analysis: clinical applications. In: Rose J, Gamble J, eds. Human Locomotion. Baltimore: William and Wilkins; 1994:139–164.
8. Inman V, Ralston H, Todd F. Human locomotion. In: Rose J, Gamble J, eds. Human Locomotion. Baltimore: Williams and Wilkins; 1994:1–22.

9. Sutherland D, Glshen R, Cooper W. The development of mature gait. J. Bone Joint Am 1980; 62:336–353.
10. Gonzalez E, Corcoran P. Energy expenditure during ambulation. In: Downey J, Myers S, Gonzalez E, Lieberman J, editors. The Physiological Basis of Rehabilitation Medicine, 2nd edn. Stoneham (MA): Butterworth-Heinemann; 1994:413–446.
11. Saunders J, Inman V, Eberhart H. The major determinants in normal and pathological gait. J. Bone Joint Am 1953; 35:543–558.
12. Nuber G. Biomechanics of the foot and ankle during gait. Clin Sports Med 1988; 7:1–13.
13. Rodgers M. Dynamic foot mechanics. J Orthop Sports Phys Ther 1995; 21:306–316.
14. Invanenko Y, Dominici N, Lacquaniti F. Development of independent walking in toddlers. Exer Sports Sci Rev 2007; 35(2):67–73.
15. Cavagna G, Franzetti P, Fuchimoto T. The mechanics of walking in children. J Physiol 1983; 343:323–339.
16. McGibbons C. Toward a better understanding of gait changes with age and disablement: Neuromuscular adaptation. Exer Sport Sci Rev 2003; 31(2):102–108.
17. Winter D, Patla A, Frank J, et al. Biomechanical walking pattern changes in the fit and healthy elderly. Phys Ther 1990; 70:340–347.
18. Devita P, Hotobagyi. Age causes redistribution of joint torques and powers during gait. J Appl Physiol 2000; 88:1804–1811.
19. Judge J, Davis R, Ounpuu S. Step length reduction in advanced age: the role of ankle and hip kinetics. J Gerontol Med Sci 1996; 51A:303–312.
20. Kerrigan D, Todd M, Croce U, et al. Biomechanical gait alterations independent of speed in the healthy elderly: evidence for specific limiting impairments. Arch Phys Med Rehabil 1998; 79:317–322.
21. McGibbon C, Krebs D. Age related changes in lower trunk coordination and energy transfer during gait. J Neurophysiol 2001; 85:1923–1931.
22. Riley P, Croce U, Kerrigan D. Effects of age on lower extremity joint moment contributions to gait speed. Gait Posture 2001; 14:264–270.
23. Hausdorff J, Rios D, Edelberg H. Gait variability and fall risk in community-living older adults: a 1-year prospective study. Arch Phys Med Rehabil 2001; 82(8):1050–1056.
24. Leetun D, Ireland M, Willson J, et al. Core stability measurements as risk factors for lower extremity injury in athletes. Med Sci Sports Exerc 2004; 36:6:926–934.
25. Bohannon R. Reference values for extremity muscle strength obtained by hand-held dynamometry from adults aged 20 to 79 years. Arch Phys Med Rehabil 1997; 78:26–32.
26. Cahalan T, Johnson M, Liu S, et al. Quantitative measurements of hip strength in different age groups. Clin Orthop 1989; 246:136–145.
27. McGill S, Childs A, Lieberman C. Endurance times for back stabilization exercises: clinical targets for testing and training form normal database. Arch Phys Med Rehabil 1999; 80:941–944.
28. Nadler S, Malanga G, Deprince M, et al. The relationship between lower extremity injury, low back pain, and hip muscle strength in male and female collegiate athletes. Clin J Sport Med 2000; 10:89–97.

29. Ferber R, McClay Davis R, Williams D. Gender differences in lower extremity mechanics during running. Clin Biomech 2003; 18:350–357.
30. Lephart S, Ferris C, Riemann B, et al. Gender differences in strength and lower extremity kinematics during landing. Clin Orthop 2002; 401:162–169.
31. Malinzak R, Colby S, Kirkendall D, et al. A comparison of knee joint motion patterns between men and women in selected athletic tasks. Clin Biomech 2001; 16:438–445.
32. Ireland M, Willson B, Ballantyne B, et al. Hip strength in females with and without patellofemoral pain. J Orthop Sports Phys Ther 2003; 33:671–676.

Chapter 5
Imaging of Hip and Pelvis Injuries

Donald J. Flemming and Eric A. Walker

CLINICAL PEARLS
- It is extremely important to provide the interpreting radiologist with a detailed and accurate history in order to avoid underappreciation of subtle findings on the requested study.
- When interpreting plain radiographs, do not focus just on the femoral head and hip joints. The scan must also include the sacroiliac joints, lumbar spine, pubic symphysis, obturator foramen, and adjacent soft tissues as well.
- If intra-articular pathology is suspected, the magnetic resonance imaging (MRI) should be performed on a high field system with a narrow field of view (as opposed to an open low field magnet).
- Magnetic resonance arthrography (MRA) is the preferred method of assessment of cartilage pathology in the hip joint.
- Stress fractures present on MR as a linear band of signal replacing normal bone marrow.
- If femoroacetabular impingement (FAI) is suspect, radiography should include a cross-table lateral view.

INTRODUCTION

Injuries of the hip and groin are not as common as those of the extremities but are important to diagnose and treat accurately because they can be associated with prolonged rehabilitation times and significant disability.[1] Imaging plays an important role in the accurate diagnosis of these injuries but should not supplant a careful history and physical examination. Many factors must be considered prior to requesting a radiologic study (i.e., age of the patient; duration, type, and location of symptoms; and likely source of injury) because the optimal exam may be different if the injured tissue is bone, muscle, cartilage, or tendon.

A physician evaluating an injured athlete has a tremendous advantage over a treatment provider compared to 30 years ago because of the relatively recent explosion of cross-sectional imaging techniques including ultrasound (US), computed tomography (CT), and, most importantly, magnetic resonance imaging (MRI). It is vital that the referring clinician understands the advantages and limitations of these various modalities to ensure that the most cost-effective and accurate diagnosis can be rendered. The importance of providing a detailed and accurate history to the interpreting radiologist cannot be over-emphasized.

MODALITIES

Radiography

Despite the proliferation of advanced imaging modalities, the radiograph continues to be an important examination for the evaluation of hip and groin pain.[2] This study is frequently referred to as a plain film, but there is nothing simple about this examination despite its humble moniker. In fact, significant findings may be under-appreciated by clinicians who are unaware of recently described subtle radiographic manifestations of important sources of hip pain such as FAI. The advantages of radiography include high spatial resolution, relative low cost, high specificity, and wide availability.

It is absolutely paramount that the examination be properly exposed and positioned. The proper examination of the hip should include an anteroposterior (AP) view of the pelvis and a lateral view of the hip. The AP view of the pelvis allows for side-to-side comparison which may aide in the detection of subtle pathology. Some authors recommend that the AP view be obtained in the weight-bearing position, and although there are potential advantages to this approach, no study has been performed to confirm the superiority of this technique over standard non-weight-bearing radiography. Regardless, the femurs should be internally rotated to optimally evaluate the femoral neck on the AP examination (Fig. 5.1a). There are two options for lateral radiography. The frog-leg lateral view (Fig. 5.1b) is preferred for general diagnostic evaluation of the hip but a cross-table lateral view (Fig. 5.1c) should be obtained if FAI is a clinical concern.

An organized approach to the evaluation of the radiograph increases the likelihood of detection of pathology. The interpreter must remember to include the sacroiliac joints, lumbar spine,

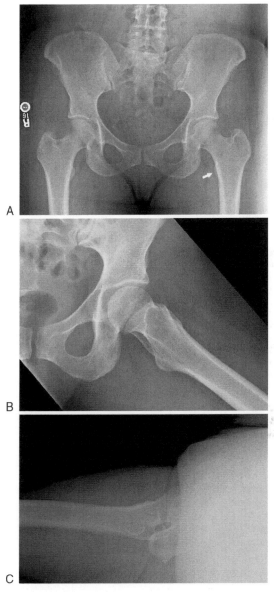

FIGURE 5.1. (A) Normal AP view of the pelvis. The curves formed by joint surface of the femoral head and the acetabulum are parallel. The femurs are internally rotated as indicated by the fact that the lesser trochanter (*white arrow*) is barely visible. (B) Normal frog-leg lateral view of the hip. (C) Normal cross-table lateral view of the hip.

pubic symphysis, obturator foramen, and soft tissues in their scan pattern and not to focus on just the femoral head and hip joints.

US

US has limited utility for evaluation of hip disease outside the pediatric population. The technique requires that the operator be knowledgeable and the learning curve can be quite steep. However, US can be used with success in the assessment of muscle and tendon pathology. For example, the diagnosis of a snapping iliopsoas tendon is rapidly and easily confirmed with US.

CT

CT is most commonly used to evaluate suspected or known fractures. However, the development of helical CT in modern scanners has led to the ability to perform reconstructed images in multiple planes. Complex oblique images are now obtainable on-the-fly on many workstations. Some investigators have taken advantage of this capability and shown that CT arthrography can yield information in patients who are not suitable for MRI evaluation regardless of the reason.

It is extremely important that referring clinicians understand that radiation dose is not insignificant with this modality. Techniques not requiring radiation should be considered before CT, particularly in young patients.

Magnetic Resonance Imaging

The introduction of clinical MRI has revolutionized the field of musculoskeletal imaging and has improved our understanding of injuries to the athlete. Although expensive and time-consuming, MRI offers a global evaluation of the hip including assessment of bone, cartilage, muscle, and tendons. The two most critical aspects leading to successful diagnosis of pathology are the quality of the examination and the experience of the interpreter.

Not all MRI examinations or scanners are equal and it is extremely important that the referring clinician has an open line of communication with the radiologist to ensure that the appropriate examination is done with the appropriate equipment. One consideration often is whether the patient should be scanned on an open low field magnet or a closed high field system. In general, if the question is fracture or muscle injury, either a low field or high field system will yield equivalent results. However, if the question pertains to intra-articular pathology such as cartilage defects or labral tears, then the examination should be performed on a high field system with a narrow field of view.

Magnetic Resonance Arthrography
MRA is the preferred examination for the assessment of cartilage pathology in the hip joint. Some investigators feel that high quality, small field of view imaging is sufficient for detection of pathology but most radiologists prefer MRA. Diagnoses can be rendered more confidently when the joint is distended by contrast. Although MRA may be superior to non-contrast examination, it does have some negative aspects. The examination is typically performed following the direct administration of contrast into the joint which requires the fluoroscopic guided introduction of a needle into the joint, which can be painful for some patients. One distinct advantage of direct arthrography is that additional diagnostic information can be obtained if anesthetic is injected into the joint at the same time as contrast. Relief of pain with provocative maneuvers following the intra-articular injection of anesthetic can go a long way toward confirming an intra-articular source of pain. Some radiologists advocate the use of indirect arthrography which involves intravenous injection of contrast with the imaging of the joint following exercise and a brief delay. While this technique is less painful, it does not distend the joint and is associated with rare but potential allergic reaction to gadolinium contrast.

A summary of recommended examinations is provided in Table 5.1.

TABLE 5.1. Recommended Examinations

Diagnosis	Radiograph	CT	US	MRI	MRA
Stress fracture	+++	−	−	+++	−
Acute fracture	+++	++	−	++	−
Arthritis	+++	−	−	+++	−
FAI	+++	+	−	++	+++
Labral tear	−	−	−	+	+++
Tendon injury	+	−	++	+++	−
Muscle injury	+	+	++	+++	−

(−) Not indicated
(+) May be useful
(++) Useful
(+++) Recommended

RADIOLOGIC DIAGNOSIS OF HIP PAIN IN ATHLETES

Osseous
Bone is an amazing organ system that develops on the basis of a combination of genetic and physical influences. Bone, despite its remarkable mechanical and physiologic properties, may fail in response to excessive acute or chronic repetitive forces.

Stress Fracture
Stress fractures are a result of excessive force being applied to bone in a chronic repetitive fashion. The normal physiologic response to new stress to a bone is for remodeling to occur, but if the osteoblastic response is outpaced by removal of bone by osteoclasts, the bone can mechanically fail. Stress fracture should be considered in the differential diagnosis of any patient who has recently changed the intensity of his or her physical activity. In addition to poor physical conditioning, risk factors for development of stress fracture includes female gender, Caucasian race, smoking, steroid use, tall/thin physique, and low sex hormones.[3,4] The basicervical portion of the femoral neck is the classic location for stress fracture to occur in the hip or pelvis, but other described locations include the pubic rami, sacrum, superior acetabulum,[5] medial femoral diaphysis,[6] and even the femoral head.[7]

Radiographs are usually the first line modality used to evaluate stress fractures. The appearance of a stress injury to bone will be dependent on the temporal nature of the injury and the bone involved. The initial radiographic examination may be completely normal because 30–50% of bone must be resorbed for a lucency to be appreciated on radiography. It is very important to make sure that the femur is properly positioned for the radiographic examination.[2] The femur should be internally rotated approximately 10–15° to ensure that the femoral neck is adequately evaluated (Fig. 5.2).

The classic radiographic findings that may be appreciated include sclerosis and periosteal reaction.[8] The initial radiographs may be normal. Sclerosis is usually in a linear pattern transverse to the long axis of the involved bone. On occasion, this sclerotic reaction and periosteal reaction can be exuberant leading to concern for tumor. The linear nature of the abnormality and the patient's history will usually be sufficient to dispel concerns about neoplasm. It is not uncommon for subtle findings to be missed, particularly when the abnormality is in an unusual location that may be obscured by bowel gas, such as the sacrum. A high degree of suspicion and careful side-to-side comparison

5. IMAGING OF HIP AND PELVIS INJURIES   93

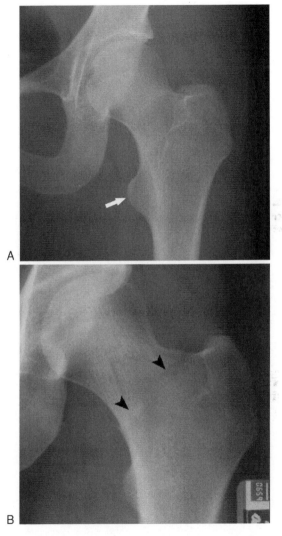

FIGURE 5.2. A 25-year-old runner with hip pain and completed stress fracture. (**A**) AP view of the hip in external rotation. The lesser trochanter (*white arrow*) is in profile indicating external rotation which foreshortens the femoral neck. (**B**) AP view of the hip in internal rotation. The fracture that was not appreciated in external rotation is now easily seen (*black arrowheads*). Note the linear lucency laterally and the condensation of trabeculae medially.

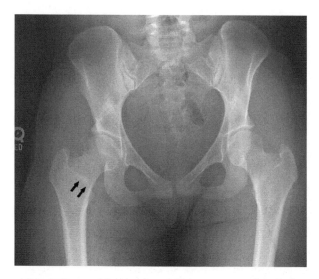

FIGURE 5.3. A 22-year-old active duty military woman with right hip pain after recent increase in miles run per week. AP view of the pelvis shows subtle band of sclerosis at the inferior basicervical portion of the femoral neck (*black arrows*) indicating stress fracture.

of the AP radiograph of the pelvis will increase the likelihood of detection of a stress injury (Fig. 5.3).

When a stress fracture is clinically likely, MRI of the hip should be ordered if the radiograph is normal. The importance of early detection has been emphasized because the prognosis is poorer if the patient progresses to a complete or displaced fracture. The MRI examination should evaluate the entire pelvis with both T1 and a fluid sensitive sequence such as a fat-suppressed T2 weighted or short-tau inversion recovery (STIR) sequence.

Stress fractures present as a linear band of signal replacing normal bone marrow.[9] On T1 weighted sequences, the normal bright signal of fat will be replaced by a linear band of low signal. On fat suppressed sequences, the normal low signal fat is replaced by bright signal that may or may not surround a thin band of low signal. The MRI presentation is usually very characteristic (Fig. 5.4).

Two recently described presentations of stress injuries deserve special mention: thigh splints[6] and subchondral stress fracture of the femoral head.[7] Patients with thigh splints present with either medial sided thigh or groin pain. This injury occurs secondary

5. IMAGING OF HIP AND PELVIS INJURIES   **95**

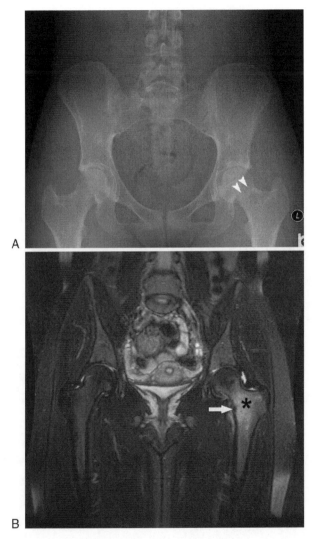

FIGURE 5.4. A 21-year-old active duty woman with left hip pain after changing physical training regimen. (**A**) AP view of the pelvis shows subtle sclerosis in the left femoral neck (*white arrowheads*). (**B**) Coronal T2 fat saturation sequence clearly demonstrates diffuse edema of the femoral neck (*) and medial callus formation (*white arrow*).

to abnormal forces at the insertion of the adductor muscles on the medial diaphysis of the femur. Radiographically, thigh splints present as solid periosteal reaction along the medial aspect of the femur. The correlate on MRI is high signal on fluid sensitive sequences medial to the cortex of the diaphysis and the femur that, unfortunately, can be easily overlooked.

Stress fracture in subchondral bone of the femoral head is a relatively newly described condition that may be confused with avascular necrosis (AVN). This diagnosis should be considered when findings mimicking AVN are seen in the femoral head of an athlete without risk factors for osteonecrosis. A correct diagnosis of subchondral stress fracture in these patients leads to the correct treatment (rest) and the prognosis is generally much better than that of AVN.

Acute Fracture

Acute hip or pelvis fracture is uncommon as a result of acute trauma in athletics, even in high energy contact sports. Children are an exception to this rule because of the inherent weakness at the physis and apophyses of growing bone.[10] Radiography with AP view of the pelvis and orthogonal view of the symptomatic hip is usually sufficient to render a diagnosis. Careful side-to-side comparison between the affected and asymptomatic side helps with identification of subtle nondisplaced fractures of the pelvis and proximal femur (Fig. 5.5).

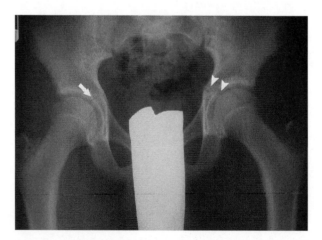

FIGURE 5.5. A 13-year-old boy with left hip pain after being tackled while playing football with fractured left acetabulum. An AP view of the pelvis shows subtle asymmetry in the triradiate cartilage, which is wider on the left (*white arrowheads*) than on the right (*white arrow*) indicating a Salter I fracture of this growth center.

Slipped capital femoral epiphysis (SCFE) is an important diagnostic consideration in the pre-adolescent or adolescent athlete. These patients are approximately 11 years of age with risk factors including obesity and black race. SCFE can present bilaterally although it is not common to see both hips symptomatically affected at the same time. Children present with either an acute or a chronic history of groin pain. Radiographs are usually abnormal (Fig. 5.6). The involved physis is usually widened and the proximal femoral epiphysis is usually displaced inferiorly and medially relative to the femoral diaphysis.[11] The displacement of the epiphysis is sometimes appreciated on the AP view of the hip if the femoral head is located below a line drawn along the superior border of the femoral neck. This line (Kline's line) should normally intersect the superior lateral aspect of the femoral head. A lateral view will confirm the displacement of the femoral epiphysis. MRI may be useful in the situation when a radiograph is normal in a patient with hip pain at risk for slipped femoral epiphysis. The MRI will reveal widening of the physis with increased signal on fluid sensitive sequences in the adjacent metaphysis.

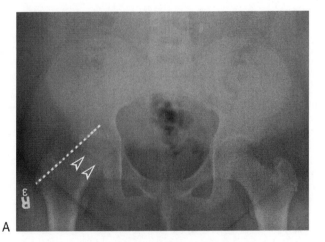

FIGURE 5.6. A 13-year-old boy with right hip pain and slipped capital femoral epiphysis. (**A**) An AP view of the pelvis shows subtle widening of the right physis (*hollow white arrowheads*) in comparison to the left hip. Note that the femoral head is below the Klein's line (*white dotted line*) drawn parallel to the superior aspect of the femoral neck, indicating the proximal femoral epiphysis is inferiorly displaced. (**B**) Frog-leg lateral view confirms posterior displacement of the femoral head.

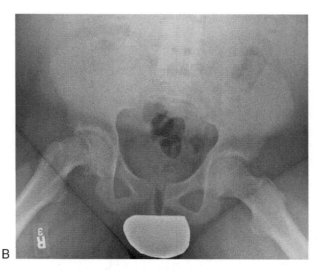

FIGURE 5.6. *Continued.*

The apophyses about the hip and pelvis are at risk for avulsion and these injuries are being diagnosed with increased frequency as children are exposed to highly competitive athletic activities that require sudden or violent muscle contraction such as soccer, hockey, gymnastics, and sprinting sports.[10] The apophyses at risk include the anterior superior iliac spine (ASIS) (sartorius origin), anterior inferior iliac spine (AIIS) (rectus femoris origin), ischial tuberosity (hamstring origin), ilium (oblique insertion), and lesser trochanter (iliopsoas insertion). Diagnosis is usually readily established with an AP radiograph (Fig. 5.7) although injuries in the ASIS and AIIS may be better appreciated on view of the pelvis oblique to the side of injury. Avulsion of an apophysis can be easily missed on MRI[12] and may be better appreciated on US or CT if confirmation is required in the setting of a normal radiograph.

Articular Pathology

There is an ever increasing body of knowledge directed at the early detection of intra-articular injuries of the hip. Although the hip is an intrinsically stable joint, it should be no surprise that cartilage structure of the hip is at risk for tears as contact forces are three to five times body weight or higher in athletes. It is very important to remember to evaluate the sacroiliac joints and the pubic symphysis for conditions such as sacroiliitis or osteitis pubis. Disease in both of these joints may present as hip or groin pain in the athlete.

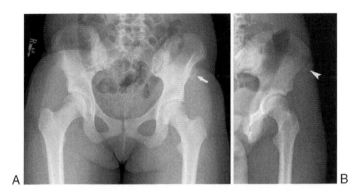

FIGURE 5.7. A 16-year-old woman with acute onset of pain in left hip and avulsion of the anterior superior iliac spine. (**A**) AP view of the pelvis shows avulsion of the ASIS (*white arrow*). (**B**) Avulsion injury is better appreciated on a left posterior oblique view of the left hip (*white arrowhead*).

Osteoarthritis

Patients with cartilage pathology present with pain that is frequently associated with locking or clicking. Both the labrum and the articular cartilage are at risk for injury. The labrum is a nerve containing fibrocartilaginous structure that is at the periphery of the joint. Its purpose is to deepen the articular socket and to help maintain the normal negative pressure of the joint. Tears of this structure can occur along its entire length but are most common anterior superiorly and increase the likelihood of damage of the articular surface.[2] Labral tears are associated with the accelerated development of osteoarthritis. While congenital and developmental anomalies of the hip are a common cause of early onset osteoarthritis, other potential causes include subclinical joint laxity, history of acetabular or femoral neck fracture, osteonecrosis, prior inflammatory arthritis, and inherited collagen production anomalies.

Osteoarthritis presents radiographically as joint space narrowing with osteophyte formation. Joint space narrowing can be subtle, but comparison to the unaffected side can increase detection of subtle alteration in joint dimensions. Joint space narrowing usually occurs at the superolateral aspect of hip. The AP view of the pelvis is usually sufficient for detection of joint space narrowing but assessment of joint dimension should also be performed on lateral views (Fig. 5.8). Posterior joint space narrowing is associated with a poor clinical prognosis and should not be overlooked on faux views of the acetabulum.[13]

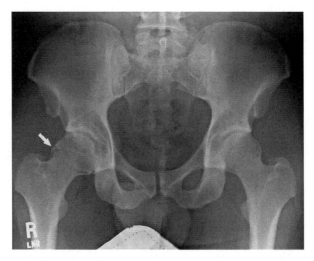

FIGURE 5.8. A 39-year-old man with right hip pain and bilateral hip osteoarthritis. AP view of the pelvis shows narrowing of the superolateral right hip joint space with osteophyte formation (*white arrow*). Subtle superolateral joint space narrowing is also seen in the left hip.

Abnormal morphology of the joint whether from prior SCFE, idiopathic AVN as a child (Legg–Calves–Perthes disease), or developmental dysplasia can lead to accelerated degenerative disease. A surprisingly large number of these conditions can escape detection at an early age and only are recognized when the patient presents with hip pain as an adult.

Developmental Dysplasia
Patients with developmental dysplasia have less osseous coverage of the femoral head than normal patients and are at increased risk for the development of labral tear and early onset osteoarthritis. Developmental dysplasia of the hip (DDH) is frequently detected in infancy but there are subclinical cases that may elude typical screening practices.

Radiographic changes of DDH may be very subtle but are extremely important to recognize. Whenever there is poor osseous acetabular coverage of the lateral femoral head, the interpreter of a radiographic examination should consider DDH as a diagnosis. Many measurements have been developed to confirm the radiographic diagnosis of DDH, but the most easily used in clinical practice is the center edge angle of Wiberg.[14] This angle is

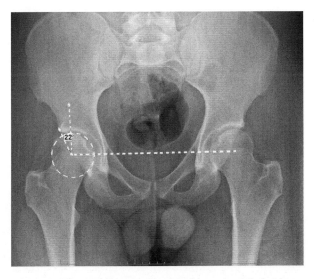

FIGURE 5.9. A 34-year-old man with right hip pain and developmental dysplasia of the hip. AP view of the pelvis shows relative lack of coverage of the lateral aspect of the femoral head that is suspicious for mild DDH. The center edge angle measures less than 25°, confirming DDH.

easily assessed electronically on images in picture archiving and communications systems (PACS). A horizontal line is drawn between the centers of the femoral heads. Perpendicular lines are drawn to this horizontal line extending through the center of the femoral head. A line is then drawn from the center of the femoral head to the lateral margin of the acetabulum. The angle formed between the perpendicular and the lateral margin of the acetabulum is known as the center edge angle and should be between 25° and 39° in the normal patient.[13,14] A center edge angle of less than 25° indicates DDH (Fig. 5.9).

Femoroacetabular Impingement

FAI has recently been recognized as an important source of hip pain.[15] Normal motion of the hip leads to impaction of the femoral neck on the acetabulum and labrum. This mechanical impaction leads to labral tears and osteoarthritis. FAI has been separated into two basic types, cam and pincer. Most patients have a combination of both types. Cam impingement is caused by an aspherical femoral head–neck junction. The pincer type of impingement is produced by excessive acetabular coverage of the femoral head.

The assessment for FAI begins with the radiograph. A properly positioned AP view of the pelvis and cross-table lateral view are used for primary evaluation.[14] These views are assessed for signs of aspherical femoral head–neck junction, acetabular over-coverage, and acetabular rim phenomenon.

The classic sign of cam type of impingement is excessive bone formation at the femoral head–neck junction that can be appreciated as flattening of the contour of the superolateral femoral neck on the AP radiograph or of the anterior superior femoral neck on the lateral view. The shape of the femoral head–neck junction can assume the shape of a pistol grip as a manifestation of asphericity. The α-angle is a measurement used to measure asphericity on the cross-table lateral view and is best performed on a PACS workstation. A circle is drawn around the femoral head and a line is drawn from the center of the femoral neck that intersects the center of this circle. A second line is drawn where the circle crosses the cortex of the anterior femoral neck junction. The resulting angle should be less than 50° in a normal patient (Fig. 5.10). Another manifestation of the same phenomenon is femoral offset. This too is measured on the cross-table lateral view.

Osseous over-coverage of the femoral head is responsible for the pincer type of FAI. Numerous measurements have been devised

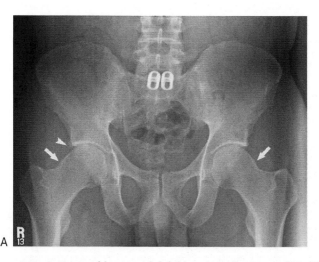

FIGURE 5.10. A 41-year-old man with left hip pain and cam-type FAI. (**A**) AP view of the pelvis shows bone formation at the superolateral aspect of the femoral neck bilaterally (*white arrows*). Ossification is present in the right acetabular labrum (*white arrowhead*). (**B**) Cross-table lateral view of the left hp shows asphericity of the femoral head with abnormally wide α-angle, which is seen in the cam type mechanism of FAI.

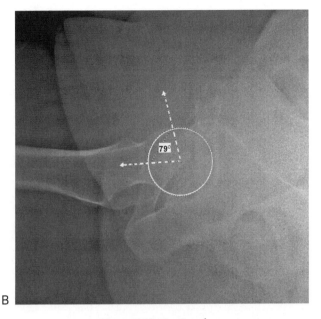

FIGURE 5.10. *Continued.*

to assess over-coverage. The simplest measurement is a center-edge angle greater than 39° (Fig. 5.11). Subtle forms of pincer impingement can occur particularly involving the anterolateral acetabular rim. All AP radiographs of the pelvis should be assessed for the "crossover" sign at the anterolateral acetabulum. The anterior acetabular wall should not project beyond the posterior acetabular wall in a properly positioned AP radiograph of pelvis. If it does, this indicates relative overgrowth of the anterior lateral acetabulum that can lead to impingement (Fig. 5.12). However, before interpreting a positive cross-over sign, one must make sure that the radiograph is properly positioned.[14] The center of the sacrum should be directed at the pubic symphysis to ensure that there is not excessive rotation of the pelvis that may be confounding. Additionally, the distance from the superior aspect of the pubic symphysis should be less than approximately 3.2 cm in men or 4.7 cm in women to correctly assess for focal acetabular over-coverage. If the pelvis is too far tilted anteriorly, this distance will widen and be associated with a false positive cross-over sign.

FAI may produce other findings that can be appreciated on radiographs including some manifestations that up until recently were discounted as normal variants. Chronic impaction may lead to separation of the rim from the remainder of the acetabulum

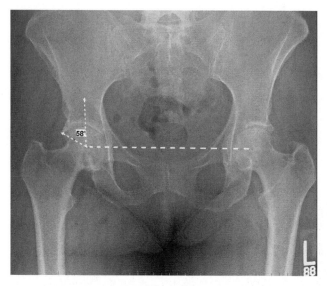

FIGURE 5.11. A 48-year-old woman with hip pain. Degenerative changes with marginal osteophytes and protrusio acetabuli lead to pincer-type FAI. In pincer-type FAI, acetabular overcoverage limits the range of motion and leads to impaction between the acetabulum and the femur.

producing what has historically been described as the os acetabulum (Fig. 5.13).[16] Impaction may also induce a focal lucency in the subcapital portion of the femoral neck (Fig. 5.14). This juxtaarticular cyst has been called a synovial herniation pit and was initially described as a normal variant to avoid confusion with neoplasm. This juxtaarticular cyst is now recognized as a manifestation of FAI particularly when it is situated in the anterior superior portion of the femoral neck.[17] Finally, chronic impaction may lead to ossification of the labrum itself.[18] This pattern of ossification is different than that of an os acetabulum but the distinction is not that important because both foci of ossification are associated with FAI.

Labral Tears

Labral tears are now widely recognized as a potential source of hip pain in athletes. Patients present with hip pain that may or may not be associated with clicking or a locking sensation. Patients with DDH are at increased risk of developing labral tears.

Labral tears are best diagnosed using high quality MRA[2] even though the diagnosis may be established by CT arthrography.

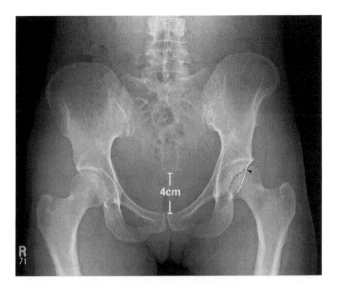

FIGURE 5.12. A 36-year-old woman with focal acetabular overcoverage and pincer-type FAI. AP view of the pelvis shows anterior wall of the acetabulum (*black dotted line*) crossing over the posterior wall (*white solid line*) superolaterally. The point of intersection is indicated by the *black arrowhead*. This is the abnormal cross-over sign indicating focal acetabular overcoverage.

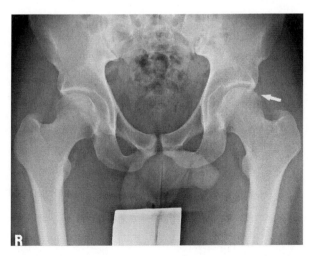

FIGURE 5.13. A 29-year-old man with left hip pain and os acetabulum. An AP view of the pelvis shows an ossicle (*white arrow*) adjacent to the left superolateral acetabulum, which is a secondary sign of FAI.

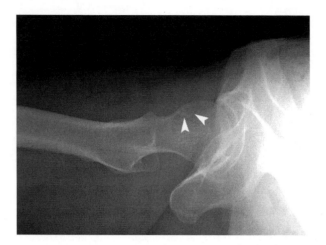

FIGURE 5.14. A 26-year-old woman with hip pain and synovial herniation pit. Cross-table lateral view shows subcortical lucency in the anterior femoral neck (*white arrowheads*) representing a secondary sign of FAI.

MRA offers a superior assessment of the surrounding soft tissues such as muscle or tendon and, therefore, may provide important additional information that cannot be obtained by CT. It is important to consult with an experienced hip arthroscopic surgeon to guide the evaluation of patients with potential hip pathology to avoid costly repeat or unnecessary imaging.

Labral pathology can present in many ways on MRA including abnormal morphology, abnormal internal signal, and detachment. Paralabral cysts are an important indicator for adjacent labral pathology because they develop from forced extrusion of joint fluid through a defect in the labrum.

Hip Ligaments

Injuries or abnormalities of ligaments and capsule are most commonly recognized in the shoulder and not really considered frequently in the hip because of the inherent stability of the joint. However, subluxation of the hip joint can occur in athletes and tears of the capsule and ligaments of the hip can transpire.[2] Subluxation events may also result in disruption of the ligamentum teres. The ligament may be thickened or torn with resulting pain. Diagnosis of capsular or ligamentous pathology is best accomplished with MR. In the acute setting, frank disruption of the capsule or ligament can be seen.

Thickening of the capsule may also be appreciated on MRI although the criteria for this diagnosis have not been widely accepted at this time. The cause of capsular thickening is not clear, but the finding is more commonly seen in patients with osteoarthritis. The relationship between capsular thickening and adhesive capsulitis has not been established in the hip, but one must wonder if there is a correlate to findings that are more commonly associated with the entity that has been well described in the shoulder.

Tendon

Multiple tendons are present around the hip that may be a source of chronic or acute hip pain. In general, tendon disease usually is not associated with radiographic findings. An important exception is calcific tendonitis. This entity, also known as hydroxyapatite deposition disease (HADD) is an idiopathic condition that is more commonly seen in the shoulder. However, the deposition of hydroxyapatite crystals into tendons about the hip can be seen and may be associated with pain (Fig. 5.15). Common locations for

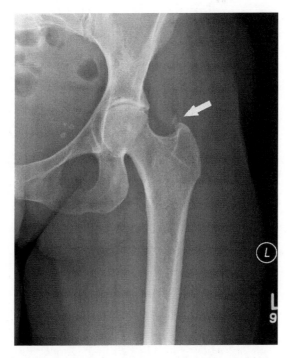

FIGURE 5.15. A 42-year-old woman with left hip pain and calcific tendinopathy of the hip abductors. AP view of the left hip shows a calcification in the hip abductor tendon immediately superior to the greater trochanter (*white arrow*).

visualization of HADD near the hip include the soft tissues lateral and superior to the greater trochanter (hip abductors) and the soft tissues posterior to the linea aspera (gluteus maximus).

Tendon degeneration or tear in the hip and groin is best evaluated on MRI. The appearance of tendon pathology on MRI is dependent on the extent of disease at presentation. Tendons are black on all sequences in the normal situation and the insertion on bone is also black. Acute avulsion or tear of a tendon is readily visible on fluid sensitive sequences (T2 weighted or STIR images) and presents as increased signal (white) at the tendon–bone interface. Increased signal may also be seen in the adjacent bone. Chronic avulsion or tear of a tendon can be subtle on imaging but is more readily appreciated if the injury is accompanied by heterotopic bone formation and retraction and atrophy of the involved muscle.

In some cases, tendon degeneration, also known as tendinopathy, may be associated with chronic pain in an athlete. Chronic disease in a tendon manifests as enlargement and internal increased signal on MRI. Chronic degeneration of a tendon can easily be overlooked on MRI and in fact, many cases of "trochanteric bursitis" actually represent tendinopathy of the hip abductors.[19]

Snapping Tendons

On occasion, a tendon may be responsible for a snapping sensation of the hip. If the snapping occurs in the groin, the iliopsoas tendon may be snapping over an osseous prominence on the superior pubic ramus. The tensor fascia lata may snap over the greater trochanter and produce lateral symptoms. Both conditions are readily confirmed with US.[20] Iliopsoas snapping can be confirmed and successfully treated with fluoroscopically guided injection of the iliopsoas bursa.[21]

Sportsman's Hernia

The so-called sportsman's hernia has recently been recognized as an important source of groin pain in athletes.[22] Patients may present with either the acute or chronic onset of pain that is worsened by twisting motions or sit-ups. Sportsman's hernia is a misnomer because a hernia is not the source of groin pain in most patients with this syndrome, and some authors prefer the term athletic pubalgia to describe this clinical complex. These patients have tears of either the adductor origin and/or the rectus abdominis insertion on the pubic symphysis probably as a result of pubic instability. Pubic instability may lead to plain film findings of osteitis pubis. Osteitis pubis presents radiographically as sclerosis with variable erosion that may simulate infection. The sportsman's hernia/

osteitis pubis complex is best visualized on MRI but can be easily overlooked by the interpreter who is not searching for the findings of this entity. Avulsion of the adductor origin or rectus abdominis insertion will manifest as increased signal on T2-weighted images at the level of the pubic symphysis[23,24] (Fig. 5.16). As with all imaging findings, the plain film or MRI results must be interpreted in conjunction with findings on physical examination because positive results in asymptomatic individuals are not uncommon.

Muscle

Muscle injuries of the lower extremities are very common. Imaging of these injuries may be required not only for confirmation but for determining treatment and prognosis. Muscle injuries have been divided into different grades for research purposes, but from a practical perspective, injuries are divided into minor requiring minimal rest and major for those injuries requiring more protracted recovery.[25,26]

Muscle injuries are usually not visible on radiographs. Heterotopic ossification is the sequela of soft tissue injury that may be visible on plain film. Recognizing heterotopic ossification on radiograph is very important to avoid confusion with tumor.[27] Many patients report a history of blunt trauma that is followed by the onset of severe pain and swelling. The initial radiographs may not show any abnormality or findings may be limited to subtle amorphous density. This will rapidly progress over weeks to a classic pattern of zonal ossification that separates this disease radiographically from neoplasm (Fig. 5.17).

Acute muscle injuries can be rapidly assessed by US when the examination is performed by an experienced user. US manifestations of injury include interruption of muscle fibers and hematoma.[28] The presence of hematoma is an indication of a higher degree of injury. Chronic injuries of muscle may be subtle on US with focal atrophy and thickening of the myotendinous junction representing indications of old trauma.

Muscle injuries are best imaged by MRI because it offers a global assessment of muscle, tendon, and bone. MRI can accurately assess and characterize both acute and chronic injuries.[29,30] Synchronous injuries are very common, so the entire extremity or pelvis should be imaged when there is a clinical concern for muscle injury. Increased signal in a muscle on T2-weighted images is an indicator of acute tear although other causes may produce the same MRI findings including contusion, delayed onset muscle soreness, and denervation. The presence of a hematoma is an indication of a high-grade injury (Fig. 5.18).

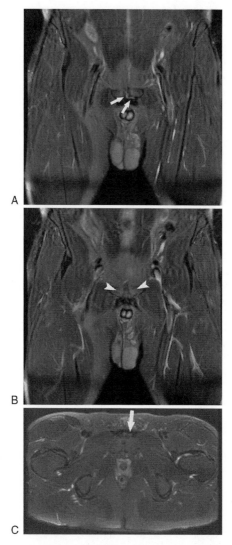

FIGURE 5.16. A 38-year-old man with left groin pain, osteitis pubis, and avulsion of adductor longus. (**A**) Coronal fat-suppressed T2-weighted image of the pelvis shows a linear cleft of high T2 signal (*white arrows*) indicating a tear of the adductor tendon origin. (**B**) Coronal fat-suppressed T2-weighted image of the pelvis shows bone marrow edema (*white arrowheads*) in the pubic symphysis indicating osteitis pubis. (**C**) Axial fat-suppressed T2-weighted image of the pelvis shows high signal (*white arrow*) replacing normal black in the left adductor longus origin indicating a tear.

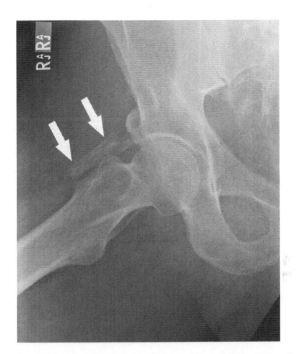

FIGURE 5.17. A 44-year-old man with right pain and myostis ossificans. Frog-leg lateral view of the right hip shows heterotopic ossification in the soft tissues posterior and lateral to the femoral neck (*white arrows*).

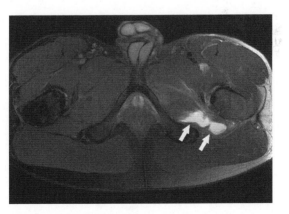

FIGURE 5.18. A 19-year-old quarterback with muscle tear and history of pop and immediate pain in left groin while playing football. Axial fat-suppressed T2-weighted image of the left hip shows a hematoma (*white arrows*) in the body of the adductor muscle indicating high grade tear.

References

1. Anderson K, Strickland SM, Warren R. Hip and groin injuries in athletes. Am J Sports Med 2001; 29:521–531.
2. Armfield DR, Towers JD, Robertson DD. Radiographic imaging of the athletic hip. Clin Sports Med 2006; 25:211–239.
3. Valimaki VV, Alfthan H, Lehmuskallio E, et al. Risk factors for clinical stress fractures in male military recruits: a prospective cohort study. Bone 2005; 37:267–273.
4. Mattila VM, Niva M, Kiuru M, Pihlajamaki H. Risk factors for bone stress injuries: a follow-up study of 102,515 person-years. Med Sci Sports Exerc 2007; 39:1061–1066.
5. Kiuru MJ, Pihlajamaki HK, Ahovuo JA. Fatigue stress injuries of the pelvic bones and proximal femur: evaluation with MR imaging. Eur Radiol. 2003; 13:605–611.
6. Anderson MW, Kaplan PA, Dussault RG. Adductor insertion avulsion syndrome (thigh splints): spectrum of MR imaging features. AJR 2001; 177:673–675.
7. Song WS, Yoo JJ, Koo KH, et al. Subchondral fatigue fracture of the femoral head in military recruits. J Bone Joint Surg Am 2004; 86A:1917–1924.
8. Dorne HL, Lander PH. Spontaneous stress fractures of the femoral neck. AJR 1985; 144:343–347
9. Lee JK, Yao L. Stress fractures: MR imaging. Radiology 1988; 169:217–220.
10. Kocher MS, Tucker R. Pediatric athlete hip disorders. Clin Sports Med 2006; 25:241–253.
11. Ozonoff MB. Pediatric Orthopedic Radiology, 2nd ed. Philadelphia: WB Saunders Co; 1992.
12. Bencardino JT, Palmer WE. Imaging of hip disorders in athletes. Radiol Clin North Am 2002; 40:267–287.
13. Tannast M, Siebenrock KA, Anderson SE. Femoroacetabular impingement: radiographic diagnosis – what the radiologist should know. AJR 2007; 188:1540–1552.
14. Delaunay S, Dussault RG, Kaplan PA, Alford BA. Radiographic measurements of dysplastic adult hips. Skeletal Radiol 1997; 26:75–81.
15. Ganz R, Parvizi J, Beck M, et al. Femoroacetabular impingement: a cause for osteoarthritis of the hip. Clin Orthop Relat Res 2003; 417:112–120.
16. Reynolds D, Lucac J, Klaue K. Retroversion of the acetabulum: a cause of hip pain. J Bone Joint Surg 1999; 81B:281–288.
17. Leunig M, Beck M, Kalhor M, et al. Fibrocystic changes at anterosuperior femoral neck: prevalence in hips with femoroacetabular impingement. Radiology 2005; 236:237–246.
18. Ito K, Leunig M, Ganz R. Histopathologic features of the acetabular labrum in femoroacetabular impingement. Clin Orthop Relat Res 2004; 429:262–271.
19. Kingzett-Taylor A, Tirman PF, Feller J, et al. Tendinosis and tears of gluteus medius and minimus muscles as a cause of hip pain: MR imaging findings. AJR Am J Roentgenol 1999; 173:1123–1126.

20. Cardinal E, Buckwalter KA, Capello WN, Duval N. US of the snapping iliopsoas tendon. Radiology 1996; 198:521–522.
21. Vaccaro JP, Sauser DD, Beals RK. Iliopsoas bursa imaging: efficacy in depicting abnormal iliopsoas tendon motion in patients with internal snapping hip syndrome. Radiology 1995; 197:853–856.
22. Kemp S, Batt ME. The "sports hernia": a complex cause of groin pain. Phys Sports Med 1998; 26:59–65.
23. Robinson P, Barron DA, Parsons W, et al. Adductor-related groin pain in athletes: correlation of MR imaging with clinical findings. Skeletal Radiol 2004; 33:451–457.
24. Cunningham PM, Brennan D, O'Connell M, et al. Patterns of bone and soft-tissue injury at the symphysis pubis in soccer players:observations at MRI. AJR 2007; 188:W291–W296.
25. Connell DA, Schneider-Kolsky ME, Hoving JL, et al. Longitudinal study comparing sonographic and MRI assessments of acute and healing hamstring injuries. AJR 2004; 183:975–984.
26. Slavotinek JP, Verrall GM, Fon GT. Hamstring injury in athletes: using MR imaging measurements to compare extent of muscle injury with amount of time lost from competition. AJR 2002; 179:1621–1628.
27. McCarthy EF, Sundaram M. Heterotopic ossification: a review, Skeletal Radiol 2005; 34:609–619.
28. Peetrons P. Ultrasound of muscles. Eur Radiol 2002; 12:35–43.
29. Boutin RD, Fritz RC, Steinbach LS. Imaging of sports-related muscle injuries. Radiol Clin North Am 2002; 40:333–362.
30. Bencardino JT, Mellado JM. Hamstring injuries of the hip. Magn Reson Imaging Clin N Am 2005; 13:677–690.

Chapter 6
Adult Hip and Pelvis Disorders

Peter H. Seidenberg

CLINICAL PEARLS

- Hip pain can originate from the hip joint, groin, surrounding musculature, sacroiliac (SI) joints, lumbar spine, abdomen, or pelvis.
- To ease in the clinical evaluation of possible etiologies of hip pain, it is helpful to divide the hip and pelvis into anterior, lateral, and posterior regions.
- Hernias should be considered in athletes with persistent hip, groin, or pelvic pain despite conservative therapy.
- Functional leg length discrepancy can result from muscle imbalances about the hip and pelvis and can further compound the biomechanical deficits.

CASE REPORT: PRESENTATION

A 29-year-old male presents to your office with a complaint of intermittent hip pain for the last 18 months, which has been progressively getting worse over the last 2 weeks. He plays softball, baseball, and runs 3–5 miles 3 days a week. He also lifts weights 2–3 days a week. He denies any history of trauma. He states the pain occurred initially only with running and heavy exertion, but now it has progressed to occur with walking as well. He admits to experiencing pain and tightness down the lateral side of his thigh to his knee. He denies weakness and tingling. He denies a snapping sensation. He denies systemic symptoms or incontinence of urine or stool. He has had no prior interventions besides rest, ice, and anti-inflammatory medication. Despite the above measures, when he returns to activity, the symptoms resurface.

Physical Examination
Physical examination reveals no erythema, edema, or ecchymosis. He has normal, pain-free full range of motion of his hip although he experiences pain with terminal flexion, abduction, and external rotation. Palpation reveals tenderness over the greater trochanter, the tensor fascia lata (TFL), and the gluteus medius. He has negative log roll, flexion abduction external rotation (FABER), Gaenslen's, Gillet, and piriformis tests. Strength is 5/5 with hip flexion, extension, and adduction. Abduction strength is 4+/5. He is neurovascularly intact with normal sensation. He has a positive Ober test, Ely's test, and Thomas test. Long sit test is normal. He has a compensated Trendelenburg on the affected side, but negative Stinchfield's, and fulcrum tests. He has mild pes planus bilaterally. No imaging studies are performed at this time.

INTRODUCTION
Hip and pelvic injuries comprise 5–6% of musculoskeletal complaints in adults. Athletic activities such as running, jumping, dancing, and playing soccer have high incidences of such injuries due to the substantial forces transferred across the joint and the extremes of movement that occur during these activities.[1] Injuries to the hip and pelvis can be frustrating for both the athlete and the treating physician. Hip pathology can result in hip pain or pain in other areas (e.g., knee). Additionally, injury and disease from surrounding structures can refer pain to the hip. This produces an extensive differential diagnosis of hip pain, which includes both musculoskeletal and non-musculoskeletal etiologies (see Table 6.1). Furthermore, the evaluation is often made difficult because injuries may involve a variety of soft tissues and bone and may be acute, sub-acute, or chronic. This chapter reviews the common musculoskeletal etiologies of pelvis and hip pain, symptoms associated with the injuries, and their treatment. In an attempt to simplify the approach to hip and pelvis pain, the chapter divides hip and pelvis pathology into anterior, lateral, and posterior causes of pain (Table 6.2). It is beyond the scope of this chapter to discuss in detail the many problems outside the hip and pelvis that refer pain to this area. The astute physician will remember to perform an examination of the abdomen, spine, and if appropriate, genitalia to rule out referred causes of hip and pelvis pain.

TABLE 6.1. Differential diagnosis of pelvic and hip pain

Hip/pelvis
  Stress fracture of the femoral neck
  Pubic ramus stress fracture
  Osteitis pubis
  Snapping hip
  Acetabular labral tear
  Bursitis (iliopectineal, trochanteric)
  Avascular necrosis
  Osteoarthritis
  Synovitis or capsulitis
  Hip dislocation
  Femoroacetabular impingement
  Gluteal strain/contusion
  Piriformis syndrome
  Coccygeal injury
  Iliac crest contusion

Low back
  Sacroileitis
  Sacroiliac dysfunction
  Sciatica
  Nerve root impingement
  Degenerative disk disease
  Lumbosacral strain

Thigh
  Muscle strains
    Adductor longus
    Rectus femoris
    Iliopsoas
    Sartorius
    Gracilis
    Tensor fascia lata
    Hamstring
  Femoral hernia
  Lymphadenopathy
  Meralgia paresthetica

Abdomen
  Lower abdominal wall strain of the rectus abdominis
  Inguinal hernia
  Ilioinguinal nerve entrapment
  Sports hernia (hockey player's syndrome)
  Abdominal organ conditions
  Abdominal aortic aneurysm
  Appendicitis
  Diverticulitis
  Inflammatory bowel disease
  Pelvic inflammatory disease
  Sexually transmitted diseases
  Ovarian cyst
  Ectopic pregnancy

TABLE 6.2. Summary of anterior, lateral, posterior hip, and pelvic pain

Anterior hip pain
  Adductor strain
  Quadriceps strain
  Quadriceps contusion
  Iliopsoas strain
  Rectus abdominis strain
  Pubic symphysis dysfunction
  Osteitis pubis
  Pubic ramus stress fracture
  Femoral neck stress fracture
  Hip dislocation
  Avascular necrosis of the femoral head
  Osteoarthritis
  Acetabular labrum tear

Continued

TABLE 6.2. *Continued*

    Femoroacetabular impingement
    Iliopsoas/iliopectineal bursitis
    Sports hernia
    Internal snapping hip

Lateral hip pain
    External snapping hip
    Hip pointer
    Tensor fascia lata syndrome
    Greater trochanteric bursitis
    Meralgia paresthetica

Posterior hip pain
    Hamstring strain
    Ischial bursitis
    Gluteus maximus strain/contusion
    Gluteus medius strain
    Sacroiliac dysfunction/sprain
    Piriformis syndrome
    Coccygeal injury

ANTERIOR HIP AND PELVIS PAIN

Adductor Strain (Groin Pull)

The adductor longus, adductor magnus, adductor brevis, pectineal, and gracilis muscles are all adductors of the hip. Adductor strains are the most common cause of groin and hip pain in athletes, with the adductor longus the most often injured in sports.[2] Adductor strain is caused by a sudden change in direction, sprinting, forced external rotation of an abducted leg, a powerful abduction stress during simultaneous adduction while performing a cutting movement, or repetitive abduction of the free leg in a skating stride. A disparity in strength between the adductor muscles and intrinsic muscle tightness can also cause strain. Adductor strains are most commonly seen in the sports of hockey and soccer. Differential diagnosis includes avascular necrosis (AVN), femoral neck stress fracture, iliopsoas/iliopectineal bursitis, osteitis pubis, osteoarthritis, pelvic stress fracture, hernia, and athletic pubalgia.

In acute injury, athletes will complain of immediate pain piercing into the groin, inability to continue the activity, swelling, and bruising. Delayed ecchymosis and soft tissue swelling may also occur. Physical examination will reveal tenderness to palpation along the subcutaneous border of the pubic ramus and along the involved adductor muscles and tendons, pain with resisted adduction, and pain with passive stretching.

Although the diagnosis is usually made clinically, radiographs can be helpful in excluding fractures or avulsions. If the diagnosis is still in question, magnetic resonance imaging (MRI) can be used to confirm muscle strain or partial or complete tendon tears. The most common site of strain is the musculotendinous junction of the adductor longus or gracilis.

Treatment depends on the severity of the symptoms. Initially, rest from aggravating factors for 1–2 weeks with ice, compression shorts, and nonsteroidal anti-inflammatory drugs (NSAIDs) provide symptomatic relief. The goal of physical therapy is to restore the range of motion, to prevent atrophy, and to regain strength, flexibility, and endurance. Therapy should be instituted as soon as pain allows and should initially include isometric contractions without resistance, followed by isometric contractions against resistance, limited by pain. Athletes can begin a stretching program after the inflammation subsides. Applying heat increases the extensibility of the collagen in the tendons and muscles and will be beneficial during this point in rehabilitation.[3] Maintaining cardiovascular fitness with aerobic exercises that do not exacerbate the pain should be encouraged. Prevention and correction of predisposing biomechanical factors should be included in the rehabilitation program. When the athlete has regained 70% of his or her strength and pain-free full range of motion, return to play may be allowed (SOR-C).[4] This return may take 4–8 weeks for acute injuries and up to 6 months for chronic strains.[5,6] Athletes with chronic adductor longus strains that have failed several months of conservative therapy have been shown to do well after surgical tenotomy and should be referred to a sports medicine orthopedic surgeon for this consideration. Complete tears of the tendinous insertion from the bone are relatively rare and generally do better with surgical repair (SOR-C).[7,8]

Rectus Femoris Strain/Quadriceps Strain

The rectus femoris is heavily recruited and frequently overused during jumping, running/sprinting, skating, and bicycling. The rectus femoris has two origins: (1) an anterior tendon from the anterior inferior iliac spine (AIIS) and (2) a posterior tendon from a brim above the acetabulum. The two combine to insert as the patellar tendon at the tibial tuberosity. The main action of the rectus femoris is to flex the hip and extend the knee. Injuries usually occur at the musculotendinous junction as a result of a heavy eccentric load.[9]

Athletes may report a feeling of a "pulling" sensation and pain in the anterior thigh. The pain often radiates to the thigh and inguinal area. Physical examination may show reproducible pain with resisted hip flexion or knee extension, tenderness to palpation, and possibly a palpable defect or mass. A rectus femoris strain is typically diagnosed clinically, but if an avulsion injury to the AIIS is suspected, radiographs should be ordered.

Initial treatment consists of rest, ice, compression, protected weight bearing, gentle range of motion, and quad set exercises. Ice massage progressing to ultrasound and ice contrast should also be started early in the rehabilitation course (SOR-C).[10] Use of NSAIDs in acute muscle injury is controversial in the first 48 h due to anti-platelet effects but is recommended for pain control after 48 h (SOR-B).[11-13] Rehabilitation goals include restoration of strength, range of motion, and sport-specific skills prior to running. Strengthening exercises are initially concentric and progress to eccentric. A good concentric exercise to start the athlete with is backward walking and running followed by progression to forward running. The athlete can return to running when his or her knee range of motion is 80% that of the unaffected side (SOR-C). Depending on the severity of the injury, return to competition is usually after 2–6 weeks. Return to running prior to full restoration of strength, flexibility, and endurance puts the athlete at risk of impaired performance and recurrent injury.[14]

A partial quadriceps tear can result in hematoma formation in the muscle. Myositis ossificans can be a complication as the hematoma resolves. Initial bleeding leads to formation of a hematoma, which later calcifies within the muscle, reducing flexibility. Keeping the muscle in a lengthened position the first 24 h after injury can help maintain flexibility and decrease bleeding through tamponade. The usual symptoms include a painful, palpable mass with progressive loss of motion. Treatment is discussed further under quadriceps contusion.

Quadriceps Contusion

Contusion to the quadriceps muscle is a common injury in contact sports and is caused by a direct blow to the thigh, which compresses the quadriceps into the femur. Examination often reveals tenderness, swelling, and a hematoma on the anterior thigh. A loss of knee flexion is often present. As in quadriceps/rectus femoris strain, myositis ossificans development may be a complication and can be reduced by immediate treatment intervention. The incidence of myositis ossificans is 9–20%.[15]

Radiographs should be taken to rule out femur fracture. A bone scan is often used to track myositis ossificans formation and to determine whether the process is still active or mature (cessation of active calcification).[16] Radiographic evidence of calcification due to myositis ossificans may not be present for weeks following injury and, therefore, a presumptive diagnosis of myositis ossificans is often made after a severe contusion does not show rapid improvement. To help differentiate late presenting myositis ossificans from a sarcoma, computed tomography (CT) scan is often utilized.

Initial treatment is essentially the same as with quadriceps strain/rectus femoris strain. It begins with immediate application of ice with a compression wrap for 10 min per waking hour for 3–5 days. Active knee flexion should be sustained only to the point of slight discomfort or as tolerated by placing a pillow underneath the knee. Weight-bearing as tolerated is allowed with active range of motion performed within the pain-free range. Deep massage, passive stretching, and ultrasound should be avoided, as these can increase muscle bleeding. Active flexion should be encouraged and continued frequently. Heat and cold contrasts and strengthening exercises are initiated after the swelling begins to decrease. Return to play may be allowed after the athlete gains quadriceps length and strength equal to 90% of the unaffected side (SOR-C).

Treatment of myositis ossificans is similar to that of quadriceps strain, with an initial short period of rest with protected weight-bearing with crutches once recognized. Loss of hip range of motion due to restricted muscle function may occur after the acute phase; therefore, early rehabilitation should include active stretching and strengthening exercises. Vigorous massage or manipulation will increase hematoma formation and formation of the calcific mass. Surgical treatment generally is not indicated, but if necessary, it should be delayed 6–12 months until the mass has matured (SOR-C).[17] Radiographic resolution is not necessary for return to play; however, rehabilitation to achieve full strength and flexibility is mandatory. Wearing protective padding over the affected area should be considered as well.

Iliopsoas Strain/Hip Flexor Strain

The iliopsoas muscle is a strong flexor of the hip and can be injured when the thigh is forced into extension or is blocked during active flexion. This injury often occurs in soccer players who are hit as they extend the leg to kick the ball. It also occurs in weight lifting, uphill running, and sit-ups.

Athletes may present with a complaint of sharp, deep groin pain. Physical examination typically reveals increased pain with active resisted hip flexion and passive external rotation or extension. Initial treatment involves rest and protection, followed by rehabilitation within the limits of pain. In adults, this injury may result in a partial or complete tear at the musculotendinous junction. With tears, it may be necessary to wait 4–6 weeks before return to play.[18]

Rectus Abdominis Strain

The rectus abdominis originates on the pubic bone, close to the origin of the adductor longus. As such, injury to the rectus abdominis may easily be confused or coexist with an adductor injury. Injury is typically caused by overzealous sit-ups or weight training.[3] Athletes typically complain of deep groin pain that is worsened with the above activities. The differential diagnosis includes abdominal pathology, sexually transmitted diseases, inguinal hernia, adductor strain, and osteitis pubis.

On physical examination, pain is reproduced by palpation of the superior pubic ramus and is exacerbated in the supine patient by a bilateral straight leg raise. Treatment includes relative rest, avoidance of provocative activities until pain subsides, and a physical therapy program that includes core stabilization.

Pubic Symphysis Dysfunction

Pubic symphysis dysfunction is an underappreciated source of pubic pain. This injury typically occurs during a high-speed cutting activity and is often present concurrently with an adductor strain. Although rare, the disorder can also be seen surrounding pregnancy, with widening of the pelvic joints occurring to allow passage of the infant through the pelvis during delivery.[19] Additionally, trauma to the pelvis or a significant axial load to the lower extremity may result in dysfunction.[20] Other etiologies in the differential diagnosis of pubic symphysis pain include osteitis pubis and pubic rami stress fracture. Athletes may complain of suprapubic pain, tenderness, swelling, suprapubic pain with urination, pain radiating to the groin, and exacerbation of symptoms with walking, climbing stairs, turning in bed, getting up from a chair, or lifting. The pain may even be accompanied by a clicking sensation.[20]

The physical examination includes evaluation of the position of the pubic tubercles by palpating their borders to assess right-to-left variation in the frontal plane. Pubic symphysis dysfunction is present if the pubic bones are not level and tension of the two inguinal ligaments is asymmetric. Pain is also evoked by a lateral compression test. Rarely, a palpable groove at the level of the symphysis may be detected. Flamingo view radiographs may be helpful and are considered positive when alternating weight-bearing views show a shift of at least 2 mm in the pubic symphysis.[20]

An elevated or depressed pubic bone may be reduced by the "adductor squeeze." This is performed by having the athlete lie in a supine position with the knees and hips flexed and abducted. The examiner places his or her forearm between the athlete's knees, and the opposite knee is grabbed with the free hand. The athlete is then asked to abduct the knees for 5 s and repeat three times. This is followed by three maximal adduction contractions for 5 s. An audible "pop" signifies reduction.[21]

If asymmetry is not detected, the injury may be treated conservatively with a short amount of bed rest; pelvic support with a brace, girdle, or compression shorts; assisted ambulation with a walker or crutches; and a graded exercise program including pelvic stabilization. NSAIDs are helpful for pain control. Adding acupuncture and symphyseal injections to conservative therapy have also been shown to relieve pain.[19,20]

Osteitis Pubis

Osteitis pubis is a painful condition that affects the pubic symphysis and surrounding tendinous attachments. It is a chronic inflammatory condition that is more commonly reported in sports requiring cutting, twisting, pivoting on one leg, excessive side-to-side motion, or multidirectional motions with frequent acceleration and deceleration – notably running, rugby, ice and field hockey, football, basketball, and soccer.[22] It is also common in exercising pregnant women and postpartum women because of the instability of this joint related to the hormone relaxin.[3] Many etiologic factors have been proposed for the development of osteitis pubis, including instability of the SI joint, repetitive adductor muscle pull at the origins of the pubic rami, overuse and microtrauma of the muscles associated with running and kicking, excessive frontal or up-and-down pelvic motion, and limitations of hip joint movement.[22] The differential diagnosis of osteitis pubis should include pubic ramus stress fracture, pubic symphysis dysfunction, hernias, and osteomyelitis.

Athletes describe a gradual onset of pain in the pubic region, which may radiate to the hip, groin, abdomen, proximal medial thigh, testicle, and scrotum, as well as perineal, suprapubic, or anterior pubic areas. The pain is often described as sharp, stabbing, or even burning and may be exacerbated by striding, pivoting (especially on one leg), twisting, climbing stairs, kicking, sit-ups, leg raises, or Valsalva maneuvers. Athletes may also describe an audible or palpable clicking sensation at the symphysis with certain activities.[22]

Physical examination reveals tenderness over the pubic symphysis and adductor origins of the inferior pubic ramus, limited rotation and pelvic obliquity due to surrounding muscle spasm of the adductors, and exaggeration of symptoms with passive hip abduction, active hip flexion, or active adduction. The lateral pelvic compression and cross-leg tests are often positive. Trendelenburg's test is often positive indicating weak hip abductors, and in severe cases, the athlete may have an antalgic gait with partially flexed hips and knees.[22]

Anterioposterior (AP) and lateral radiographs of the pelvis should be obtained. It is important to note that radiographs can lag behind clinical symptoms by as much as 4 weeks. As the disease progresses, reactive sclerosis of the adjacent pubic bones, erosion and resorption of the symphysis margins, and widening of the joint space may appear on the X-ray.[22] If the pain is long-standing, a bone scan or MRI should be performed.[23] They often reveal symmetric involvement of the pubic symphysis, which is in contrast to tumors, tendonitis, strains, or pelvic fractures. If instability is suspected, one-legged standing flamingo views should be performed. Instability is defined as greater than 2 mm height difference between the superior rami of the symphysis.[22]

Various treatment options have been suggested, but initially, the goal is to reduce inflammation and remove the provocative activity by modifying training – decrease mileage, prevent overstriding, and eliminate downhill running. NSAIDs and ice should be used for symptom reduction. Oral corticosteroids can be used if the athlete demonstrates intense pain from inflammation.[22] Corticosteroid injection into and around the pubic symphysis may be considered in athletes with refractory symptoms.[24] However, prior to injection, blood tests to assess for leukocytosis should be performed to rule out osteomyelitis as a possible cause (SOR-C).[3]

A structured physical therapy program should begin when pain and inflammation are reduced. Modalities such as ultrasound and phonophoresis may assist with pain control. Leg length discrepancy should also be corrected if found. A graduated exercise program should be utilized with the goal of returning the athlete to a pre-injury level of participation. However, patience is required, as this may take from 3 to 6 months or longer.

Pubic Ramus Stress Fracture

Pubic ramus stress fractures account for a small percentage of the stress fractures experienced by athletes. The etiology of pubic ramus stress fractures has not been determined, but one common thought is that it often starts with a periosteal reaction at the adductor muscle origin on the pubis as a result of the tensile forces produced by these muscles. This type of stress fracture is usually seen in distance runners undergoing a rapid change in distance or speed. Athletes complain of an insidious onset of pain that is exacerbated by activity and relieved by rest. It may be localized to the inguinal, peroneal, or adductor region.[12,25]

Physical examination reveals tenderness on the inferior aspect of the pubic rim, an antalgic gait, and a positive standing sign (frank pain or inability to stand unsupported on the affected leg). Hip range of motion is often normal. Radiographs may not be positive for several weeks after the initial injury and, if obtained late in the healing phase, can show abundant callus that can be confused with malignancy.[12] If the X-ray is negative and a stress fracture is still suspected, then advanced imaging is indicated. The most sensitive tests in early diagnosis of stress fractures are the bone scan and MRI.[26] Treatment consists of avoiding pain-inducing activities for 4–6 weeks. The athlete should focus on non-weight-bearing activities and stretching of the adductor muscle group and hip joint capsule. This is followed by a gradual functional progression to activity. Most athletes will show a response to treatment in 3–5 months. In addition, evaluation of the athlete's nutritional intake, estrogen status, and training program is warranted.

Femoral Neck Stress Fracture

If the diagnosis of a femoral neck stress fracture is delayed or missed, it can be a potentially career-ending injury with serious complications including AVN, nonunion, and varus deformity. As such, the clinician needs to maintain a high index of suspicion for this injury. This type of fracture often occurs in distance runners and is usually preceded by a recent change in mileage or intensity. It also can be caused by overuse, impaired bone metabolism, and a loss of shock absorption due to muscle fatigue. Other risk factors include training errors, inadequate footwear, running on poor surfaces, and coxa vara.[27,28] The differential diagnosis includes AVN, hip flexor tendonitis or bursitis, hernia, and osteitis pubis.

The athlete may describe an aching pain sensation in the groin, hip, thigh, or knee, which abates shortly after cessation of activity. Nocturnal pain is also common. Pain is frequently associated with exertion and weight-bearing. The athlete often notes a progressive limitation of activity because of the pain.

Physical exam findings include pain with internal rotation and with hopping, limitation of hip motion secondary to regional muscle guarding, pain with axial compression, pain with percussion over the greater trochanter, positive log roll, pain with FABER test, and an antalgic or painful Trendelenburg gait. Pain is also often present at the end range of hip motion. Many feel that a single leg hop test should not be performed in a patient suspected of having a femoral neck stress fracture for fear of completing the fracture (SOR-C).

If a femoral neck stress fracture is suspected and physical exam findings are suggestive, then it should be considered to be present until proven otherwise. Distinct radiographic findings may not develop until 2–4 weeks after the initial injury. Bone scan is the most sensitive test in early diagnosis and is indicated if pain has been present for less than 3 weeks. However, bone scans have a poor specificity, with a positive predictive value of only 68%.[29] MRI has the advantage of greater localization and grading of injury severity and in differentiating stress fracture from other bone and soft tissue conditions.[12] Additionally, studies have found MRI for the diagnosis of femoral stress fracture to be both 100% sensitive and specific.[29,30]

Femoral neck stress fractures can be classified as tension, compression, or displaced fracture. Tension stress fractures, also known as distraction fractures, are more common in older patients and occur on the superolateral side and have a high likelihood of displacement with continued stress. These should be referred immediately to an orthopedic surgeon (SOR-C).

Compression fractures are more common in younger patients and occur on the inferomedial or compression side of the femoral neck. If the fracture involves less than 50% of the width of the femoral neck, there is low risk for displacement, and it can be treated with prolonged non-weight-bearing until pain free. Some patients may even require a short time on bed rest. The athlete should not progress from non-weight-bearing with crutches until there is evidence of radiographic healing. Frequent radiographs, as often as weekly, should be performed until complete healing is documented. Supervised gradual return to activity can than occur. Recurrence of pain requires rest for 2–3 days, and then resumption of activity at the last tolerated level. Progression of the fracture is an indication for immediate orthopedic referral.[12]

A displaced fracture is a combination of both the tension and compression fractures, which results in displacement of the femoral head. This type of femoral neck stress fracture is an orthopedic emergency requiring immediate surgical reduction and internal fixation. Postoperatively, the athlete is kept non-weight-bearing for the first 6 weeks, then partially weight-bearing for another 6 weeks, at which time a progressive activity and weight-bearing rehabilitation program is started.[31] Exact time lines for return to activity depend upon the nature of the fracture, type of fixation utilized, and surgeon's preference.

The primary goal in management of femoral neck stress fractures should be to prevent complications through early diagnosis and careful treatment. Athletes must be told that stress fractures of the femoral neck are serious injuries that can compromise their careers. If a stress fracture is suspected, the athlete should remain non-weight-bearing on the affected leg until a stress fracture is ruled out. Return to play or normal activities following a stress fracture can take as long as 4–5 months.

Hip Dislocation

The hip joint is an extremely stable joint, and great force is usually required to dislodge it (except in the elderly or those with osteoporosis). A trauma with high energy directed along the axis of the femur when the hip is in the extremes of its normal range of motion is required to cause a dislocation. Hip dislocations can be anterior, posterior, or central. Posterior dislocations account for 90% and anterior dislocations account for only 8–15%.[32,33] At least 70% of posterior hip dislocations occur as a result of a motor vehicle collision.[1,34] Because of the large amount of force required to produce a hip dislocation, the clinician must maintain a high index of suspicion of associated injuries, such as fractures of the femoral neck, femoral head, and/or acetabulum.

When a hip dislocation occurs, the athlete is immediately disabled and complains of extreme pain. Attempts to move the hip will increase discomfort. Posteriorly dislocated hips are characteristically held in adduction, internal rotation, and slight flexion. The femoral head may be palpable posteriorly.

Hip dislocations are orthopedic emergencies. Attempts at reduction should not be performed on the playing field; however, it is critical to perform an on-field neurovascular examination because sciatic nerve injury is observed in 10–14% of patients with posterior dislocations. The athlete should be immobilized and transported to the emergency room for definitive evaluation and treatment.[33,35] A hip trauma series of radiographs should be obtained in the emergency room, including AP and oblique views of the pelvis. CT scans are not routinely obtained prior to reduction because of the need for rapid treatment. This is usually obtained post reduction.

Prompt reduction using proper technique is the most important factor in decreasing the incidence of late sequelae, including AVN of the femoral head, sciatic nerve injury, future degenerative joint disease, and chondrolysis. The blood supply to the femoral head reaches a minimum level after 24 h, and reduction after 24 h has been shown to cause an increase in osteonecrosis and post-traumatic arthritis. A reduction within 6 h enhances early and complete recovery of the vascularity to the femoral head. For this reason, delays of more than 6 h should be avoided (SOR-B).[36]

Reductions of hip dislocations are usually performed under general anesthesia to allow adequate muscle relaxation and to reduce the amount of trauma associated with reduction. Some of the hip reduction techniques used include Bigelow, Stimson, Allis, and Whistler methods. Detailed discussion of hip reduction is beyond the scope of this chapter.

AVN of the Femoral Head

AVN of the femoral head in adults is a poorly understood condition in which the circulation to the femoral head is disrupted resulting in bone death and osteophyte formation. The segment that has lost blood supply usually collapses and causes progressive arthritis of the hip joint. There are both traumatic and nontraumatic causes of AVN. Traumatic causes include displaced fractures of the femoral neck and hip dislocation. Nontraumatic causes are not as well defined, but the most common underlying factors include systemic corticoid steroid use (typically high dose) and heavy alcohol intake, which are retrospectively present in 80% of cases.[37]

Athletes usually present with nonspecific groin or hip pain that gets worse with weight-bearing and nonspecific hip motion. Rest and night pain also occur. Hip range of motion and gait are usually normal unless the process is advanced. AP and lateral X-rays of both hips are essential. Films taken at the time of injury are normal unless a fracture is present. The earliest changes on X-ray are not evident until 3 months after the initial injury. Osteopenia or a mottled appearance of the AP aspect of the femoral head consisting of patchy areas of sclerosis and lucency is the earliest X-ray finding. As the injury progresses, collapse of the involved segment and secondary degenerative changes and arthritis occur. If the disease is suspected and radiographs are normal, an MRI or bone scan should be ordered as these are the gold standard diagnostic studies for AVN.[38,39] MRI has a sensitivity of greater than 90% with a high specificity as well. The use of gadolinium increases the likelihood of detection early in the course of the disease. This is in contrast to radionuclide scan which has decreased sensitivity in the settings of early or bilateral disease (SOR-B).[38]

Management depends on the stage of the disease and should be coordinated with an orthopedic surgeon. The most important factors in making the diagnosis of AVN are a high index of suspicion and awareness to predisposing history.

Osteoarthritis

Osteoarthritis of the hip is the end stage of many different disorders. It is the main cause of anterior hip pain in patients over 50 years of age.[40] It may also be a source of hip pain in runners. For a more complete discussion of osteoarthritis, see Chap. 14.

Acetabular Labral Tear

Like the shoulder, the hip has a labrum consisting of a fibrocartilaginous rim that serves to deepen the acetabulum. Tears of the labrum typically present after an athlete has experienced some form of trauma such as slipping, twisting, or dislocation. Labral tears can also be associated with osteoarthritis. The differential diagnosis includes external and internal snapping hip, osteonecrosis, and synovial chondromatosis.

Classic symptoms of a labral injury include painful catching or clicking, episodes of sharp pain precipitated by pivoting or twisting, worsening pain with extension, and a feeling that the hip is "giving way." Physical exam reveals palpable clicking on Thomas flexion-to-extension, which frequently correlates with the finding of labral tears at arthroscopy (SOR-B).[41] Bringing the hip from full flexion, external rotation, and abduction into extension with internal rotation and adduction is useful in diagnosing anterior labral tears; and bringing the hip from full flexion, adduction, and internal rotation to extension with abduction and external rotation is reported by some experts as useful for posterior labral tears. However, Browder et al. found an inter-examiner reliability of only 48% (SOR-B).[42]

Plain radiographs are essential in that they can show other sources of intra-articular disease that can account for the symptoms. MRI can be useful in further screening for osteonecrosis, synovial chondromatosis, and other diseases. Injection of local anesthetic into the joint guided by fluoroscopy can also be useful in diagnosing labral tears. If the symptoms resolve after injection, an intra-articular etiology is more likely (SOR-C).[43] Hip arthroscopy or magnetic resonance arthrography (MRA) are the diagnostic investigations of choice in acetabular labral tear diagnosis. MRA has reported sensitivities greater than 90% (SOR-B).[44]

Conservative management with anti-inflammatory medications and physical therapy may be useful. Once the diagnosis is made, some authors recommend protected weight-bearing for 4 weeks. However, this intervention only resulted in symptom resolution in approximately 13% of patients.[43] Subsequently, if conservative measures fail, surgical intervention by hip arthroscopy should be offered. This is also the preferred method of treatment for many experts (SOR-C).[45]

Femoroacetabular Impingement

Femoroacetabular impingement (FAI) is caused by impingement of the anterior femoral head–neck junction against the adjacent anterosuperior labrum. Recognition of FAI can be clinically and radiologically difficult. However, familiarity with this disorder is essential, as it is thought to lead to osteoarthritis in young adults despite having normal anatomy and intra-articular pressures.[46,47] Clinically, patients present with groin pain or pain over the greater trochanter[46] as well as grinding or popping. Patients report pain with flexion and internal rotation and after prolonged sitting. On examination, there is a decrease in internal rotation that appears out of proportion to the loss of other ranges of motion. The impingement test, elicited by 90° flexion, adduction, and internal rotation of the hip, is almost always positive (SOR-C).[47]

The imaging findings of FAI can be seen on plain radiographs, CT scan, MRI, or MRA. Some of the abnormalities seen include an abnormal lateral femoral head/neck offset seen as a lateral femoral neck bump, os acetabulae, synovial herniation pits, acetabular over-coverage, hyaline cartilage abnormalities, and labral tears. One study found that 100% of patients with FAI had evidence of labral pathology (SOR-C).[48] Treatment of FAI has traditionally been surgical.[49]

Iliopsoas/Iliopectineal Bursitis

Bursitis is an inflammation of the saclike cavities associated with joints and bony prominences. In the hip and pelvis, the ischial, iliopectineal, and greater trochanteric bursae are commonly injured. Ischial and greater trochanteric bursitis will be discussed with posterior and lateral hip pain, respectively. There are generally two mechanisms of hip bursitis; inflammation due to excessive friction (most common) and post-traumatic injury. Direct blows and contusions can cause bleeding into the bursa and may result in hematoma formation. The iliopsoas/iliopectineal bursa is the largest bursa in the body and communicates with the hip joint in 15% of athletes.[50] This bursitis is associated with sports requiring extensive use of the hip flexors (i.e., soccer, ballet, uphill running, hurdling, jumping) and may be particularly disabling for athletes.

Athletes may present with severe, acute, deep groin pain radiating to the anterior hip or thigh. The pain may be great enough to disrupt normal gait and cause a limp, and it is often associated with a snapping sensation. Athletes will assume a position of hip flexion and external rotation to obtain relief.[51] Pain is often related to the iliopsoas tendon snapping over the iliopectineal eminence. Symptoms may be exacerbated by hip extension (stretching of the iliopsoas) or when the supine athlete raises his or her heels off the table approximately 15°, thereby isolating the iliopsoas.[52] Deep palpation of the femoral triangle where the musculotendinous junction of the iliopsoas lies elicits pain.[50] MRI reveals a collection of fluid coursing adjacent to the muscle with iliopsoas/iliopectineal bursitis.[53]

Treatment is almost always nonoperative and consists of rest, ice, NSAIDs, and stretching of the iliopsoas. If symptoms are recalcitrant to conservative therapy, corticosteroid injection or even release of the iliopsoas tendon near its insertion on the lesser trochanter and/or excision of the bursa may be necessary.[50]

Athletic Pubalgia (Sports Hernia)

Athletic pubalgia is a controversial injury. Some authors distinguish hockey player's syndrome, Gilmore's groin, sports hernia, and athletic pubalgia from each other. However, for the purpose of brevity, the author has chosen to label all of these as sports hernia. Sports hernia involves injury to the posterior wall of the inguinal canal and can appear as a tear of the transverses abdominis muscle or as a disruption to the conjoined tendon (tendon of insertion of the internal oblique and transverses abdominis muscles). The internal oblique muscle and external oblique aponeurosis of the internal inguinal wall may also be involved.[3,54–56] This injury is more common in men than women and typically occurs in fast-moving sports that involve twisting and turning, like soccer, football, rugby, and ice hockey. Because only the posterior abdominal wall is injured, the sports hernia differs from the more common inguinal hernia in that it does not involve a clinically detectable hernia. Differential diagnosis includes adductor strain, osteitis pubis, or a true inguinal or femoral hernia.

Athletes may present with unilateral groin pain exacerbated by exercise. In chronic cases, the athlete may have pain with activities of daily living. It is usually insidious in onset and may radiate to the hip. Sudden movements, sit-ups, and increases in intra-abdominal pressure also exacerbate the pain. Examination is usually performed by inverting the scrotal skin with a finger and palpating for pain over the conjoined tendon, pubic tubercle, and mid-inguinal region. Radiographs are important to rule out other injuries.[3]

Treatment of this group of disorders is controversial. The simplest initial maneuver is rest followed by slow resumption of physical activity with supervised physical therapy consisting of core and pelvic stabilization, strengthening, and flexibility training. The athlete should avoid sudden, sharp, cutting movement. Those who insist on continuing activity will take considerably longer to heal. Supplemental administration of NSAIDs and application of ice packs 3–4 times a day for 20–30 min may also be beneficial (SOR-C). Athletes who fail conservative treatment should be referred to a surgeon for evaluation.[57-59]

Internal Snapping Hip

Snapping hip syndrome is a clinical condition with a painful, audible snap occurring during hip flexion and extension. The cause of snapping hip can be divided into external and internal, with internal being further subdivided into intra- and extra-articular. Snapping hip is most commonly seen in individuals in their late teens and twenties who are active in dance and running (particularly hurdlers) and have no specific history of trauma.[60] External snapping is discussed in the *Lateral Hip and Pelvis Pain* section.

Extra-articular internal snapping typically involves pathology related to the iliopsoas tendon. The iliopsoas muscle is a confluence of the iliacus, which originates mainly from the ilium and sacral ala, and the psoas, which originates from the vertebrae and intervertebral disks of T-12 to L-5. The tendinous portion of the iliopsoas passes through a groove on the bony pelvis that is bordered laterally by the AIIS and medially by the iliopectineal eminence. An anteromedial bony prominence lies adjacent to the lesser trochanter, over which the tendinous portion of the iliopsoas passes before its insertion on the lesser trochanter. The iliopsoas bursa lies over the anterior hip capsule and deep to the portion of the iliopsoas tendon.[61-63] When the hip is flexed, abducted, and externally rotated, the tendinous portion lies lateral to the anterior aspect of the femoral head and hip capsule. It passes over the femoral head and hip capsule to a more medial position with hip extension, adduction, and internal rotation, causing snapping.[60] Other causes include the iliopsoas tendon snapping over the iliopectineal eminence and the bony ridge of the lesser trochanter, movement of the iliofemoral ligaments over the anterior hip capsule, and the origin of the long head of the biceps femoris moving over the ischium. Iliopsoas bursitis can also lead to painful snapping.

Intra-articular snapping hip is most often caused by loose bodies that may arise from labral disease, acetabular or femoral head chondral lesions, idiopathic recurrent hip subluxation, and synovial chondromatosis.[61]

Athletes may complain of an audible, often painful, snap with motion of the hip. The location of the snap is in the groin or anterior hip with the internal type. In extra-articular snapping, the pain is usually insidious in onset and is caused by inflammation of the iliopsoas bursa. Athletes are usually able to voluntarily reproduce the snapping with certain hip motions. Performance is rarely impaired. This is in contrast to the intra-articular type. Here, athletes report a sudden onset of snapping or clicking after trauma, and more often report a click rather than a snap. Reproduction of the snapping is more difficult, and performance may or may not be inhibited.

The physical examination in internal snapping is performed by placing the athlete in a supine position and passively extending, internally rotating, and adducting a flexed, externally rotated, and abducted hip to reveal snapping as the iliopsoas tendon passes from lateral to medial over the femoral head and joint capsule. If the source is extra-articular, snapping may be prevented by placing significant pressure on the iliopsoas tendon and anterior hip.[61,64,65] Intra-articular snapping may be uncovered with a scour test.

Plain radiographs, including AP, frog leg, and lateral views, are often normal in athletes with snapping hip. However, they are imperative to rule out less common etiologies such as fractures, loose bodies, dysplasia, and synovial chondromatosis. MRI with intra-articular contrast may be used to evaluate intra-articular causes of snapping hip including labral tears, osteochondral fractures, and loose bodies. In extra-articular snapping, the MRI (without intra-articular contrast) will show iliopsoas tendon thickening and inflammation of the iliopsoas bursa. Static and dynamic ultrasound can also be helpful in the diagnosis of internal snapping hip. Static ultrasound demonstrates iliopsoas tendon thickening, enlarged bursa, and peritendinous fluid collections, while dynamic ultrasound reveals abnormal jerking motion of the tendon corresponding to the athlete's painful sensation and to palpable audible snapping.[66,67] Bursography and tenography have also been used to diagnose internal and external snapping hip, but are operator-dependent and therefore not often used.[61]

The mainstay of treatment for extra-articular internal snapping hip is nonoperative and involves rest, activity modification, NSAIDs, and physical therapy. Hip flexor stretching and strengthening, pelvic and peripelvic mobilization, and alignment exercises help relieve the pain of internal snapping hip. Core stabilization and pelvic tilt should also be addressed, as an increased anterior tilt may cause tightening of the hip flexor tendons.[61] Other modalities include corticosteroid injection of the bursa and biofeedback to teach the patient how to avoid repetitive hip snapping. If conservative therapy does not relieve symptoms, surgical intervention may be necessary. Surgical intervention in extra-articular internal snapping involves release or lengthening of the iliopsoas tendon.

For intra-articular etiologies, hip arthroscopy can be used to debride a torn acetabular labrum, remove loose bodies, or repair an osteochondral defect.[68,69]

LATERAL HIP AND PELVIS PAIN

External Snapping Hip

Like internal snapping, external snapping hip is also most commonly seen in runners and dancers in their teens to twenties with no history of trauma. The etiology is unclear but is typically caused by friction on the greater trochanter by the iliotibial band (ITB), the anterior border of the gluteus maximus, or the posterior border of the TFL.

The ITB is thought to be the most common cause. It originates from the gluteus maximus and TFL. Most of the ITB inserts at the proximal lateral aspect of the tibia at Gerdy's tubercle, and some fibers insert on the lateral aspect of the distal knee, including the lateral femoral condyle and the lateral patella. A large bursa overlies the greater trochanter separating the trochanter from the ITB. Normally, the ITB remains taut throughout hip range of motion. When the hip is extended, the band lies posterior to the greater trochanter. It moves anteriorly when the hip is flexed. Ordinarily, the ITB glides smoothly over the greater trochanter with assistance from the underlying bursa. If the posterior aspect of the ITB band or the anterior aspect of the gluteus maximus is thickened, it rubs over the greater trochanter causing a snapping sensation. The bursa may also become painful and inflamed. Other proposed causes of external snapping hip relate to alteration of hip mechanics: decreased angulation of the femoral neck (coxa vara), fibrotic scar tissue after intramuscular injection or total hip replacement, narrow bi-iliac width, increased distance between the greater trochanters, prominent greater trochanters, and lateral patellar release.[61,70,71]

Athletes may complain of an audible, often painful snap over the greater trochanter with motion of the hip. The athlete can often voluntarily reproduce the snapping. Ober testing during physical examination will reveal snapping when the affected leg is taken from full extension to 90° of flexion. The examiner's hands should be placed posterior to the greater trochanter in order to feel the snap. If enough force is applied to the greater trochanter to keep the ITB reduced behind the trochanter, the snapping will stop.

Plain radiographs are typically normal. In external snapping, MRI (without intra-articular contrast) will show inflammation of the greater trochanteric bursa or thickening of the ITB or gluteus maximus. Ultrasound has also been used in external snapping to visualize the ITB or gluteus maximus muscle snapping over the greater trochanter.[61]

The mainstay of treatment for external snapping hip is nonoperative and involves rest, activity modification, NSAIDs, and physical therapy. Physical therapy should include stretching of the ITB, core stabilization, and correction of functional pelvic tilt. Corticosteroid injection of the greater trochanteric bursa can be performed if these measures are unsuccessful. If conservative therapy does not relieve symptoms, surgical intervention may be necessary. Surgical intervention involves excision of the greater trochanteric bursa and resection of a portion of the ITB.[60,70,71]

Hip Pointer (Iliac Crest Contusion)

A hip pointer typically occurs in contact sports from a direct blow to an unprotected iliac crest. These injuries include contusions, muscle avulsions from violent contractions, and periostitis from repetitive abdominal muscular contractions. The term "hip pointer" is used to describe an iliac crest contusion that is associated with a subperiosteal hematoma.[37,71]

Athletes may complain of pain with rotation and side-bending away from the injured side and numbness or decreased sensation in the lateral buttock and hip. Physical examination may reveal swelling and ecchymosis, tenderness on and superior to the iliac crest extending superiorly into the internal and external oblique muscles. A palpable defect would indicate an avulsion injury. Numbness and decreased sensation in the lateral buttock and hip indicate damage to the cutaneous nerve branches (T12 to L3). Radiographs are generally unnecessary at the time of diagnosis, but AP and oblique pelvis radiographs are indicated to rule out avulsion fracture, periostitis, or an acute fracture of the iliac wing in athletes with prolonged or increasing symptoms.

Treatment is initiated with ice packs for 20 min every 1–2 h initially until the swelling subsides. After 3–4 days, moist heat should be applied for 10 min followed by ice packs (SOR-C). Abdominal muscle, low back, and flank stretching and strengthening are performed as tolerated. Local modalities such as ultrasound or anesthetic/corticosteroid injections may be utilized to reduce pain and tolerance for therapeutic exercise, thereby speeding return to play (SOR-C).[71–73] Trunk range of motion must be pain free and the athlete should be adequately padded before returning to contact sports (SOR-C).

TFL Syndrome

TFL syndrome is common in runners and cyclists and is caused by inflammation of the TFL as it passes over the greater trochanter.

Athletes usually complain of a gradual onset of anterolateral hip pain coinciding with a change in a training program and a "snapping" sensation during hip flexion and extension. Other risk factors include leg length discrepancy (with the long side being most often affected) and improperly adjusted seating and shoe systems in cyclists. Differential diagnosis includes femoral neck stress fracture, greater trochanteric bursitis, and snapping hip.[74,75]

Physical examination reveals tenderness over the TFL, positive Ober test, and palpable snapping over the greater trochanter with hip flexion and extension. If a femoral neck fracture is suspected, then radiographs, bone scan, and/or MRI should be obtained. Otherwise, treatment should begin with training modification (decrease mileage, decrease speed, and eliminate hills), short-term use of NSAIDS, and ice and heat contrast with phonophoresis to reduce inflammation (SOR-C). A stretching program for the TFL and hip abductor muscle strengthening should be implemented. Leg length and other biomechanical discrepancies should be corrected to prevent recurrence.[71]

Greater Trochanteric Bursitis

Greater trochanteric bursitis can often be difficult to distinguish from TFL syndrome. In greater trochanteric bursitis, the pain is usually felt more posterior to the greater trochanter and can often radiate into the lateral buttock. Irritation of the bursa by a tight overlying ITB, a broad pelvis, leg length discrepancy, and excessive pronation of the foot are all risk factors for developing greater trochanteric bursitis.[76] Athletes may complain of pain with prolonged standing, lying on the ipsilateral side, climbing stairs, or running. In runners, it is commonly a result of overuse rather than direct trauma. The differential diagnosis should include radiation from the SI joint and radicular symptoms of lumbar origin.

On physical examination, pain may be exacerbated by external rotation, adduction, and abduction of the hip, as well as by resisted abduction. The hip abductors are often found to be weak, the ITB is tight, Patrick's test (FABER) causes lateral hip pain, and palpation of the greater trochanter elicits pain. Initial treatment should begin with ice massage and heat contrasts. NSAIDs and local treatment modalities such as phonophoresis help control local inflammation. TFL and ITB flexibility as well as gluteal, hip abductor, and core strengthening exercises should also be included in the rehabilitation program. In cases not responsive to conservative therapy, local corticosteroid injection may be necessary (SOR-C).[76] If greater trochanteric bursitis is refractory to the above, operative release of the ITB and/or bursectomy may be required.[71]

Meralgia Paresthetica (Lateral Femoral Cutaneous Nerve Entrapment)

Meralgia paresthetica is an entrapment of the lateral femoral cutaneous nerve that was initially reported to follow operative interventions such as iliac crest bone grafting, appendectomy, pelvic osteotomy, and total abdominal hysterectomy.[37] It is also seen in diabetic and obese patients or in those wearing tight pants, belts, or girdles.[76]

Most athletes will describe pain, numbness, tingling, and/or burning pain over the anterolateral thigh. Important predisposing factors such as recent weight gain or previous surgical procedure should be obtained. In athletes, prolonged flexion (marksmen), increased muscle mass (weight lifters), or constrictive clothing may play a role. However, in the athletic population, it is not unusual for no identifiable cause to be found.[76] Diagnosis is based on sensory symptoms in the lateral femoral cutaneous nerve distribution. On physical examination, a positive Tinel's sign is usually present 1 cm medial and inferior to the anterior superior iliac crest. Radiography and MRI of the hip and pelvis are useful to rule out intra-pelvic causes of compression on the nerve and intra-articular derangement. Nerve conduction studies often demonstrate prolonged latency or decreased conduction velocity consistent with compression.[37]

Nonoperative treatment is the mainstay of therapy. A local nerve block has been shown to temporarily relieve symptoms and is a useful diagnostic tool and excellent predictor of benefit from surgical decompression (SOR-C).[77] Heat, physical therapy, local steroid injections, and NSAIDs have been shown to be effective. If symptoms are persistent and disabling despite conservative therapy, surgical intervention to perform a nerve decompression may be warranted. Another intervention is transection of the nerve, but this often times results in hypoesthesias and possible neuroma development.[37,76,77]

POSTERIOR HIP AND PELVIS PAIN

Hamstring Strain

The hamstring is made up of the semitendinosus, semimembranosus, and the long head of the biceps femoris. The three muscles have a common origin at the ischial tuberosity. Because the hamstring muscle group spans two joints, it is highly susceptible to injury. The biceps femoris is the most frequently injured muscle of the hamstring group. The injury usually extends longitudinally within the muscle rather than in a single cross-sectional area and typically occurs during the swing phase, when the hamstrings are working eccentrically, or early during stance phase, when there is a large concentric burst, such as in jumping or sprinting motions.[78] Complete tears are rare, but have been reported in water skiers, runners, dancers, and power lifters. Risk factors for hamstring injury include leg length discrepancy, muscle imbalances, poor flexibility, insufficient preactivity stretching, prior hamstring injury, and poor technique.[79] The differential diagnosis includes radicular pain of lumbar origin, referred pain from the SI joint, and avulsion fracture of the ischial tuberosity.

The athlete usually self diagnoses the injury at the time it occurs. They report a "pop" or pulling sensation in the posterior thigh. Physical examination may show edema and ecchymosis over the muscle belly which usually occurs within 2 and 48 h, respectively. The examiner should palpate the ischial tuberosity and follow the muscle inferiorly to locate the area of maximal tenderness and to determine whether there is a palpable defect in the muscle. If the ischial tuberosity is extremely tender, then an avulsion fracture should be suspected. Symptoms typically increase with resisted knee flexion, and the athlete is often unable to straighten his or her knee during the terminal swing phase. Athletes with a large amount of swelling and ecchymosis associated with knee flexion weakness may have a complete rupture.[14]

Radiographs should be ordered in athletes with suspected ischial tuberosity avulsion fractures. An MRI is unnecessary unless the clinician is entertaining the possibility of complete rupture. The diagnosis is primarily made clinically, as Verrall et al. found MRI to have a false negative rate of 18%.[80]

There are no evidence-based treatment guidelines for hamstring strains. As such, recommendations are based upon expert opinion and personal experience. Initial treatment should consist of ice packs or ice massage, compression wraps, and possibly protected weight-bearing. This is then followed by passive hamstring stretches in the pain-free range and then ice massage. As symptoms resolve, the athlete progresses to active hip and knee range of motion exercises and contract–relax techniques to the hamstring, followed by hamstring isometrics. The final rehabilitation phase consists of active strengthening emphasizing eccentric exercises and speed exercises. For part of the speed work, some advocate including running backward, which helps stretch the hamstrings.[81,82] It has been suggested that concentric exercises may actually be detrimental as opposed to eccentric training and sprinting, which better prepare the athlete for return to play.[14]

Ischial Bursitis

Ischial bursitis occurs after a direct blow to or contusion of the ischial tuberosity or may occur as a complication from an injury of the hamstring insertion on the ischial tuberosity. Inflammation of the ischial bursa with associated pain and tenderness occurs as a result of scar and hematoma formation. Athletes may complain of pain while sitting.[83] On physical examination there will be localized tenderness. Ultrasound or MRI can be used to confirm the diagnosis.[53] Treatment consists of rest, ice, NSAIDS, hamstring stretching and strengthening, and protection; often a doughnut cushion will help alleviate pain while sitting. In recalcitrant cases, aspiration of the bursa and injection of corticosteroid should be considered (SOR-C). If the athlete continues to have persistent pain and disability despite conservative therapy, surgical excision of the bursa is indicated.[84]

Gluteus Maximus Strain

Compared to hamstring injuries, isolated strains of the gluteus maximus are uncommon but can occur in sprinters. More often, this muscle is injured through direct trauma.[85] The hip, lumbar spine, and SI joints should be examined in athletes reporting buttock pain. If no tenderness is elicited in any of these areas, then a gluteus maximus strain is suspected. The athlete may report a sudden, sharp pain in the buttock during a burst of speed or sudden change in direction. If the SI joint or lumbar spine is involved, then a rehabilitation program that is specific for these areas should be implemented. Otherwise, treatment of a gluteus maximus strain involves rest, ice, and compression to reduce pain and inflammation. After the range of motion begins to normalize, strengthening should be performed.[72,73] Return to full participation can occur once the athlete is pain-free and is able to do sports-specific activities (SOR-C).

Gluteus Medius Strain

The gluteus medius functions as a hip abductor. Injuries to this muscle are common in runners. The patient often complains of lateral thigh pain near the greater trochanter and is often mistaken for greater trochanteric bursitis. The pain will be reproduced by palpation just proximal to the tendon insertion on the greater trochanter[72] and often in the muscle belly itself. Resisted abduction of the hip will also provoke pain. Treatment follows the same principles as gluteus maximus strain, with additional emphasis placed upon core strengthening.[71]

SI Joint Dysfunction/SI Sprain

SI joint dysfunction/sprain is a controversial diagnosis; therefore, pain and injury to the SI joint is commonly overlooked. The SI articulation is formed by the sacrum and the ilia separated by a synovial cavity. The anterior and posterior SI ligaments, the interosseous SI, and the sacrotuberous ligaments are the major ligaments supporting the joints. Although uncommon, painful tearing and stretching of any of these ligaments can occur. Sudden, violent contraction of the hamstrings or the abdominal muscles; sudden torsion; a severe, direct blow to the buttocks; or forceful straightening from a crouched position can generate enough force to produce injury to these ligaments. Sports that that involve repetitive unidirectional pelvic shear and torsional forces (e.g., skating, gymnastics, bowling) also put the athlete at risk of SI dysfunction.[86] Movements that occur between the sacrum and ilia are rotatory, translatory, or a combination of both. Loss of motion in the SI joint or sustained contraction of the overlying muscles may cause pain. SI dysfunction can also cause low back, thoracic, and even cervical pain.[87] The differential diagnosis should include radicular pain, piriformis syndrome, gluteus medius strain, ankylosing spondylitis, Reiter's syndrome, and other spondyloarthropathies. Autoimmune etiologies should especially be considered if both SI joints are involved and/or if the athlete is not responding to conservative therapy.

The athlete typically presents with traumatic or insidious onset of pain over one SI joint. The pain may radiate to the low back, groin, posterolateral hip, and thigh. The pain pattern may mimic radicular pain from a herniated nucleus pulposus or lateral spinal stenosis. The lack of nerve root tension signs and absence of motor, reflex, or sensory deficits help distinguish SI joint dysfunction from nerve root compression lesions.

Physical examination shows unilateral tenderness over the affected posterior superior iliac spine (PSIS) and along the sacral sulcus. FABER, piriformis, and Gaenslen's tests may be positive. Straight leg raise may cause SI pain. Pain is also exacerbated by forward flexion of the trunk with knees extended. A positive one-legged stork test (Gillet test) indicates a lack of mobility on the affected side. Sacral compression medial to the PSIS often causes localized pain. The athlete should also be evaluated for a leg length discrepancy.[87]

The goal of treatment is restoration of normal movement. Treatment consists of ice, NSAIDS, ice massage, and heat. After the acute phase, a corset, constricting elastic bandage, or SI belt may provide relief. Progressive protected motion for 5–6 weeks may be necessary before healing occurs. Treatment should also consist of pelvic stabilization exercises and exercises to stretch and strengthen the piriformis muscle (SOR-C).

Multiple dysfunctions of the SI joint have been identified. Two of the most common ones are anterior innominate dysfunction and posterior innominate dysfunction. Anterior innominate dysfunction is diagnosed when the athlete has a positive Gillet test and an anterior superior iliac spine (ASIS) that is relatively inferior to the contralateral ASIS. Posterior innominate dysfunction is diagnosed by a positive Gillet test and a superior ASIS on the affected side. Treatment of anterior and posterior innominate dysfunction should be by a physician skilled in manual medicine. See Chap. 11 for a more in-depth discussion on this topic.

Piriformis Syndrome

The piriformis muscle originates on the anterolateral aspect of the sacrum and inserts on the upper border of the greater trochanter and femur. It lies deep to the gluteus maximus muscle. Spasm of the muscle can result from a twisting injury sustained during a single-legged stance and often occurs in runners. Differential diagnosis includes hip joint disease, SI joint dysfunction, nerve root irritation, lateral stenosis, and lumbar herniated nucleus pulposus.

Athletes usually present with a history of blunt trauma to the gluteal or SI region. They complain of pain in the lower SI joint, the greater sciatic notch, and piriformis muscle radiating down the posterior buttock, hip, and thigh. The pain may be described as cramping or a feeling of tightness in the hamstring muscles. It is frequently exacerbated by stooping or lifting.

On examination, athletes may have a tender, palpable fullness of the piriformis muscle, point tenderness of the muscle belly, and buttock pain exacerbated by hip flexion and passive internal rotation. Straight leg raise is occasionally positive with referred pain down the posterior thigh and calf. Resisted hip abduction and external rotation exacerbate the symptoms. Passive hip extension should relieve the symptoms. A loss of hip internal rotation may also be present.[86] Patients will often have a positive piriformis and Gaenslen's test. The FAIR test (flexion, adduction, internal rotation) has been shown to have a sensitivity of 88% and a specificity of 83% (SOR-B).[88] Radiographs, MRI, and CT scanning provide little information and are not needed to make the diagnosis. Neurophysiologic testing has been shown to be effective in confirming the diagnosis.[86,89,90]

Treatment of piriformis syndrome includes ice massage, ultrasound and/or electrical stimulation, physical therapy to stretch and massage the piriformis, NSAIDs, muscle relaxants, and local anesthetic or steroid injections.[86,91] Osteopathic manipulative treatment has also been shown to be helpful.[92] Athletes can also stretch the piriformis muscle themselves by lying supine and pulling the knee on the affected side toward the opposite shoulder. To prevent recurrence, lumbosacral dysfunction and imbalances in the surrounding musculature must be concurrently treated. If conservative therapy fails or if the patient develops foot drop or gluteal muscle atrophy, referral to orthopedics for operative release of the piriformis muscle, fibrous bands, and/or compressing vessels may be considered.[86,91]

Coccygeal Injury

The coccyx is joined to the sacrum by cartilage which forms a synchondrosis. It is susceptible to injury during a fall on the buttocks, being struck from behind, or during a difficult vaginal delivery. Physical examination reveals localized tenderness, pain in the coccygeal region (coccydynia), localized swelling or ecchymosis, and pain exacerbated by sitting. X-rays are required to rule out an inferior sacrum fracture and to determine whether the coccyx is dislocated or displaced. If there is no history of trauma, rectal examination and lower gastrointestinal evaluation are indicated. Although controversial, the examiner can reduce a dislocated or displaced coccyx by inserting a lubricated index finger into the rectum so that the palmar surface rests against the anterior aspect of the coccyx. He or she then palpates the posterior aspect of the coccyx externally, applies a gentle traction on the coccyx, and glides the coccyx into its normal position. If successful, pain relief is usually immediate. However, there is no conclusive evidence as to the efficacy of this approach. Successful treatment of chronic coccydynia has been reported with pelvic relaxation exercises, pelvic floor strengthening, biofeedback, local corticosteroid injection, botulin toxin injection, and coccygectomy.[93–96]

Other

Leg Length Discrepancy

Pain originating in the pelvis, low back, and hip region can be caused or exacerbated by a disparity in leg length. The evaluation of atraumatic and nonacute traumatic hip and pelvis pain should always include screening for a leg length discrepancy (SOR-C).[97–99] There are two types of leg length discrepancies: true and functional (or apparent). In a true leg length discrepancy, the actual length of the two lower extremities is different when measured from the femoral heads to the plantar surfaces of the feet. In a functional leg length discrepancy, the athlete's two lower extremities are, in fact, the same length. However, pelvic obliquity gives the appearance of a discrepancy. The true leg length discrepancy is caused by one of the bones of the lower limb actually being longer or shorter than the other side.[97] This may be the result of a varus or valgus deformity of the femoral neck, congenital anomalies of the femur or tibia, or growth disturbances of the femur or tibia. Possible causes of a functional leg discrepancy include contractures at the lumbosacral junction due to scoliosis, post-traumatic deformities of the pelvis, somatic dysfunction of the pelvis and/or SI joints, and muscle contractures about the hip and knee. The physical examination and osteopathic manipulation chapters discuss the evaluation of leg length in greater detail.

A more precise measurement of leg length is obtained with a standing AP radiograph film of the pelvis down to the feet. This view should include the upper lumbar spine and the femoral heads. The athlete should stand with his or her feet shoulder width apart with equal weight distribution while the X-ray is being taken. Lines are then drawn on the radiograph at the superior sacral ala bilaterally to form a sacral base and at the superior margin of each femoral head. The examiner then draws a line from the sacral base and femoral heads to the base of the film. This method is recommended if the standing measurements have not been accurate. Instead of plain radiographs, some facilities are now using a quick computer tomography scan from the upper lumbar spine to the feet and then comparing measurements from the medial malleolus to the superior margin of the femoral head on each side.

CONCLUSION OF THE CASE

The patient was diagnosed with greater trochanteric bursitis and ITB syndrome. He was instructed to take NSAIDs twice a day with food for 7 days, and then as needed. He was also given a referral for physical therapy for gluteus medius, quadriceps, hamstring, and ITB stretching and strengthening program with modalities (ultrasound, electrical stimulation, iontophoresis, or phonophoresis) as needed. A core stabilization program was also emphasized. Additionally, over-the-counter orthotics were recommended for the pes planus with hyperpronation.

References

1. Vitanzo PC, McShane JM. Osteitis pubis: solving a perplexing problem. Phys Sports Med 2001; 29(7):33–40.
2. Cunningham PM, Brennan D, O'Connell M, et al. Patterns of bone and soft-tissue injury at the symphysis pubis in soccer players: observations at MRI. AJR Am J Roentgenol Mar 2007; 188(3): W291–W296.

3. King JB. Treatment of osteitis pubis in athletes: results of corticosteroid injections. Am J Sports Med 1996; 24(2):248.
4. Pavlov H, Nelson TL, Warren RF, et al. Stress fractures of the pubic ramus: a report of twelve cases. J Bone Joint Surg (Am) 1982; 64(7):1020–1025.
5. Deutsch AL, Coel MN, Mink JH. Imaging of stress injuries to bone: radiography, scintigraphy, and MR imaging. Clin Sports Med 1997; 16(2):275–290A.
6. Markey KL. Stress fractures. Clin Sports Med 1987; 6(2):405–425.
7. Malanga GA, Jasey NN, Solomon J. Femoral neck fracture. At: www.emedicine.com/sports/TOPIC36.HTM. Accessed 2 December 2008.
8. Shin AY, Morin WD, Gorman JD, et al. The superiority of magnetic resonance imaging in differentiating the cause of hip pain in endurance athletes. Am J Sports Med 1996; 24(2):168–176.
9. Quinn SF, McCarthy JL. Prospective evaluation of patients with suspected hip fracture and indeterminate radiographs: use of T1-weighted MR images. Radiology 1993; 187(2):469–471.
10. Fullerton LR, Snowdy HA. Femoral neck stress fractures. Am J Sports Med 1988; 16:365.
11. Scudese BA. Traumatic anterior hip redislocation. Clin Orthop 1972; 88:60.
12. Walsh ZT, Micheli LJ. Hip dislocation in a high school football player. Phys Sports Med 1989; 17:112.
13. Wolfe MW, Brinker MR, Cary GR, et al. Posterior fracture-dislocation of the hip in a jogger. J South Orthop Assoc 1995; 4:91–95.
14. Nishina T, Saito S, Ohzono K, et al. Chiari pelvic osteotomy for osteoarthritis: The influence of the torn and detached acetabular labrum. J Bone Joint Surg Br 1990; 72:765.
15. Hougaard K, Thomsen PB. Traumatic posterior dislocation of the hip – prognostic factors influencing the incidence of avascular necrosis of the femoral head. Arch Orthop Trauma Surg 1986; 106:32–35.
16. Nuccion S, Hunter DM, Finerman GAM. Hip and pelvis: adult. In: DeLee JC, Drez D Jr, Miller MD, eds. DeLee & Drez's Orthopaedic Sports Medicine: Principles and Practice, 2nd ed. Philadelphia: WB Saunders; 2003:1443–1480.
17. Imhof H, Breitenseher M, Trattnig S. Imaging of avascular necrosis of bone. Eur Radiol 1997; 7(2):180–186.
18. Tofferi JK, Gilliland W. Avascular necrosis. At: www.emedicine.com/Med/topic2924.htm. Accessed 2 December 2008.
19. Roberts WN, Williams RB. Hip pain. Prim Care 1988; 15:783–793.
20. McCarthy JC, Busconi B. The role of hip arthroscopy in the diagnosis and treatment of hip disease. Orthopedics 1995; 18:753–756.
21. Browder D, Enseki K, Fritz J. Intertester reliability of hip range of motion measurements and special tests. J Orthop Sports Phys Ther 2004; 34:A1.
22. Byrd JW. Labral lesions: an elusive source of hip pain: case reports and literature review. Arthroscopy 1996; 12:603–612.
23. Czerny C, Hoffmann S, Urban M, et al. MR arthrography of the adult acetabular capsular–labral complex: Correlation with surgery and anatomy. AJR Am J Roentgenol 1999; 173:345.

24. Lage L, Patel J, Villar R. The acetabular labral tear: An arthroscopic classification. Arthroscopy 1996; 12(3):269–272.
25. Beal DP, Sweet CF, Martin HD, et al. Imaging findings of femoroacetabular impingement syndrome. Skeletal Radiol 2005; 34: 691–701.
26. Ganz R, Parvizi J, Beck M, et al. Femoroacetabular impingement. A cause for osteoarthritis of the hip. Clin Orthop 2003; 417:112–120.
27. Kassarjiam A, Yoon LS, Belzile E, et al. Triad of MR arthrographic findings in patients with Cam-type femoroacetabular impingement. Radiology 2005; 236:588–592.
28. Manaster BJ, Zakel S. Imaging of femoral acetabular impingement syndrome. Clin Sports Med 2006; 25(4)635–657.
29. Johnston CA, Wiley JP, Lindsay DM, Wiseman DA. Iliopsoas bursitis and tendonitis. Sports Med 1998; 25(4): 271–283.
30. Fricker PA. Management of groin pain in athletes. Br J Sports Med 1997; 31(2):91–101.
31. Heolmich P. Adductor-related groin pain in athletes. Sports Med Arthroscopy Rev 1997; 5(4):285–291.
32. Karlsson J, Jerre R. The use of radiography, magnetic resonance, and ultrasound in the diagnosis of hip, pelvis, and groin injuries. Sports Med Arthroscopy Rev 1997; 5(4):268–273.
33. Lacroix VJ, Kinnear DG, Mulder DS, et al. Lower abdominal pain syndrome in National Hockey League players: a report of cases. Clin J Sports Med 1988; 8(1):5–9.
34. Hackney RG. The 'sports hernia' a cause of groin pain. Br J Sports Med 1993; 27(1): 58–62.
35. Kemp S, Batt ME. The 'sports hernia': a common cause of groin pain. Phys Sportsmed 1998; 26(1):36–44.
36. Ahumada LA, Ashruf S, Espinosa-de-los-Monteros A, et al. Athletic pubalgia: definition and surgical treatment. Ann Plast Surg 2005; 55(4):393–396.
37. Meyers WC, Foley DP, Garrett WE, et al. Management of severe lower abdominal or inguinal pain in high-performance athletes. Am J Sports Med 2000; 28(1):2–8.
38. Srinivasan A, Schuricht A. Long-term follow-up of laparoscopic preperitoneal hernia repair in professional athletes. J Lapar Adv Surg Tech 2002; 12(2):101–106.
39. Jacobson T, Allen WC. Surgical correction of the snapping iliopsoas tendon. Am J Sports Med 1990; 18(5): 470–474.
40. Idjadi J, Meislin R. Symptomatic snapping hip: targeted treatment for maximum pain relief. Phys Sport Med 2004; 32(1):25–31.
41. Schaberg JE, Harper MC, Allen WC. The snapping hip syndrome. Am J Sports Med 1994; 12(5):361–365.
42. Harper MC, Schaberg JE, Allen WC. Primary iliopsoas bursography in the diagnosis of disorders of the hip. Clin Orthop 1987; 221(Aug):238–241.
43. Allen WC, Cope R. Coxa saltans: the snapping hip revisited. J Am Acad Orthop Surg 1995; 3(5):303–308.
44. Larsen E, Johansen J. Snapping hip. Acta Orthop Scand 1986; 57(2): 168–170.

45. Wunderbaldinger P, Bremer C, Matuszweski L, et al. Efficient radiological assessment of the internal snapping hip syndrome. Eur Radiol 2002; 11(9):1743–1747.
46. Pelsser V, Cardinal E, Hobden R, et al. Extraarticular snapping hip: sonographic findings. AJR Am J Roentgenol 2001; 176(1):67–73.
47. Gruen GS, Scioscia TN, Lowenstein TE. The surgical treatment of internal snapping hip. Am J Sports Med 2002; 30(4):607–613.
48. Frich LH, Lauritzen J, Juhl M. Arthroscopy in diagnosis and treatment of hip disorders. Orthopedics 1989; 12(3): 389–392.
49. Zoltan DJ, Clancy WG, Keene JS. A new operative approach to snapping hip and refractory trochanteric bursitis in athletes. Am J Sports Med 1986; 14: 201–204.
50. Farber AJ, Wilckens JH, Jarvis CG. Pelvic pain in the athlete: In: Seidenberg PH, Beutler AI, eds. The Sports Medicine Resource Manual. Philadelphia: Saunders Elsevier; 2008:306–327.
51. Boyd KT, Peirce NS, Batt ME. Common hip injuries in sport. Sports Med 1997; 24(4):273–288.
52. Anderson K, Strickland SM, Warren R. Hip and groin injuries in athletes. Am J Sports Med 2001; 29(4):521–523.
53. Fredericson M, Cookingham CL, Chaudhari AM, et al. Hip abductor weakness in distance runners with iliotibial band syndrome. Clin J Sport Med 2000; 10:169–175.
54. Holmes JC, Pruitt AL, Whalen NJ. Lower extremity overuse in bicycling. Clin Sports Med 1994; 13:187–205.
55. Seidenberg PH, Childress MA. Managing hip pain in athletes. J Musculoskel Med 2005; 22(5):246–254.
56. Williams P, Trzil K. Management of meralgia paresthetica. J Neurosurg 1991; 74:76.
57. Woods C, Hawkins RD, Maltby S, et al. The football association medical research programme: an audit of injuries in professional football – analysis of hamstring muscle strain. Br J Spots Med 2004; 38(1):36–41.
58. Gabbe BJ, Finch CF, Bennell KL, et al. Risk factors for hamstring injuries in community level Australian football. Br J Sports Med 2005; 39(2):106–110.
59. Verrall GM, Slavotinek JP, Barnes PG, et al. Diagnostic and prognostic value of clinical findings in 83 athletes with posterior thigh injury: comparison of clinical findings with magnetic resonance imaging documentation of hamstring muscle strain. Am J Sports Med 1992; 20(6):640–643.
60. Bates BT, McCaw ST. A comparison between forward and backward locomotion. Human Locomotion IV, Proceedings of the Biennial Conference of the Canadian Society for Biomechanics (CSB), Montreal, Quebec, Canada; 1986: 307–308.
61. Bates BT, Morrison E, Hamill J. Differences between forward and backward running. In Adrian M, Deutsch, eds. Proceedings: The 1984 Olympic Scientific Congress. Eugene, Oregon: University of Oregon Microform Publications; 1986:127–135.
62. Roos HP. Hip pain in sport. Sports Med Arthrosc Rev 1997; 5(4):292–300.

63. Waters PM, Millis MB. Hip and pelvic injuries in the young athlete. Clin Sports Med 1988; 7(3):513–526.
64. Armfield DR, Kim DH, Towers JD, et al. Sports-related muscle injury in the lower extremity. Clin Sports Med 2006; 25(4): 803–842.
65. Webb CW, Geshel R. Thoracic and lumbar spine injuries. In Seidenberg PH, Beutler AI, eds. The Sports Medicine Resource Manual. Philadelphia: Saunders Elsevier; 2008:285–305.
66. Prather H. Pelvis and sacral dysfunction in sports and exercise. Phys Med Rehabil Clin North Am 2000; 11(4):805–836.
67. Fishman L, Dombi G, Michaelson C, et al. Piriformis syndrome: diagnosis, treatment and outcome – a 10 year study. Arch Phys Med Rehabil 2002; 83:295–301.
68. Robinson DR. Pyriformis syndrome in relation to sciatic pain. Am J Surg 1947; 47:355–358.
69. Fishman L, Zybert P. Electrophysiologic evidence of piriformis syndrome. Arch Phys Med Rehabil 1992; 73:359–364.
70. Papadopoulos EC, Khan SN. Piriformis syndrome and low back pain: a new classification and review of the literature. Orthop Clin North Am 2004; 35(1):65–71.
71. Steiner C, Staubs C, Ganon M, Buhlinger C. Piriformis syndrome: pathogenesis, diagnosis, and treatment. J Am Osteopath Assoc 1987; 87(4):318–323.
72. Hodges SD, Eck JC, Humphreys SC. A treatment and outcomes analysis of patients with coccydynia. Spine J 2002; 4:138–140.
73. Jarvis SK, Abbott JA, Lenart MG, et al. Pilot study of botulinum toxin type A in the treatment of chronic pelvic pain associated with spasm of the levator ani muscles. Aust N Z J Obstet Gynaecol 2004; 44:46–50.
74. Perkins R, Schofferman J, Reynolds J. Coccygectomy for severe refractory sacrococcygeal joint pain. J Spinal Disord Tech 2003; 16:100–103.
75. Doursounian L, Maigne JY, Faure F, Chatellier G. Coccygectomy for instability of the coccyx. Int Orthop 2004; 28:176–179.
76. Seidenberg PH, Childres MA. Physical examination of the hip and pelvis. In: Seidenberg PH, Beutler AI, eds. The Sports Medicine Resource Manual. Philadelphia: Saunders Elsevier; 2008:110–122.
77. Geraci MC Jr, Brown W. Evidence-based treatment of hip and pelvic injuries in runners. Phys Med Rehabil Clinc N Am 2005; 16(3):711–747.
78. McGrory BJ. Stinchfield resisted hip flexion test. Hosp Physician 1999; 35(9):41–42.

Chapter 7
Hip and Pelvis Injuries in Childhood and Adolescence

Christopher S. Nasin and Marjorie C. Nasin

CLINICAL PEARLS
- Ultrasound as a screening tool for developmental dysplasia of the hip (DDH) prior to 6 weeks of age is considered overly sensitive; monitor at-risk infants with biweekly physical exams until that time.
- Legg–Calvé–Perthes disease (LCPD) tends to be a self-limited process involving natural hip remodeling. Severe cases may benefit from surgical intervention.
- Transient synovitis is the most common cause of limp and hip pain in children.
- Slipped capital femoral epiphysis (SCFE) is the most common hip disorder of the adolescent and should be considered in all children between ages of 10–16 years who present with hip pain or limp.
- The vast majority of pelvic apophyseal injuries are treated without surgical intervention.

CASE STUDY
A 12-year-old boy is brought in by his mother with worsened right-sided knee pain, which began without trauma several weeks earlier. The mother notes that the boy has been complaining of worsening pain with running, which suddenly became worse today after he tripped on a curb. The patient is found to have a body-mass index greater than the 95th percentile for age and appears uncomfortable sitting on the exam table. Flexion and internal rotation of the right hip exacerbate the pain. The patient is sent to X-ray in

a wheelchair as he now refuses to ambulate. The radiologist calls your office and reports that the patient has an SCFE.

INTRODUCTION

The approach to the child with hip pathology is unique and necessitates an understanding of the anatomy and physiology of normal hip development. Not all hip disorders of childhood are painful at that joint; often children will complain of pain below the hip or will present with a painless limp. The differential diagnosis of hip pain and limp changes as children grow. It is the duty of the physician to understand all possible conditions that affect the pediatric hip at different stages of development in order to take the appropriate history, perform a competent examination, and order the appropriate tests. Several common pediatric and adolescent hip maladies will be highlighted throughout this chapter. Of note, infections of the hip, thigh, and pelvic structures are not discussed in this chapter and are vital in the differential diagnosis of hip pain in a child who demonstrates any signs of illness. The injuries described below occur in otherwise healthy children.

DEVELOPMENTAL DYSPLASIA OF THE HIP

DDH, similarly termed congenital hip dysplasia, describes a variety of conditions present at birth which result from an interruption to the normal growth and development of the hip joint. This spectrum can range from mild acetabular change to complete dislocation, but does not include anatomically stable hips with clicking ligaments that primary care providers will note much more commonly in newborns.[1] Of utmost importance then is the early distinction between those two entities in order to establish for the patient with DDH, a postnatal hip position which will foster the development of the acetabulum and femoral head and minimize the predisposition to degenerative changes and osteoarthritis (Fig. 7.1).[2] Published incidence of DDH is highly variable, ranging from 1 to 10 per 1,000 live births.

Both genetic and mechanical risk factors have been identified: female gender, firstborn status, family history, North American Indian race (which perhaps may not be genetic but rather due to postnatal cultural positioning of the infant), and intrauterine conditions such as oligohydramnios or breech positioning. Eighty percent of children with DDH are female, presumably because of the estrogen effect on ligamentous laxity. The left hip is affected in the majority of cases (60%), likely due to intrauterine positioning, while the right hip is affected 20% of the time, and both hips are involved the remaining 20% of the time.

7. HIP AND PELVIS INJURIES IN CHILDHOOD AND ADOLESCENCE   151

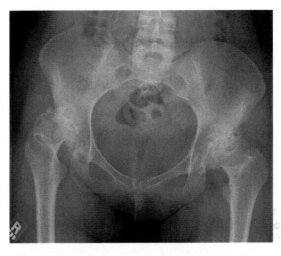

Figure 7.1. AP radiograph of the pelvis demonstrating the outcome of a chronic missed developmental dysplasia of the hip (DDH). Note the superolateral subluxation of the hips bilaterally with severe degenerative changes (Courtesy of Dr Michael Gibson, National Naval Medical Center).

Diagnosis

Diagnosis of DDH can be made by physical exam or, definitively, by ultrasound. Currently, the American Academy of Pediatrics recommends ultrasound study (after 6 weeks of age) for any infant with risk factors for DDH or evidence of DDH on physical exam (SOR-C). Radiographs prior to 4 months will be of limited value since the femoral head and majority of acetabulum are not yet ossified. However, prior to 6 weeks of age, ultrasound as a screening tool can be overly sensitive, so it is best to wait to achieve an optimal study. But, if there is clinical evidence of dislocation, the study can be ordered in a timely fashion. Although it is debatable whether selective screening (based on risk factors) can truly have an impact on the incidence of the late development of DDH (which carries with it the most morbidity), universal postnatal ultrasound screening is not considered a cost-effective measure at this time.[3,4] After 4–6 months of age, if DDH is suspected, plain radiographs are the preferred imaging modality.

Clear and repetitive instruction in residency training programs on diagnostic physical exam maneuvers for DDH emphasize the recommendation for multiple neonatal hip exams to be performed on every neonate (SOR-C). The clinician who examines infants should become comfortable with the visual and sensory cues of the Ortolani and Barlow maneuvers (which attempt to relocate and dislocate the femoral head, respectively) as well as with assessing the symmetry and muscular tone of an infant. These maneuvers must be done on each hip separately. The sensitivity of the Ortolani maneuver decreases with the age of the patient, making careful attention to the exam during the first 60 days of life essential.[5] Asymmetric inguinal or thigh skin folds, knee height difference in the supine position with hips flexed and soles on the exam table (Galeazzi sign), and limitation of hip abduction are additional physical exam findings that may be useful. If diagnosis is confirmed with radiographic tests, referral to an orthopedist should be initiated at that time.

Treatment

In the very young infant as well as in infants who are known to have subluxation only, observation is usually the first line of treatment. Often, the subluxation will resolve within 2 weeks and no further instability will be noted. In these cases, more extensive treatment regimens are not required. However, if evidence of instability remains beyond 2 weeks, if true dislocation is present, or if the infant is beyond the neonatal period, bracing is usually considered (SOR-3).

Bracing with a Pavlik harness, which is a technique generally reserved for infants less than 6 months of age, allows consistent placement of the femoral head into the acetabulum by positioning the hips in flexion and abduction while still allowing some movement. Typically, a dislocated femoral head should be relocated by the harness within 3 weeks, with the average length of bracing generally lasting 6 weeks full time and an additional 6 weeks part time for infants. With the femoral head in position, further normal growth and development of the hip joint can occur throughout childhood. Complications of the harness can include failure of treatment, skin breakdown, avascular necrosis (AVN) of the femoral head, and femoral nerve palsy. Late diagnosis or failure of Pavlik harness permits time for abnormally vectored growth to occur, often requiring closed reduction with spica casting or open surgical reduction (SOR-C).

LEGG-CALVE-PERTHES DISEASE

LCPD was described nearly a century ago by the three physicians whose names were joined to entitle the complex cycle of femoral head AVN, resorption, and collapse, followed by subsequent repair and remodeling. Often simply called Perthes disease, this condition is most often diagnosed between the ages of 4 and 8 (range: 2 to teenage years), with an incidence of 1 in 1,200 and a male predominance of 4:1.[6] Unilateral hip involvement is most common, and the 10–20% of cases that are found to be bilateral overwhelmingly occur in girls. If bilateral, hips tend to be affected sequentially, following independent diseases courses. Perthes disease diagnosed as truly a bilateral, concurrent phenomenon is a rare event, and should prompt a further workup for systemic illness or skeletal dysplasia.

The etiology of this disease remains elusive; although interruption of the blood supply to the femoral head is one of the initial events in the cycle, the risk factors for this event remain debated. There has been an association between low birth weight, mildly short stature, and even some medical conditions (hypothyroidism), particularly with bilateral disease. However, there remains considerable discussion as to whether the necrosis occurs as a result of a separate primary disorder altogether such as a coagulation defect or disorder of intracapsular hip pressure.[7,8] The literature does not strongly support these theories, but both topics represent the ongoing pursuit to understand LCPD more completely. There is a family history of LCPD in approximately 10% of cases.[9]

Diagnosis

Presentation most commonly occurs with a painless limp or difficulty walking. It is not associated with an illness or fever, or generally with known trauma, although the younger child routinely has so many minor falls that parents may "explain" as due to a limp by citing an unrelated event.

Physical exam reveals a limp – the chief complaint of the otherwise well-appearing child. And while a lengthy differential diagnosis for the limping child can be formulated, if the clinician has ruled out an infectious process through an appropriate physical exam, the biggest challenge will be differentiating between an irritable hip from transient synovitis and the acute symptoms of LCPD.[10] If not painless, LCPD will cause a mildly painful or intermittently painful limp, often with the pain referred down the inner aspect of the thigh or to the knee. Activity worsens these symptoms, as opposed to the limp of transient synovitis, which is improved with activity, as if the joint is being "loosened up."

Even early in the disease process, decreased hip abduction and internal rotation due to muscle spasm and synovitis are noted. If more damage has occurred to the femoral head, the limitation of movement may be due to bony impingement of the femoral head on the acetabulum. Pain is more likely to be elicited at the end range of motion, with less painful midrange motion.[11] Examination of the buttocks, thigh, and calf of the affected side should be performed for evidence of atrophy. Leg length discrepancy is a relatively late finding, since it represents collapse of the femoral head – the third step in the disease cycle. The Thomas test and Trendelenburg test are often positive. If a child has bilateral Perthes disease, her upper body would sway toward the more affected, or weaker, side during Trendelenburg testing.

Radiographs remain the mainstay of diagnosis, classification, and follow-up of Perthes disease. Initial findings may include only an increase in the affected hip's joint space, although this is a nonspecific finding. With disease progression, subarticular lucencies become evident within the femoral capital epiphysis, which may then become flattened, sclerotic, and fragmented (Fig. 7.2). Early changes may be evident only on frog leg views, and these should be performed during the initial evaluation. Very early in the course of the illness, radiographs may be normal. If clinical suspicion for LCPD remains high, magnetic resonance imaging (MRI) or scintigraphy may be useful to establish the diagnosis. Scintigraphy has been shown to reveal focal areas of increased uptake seen within the femoral head, while MRI may reveal areas of low signal intensity within the femoral head on T-1-weighted images.[12]

Treatment

Once diagnosed, the two classification schemes most commonly used are Catterall and Herring. The Catterall classification divides involvement of the femoral epiphysis into quarters ($1 = 25\%$ through $4 = 100\%$ involvement). The Herring classification uses the degree of collapse of the lateral epiphyseal pillar during the fragmentation phase, divided into three groups ($A = 1/3$ or less collapse, $B = 2/3$, $C =$ up to full collapse). The Herring classification scheme is considered a more accurate predictor of long-term outcome. However, regardless of classification, whether treated by conservatively or surgically, results are highly variable and largely dependent on age of onset and degree of femoral head involvement.[13] Presentation at a young age is protective for a good outcome, presumably because the hip has a longer time period of natural growth and development to remodel naturally.

The role of surgical intervention and its impact on clinical outcome is controversial and widely debated within the literature. Unfortunately, identifying those patients who are believed to be the best surgical candidates would require being able to predict the natural course of a given patient's disease very early on. Although such predictions are not generally possible, at the time of this writing, there is one promising study which suggests that patients with hand bone age delays of greater than 2 years at time of diagnosis

7. HIP AND PELVIS INJURIES IN CHILDHOOD AND ADOLESCENCE   155

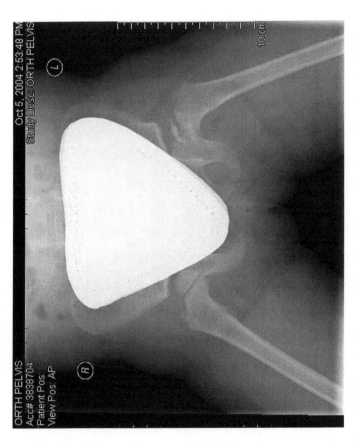

FIGURE 7.2. AP radiograph of the pelvis demonstrating Legg–Calvé–Perthes disease (LCPD) in the left hip in a 5-year-old female. Although the right hip is normal in this study, the patient went on to develop bilateral disease.

can be predicted to go on to develop severe hip disease.[14] Goals of any intervention are maintenance of hip motion, pain relief, and containment of the femoral head in the acetabulum (SOR-C). For severe disease, surgical intervention appears preferable to nonoperative treatment, although there are lack of conclusive data regarding indications for and benefits of specific surgical interventions.[15] The two most widely used surgical techniques for LCPD are varus osteotomy and the Salter innominate osteotomy.

A facility- or home-based physiotherapy program emphasizing stretching, strengthening, and range of motion can address all three of the above treatment goals. There are only limited published data scientifically evaluating the efficacy of such a program, but it is believed to be beneficial (SOR-C).[16] Relative activity restriction, appropriate for the child's age and degree of disease, may be recommended during the necrosis, resorption, and collapse phases of the cycle (SOR-C).

TRANSIENT SYNOVITIS

Transient synovitis is a self-limited unilateral inflammatory synovitis, typically of the hip joint, which represents the most common cause of hip pain in children aged 3–10 years. Although self-limited and treated symptomatically, it is crucial to differentiate this condition from septic arthritis, which requires treatment with surgical drainage and parenteral antibiotics.[17] Although the incidence of this condition in the United States is unknown, it is frequently referred to as the most common cause of hip pain in children, with boys affected twice as often as girls.[18] The annual incidence in one study of Swedish children was 0.2%.[19]

The etiology of transient synovitis remains unknown. Histologic examination of the synovium reveals nonspecific inflammation. Many children are noted to have had a recent or concurrent respiratory or gastrointestinal viral infection, and many authors believe that transient synovitis may represent a self-limited infection of the synovium or a postinfectious inflammatory response.[20] In one study, increased antibody titers against Epstein–Barr, rubella, enterovirus, or mycoplasma were demonstrated in 67 children out of 80 with transient synovitis, but all synovial viral cultures were negative.[21] Finally, an association between transient synovitis and a positive throat culture for Group A *Streptococcus*, a positive antistreptolysin O titer, or both has been demonstrated.[22]

Diagnosis

Clinically, transient synovitis presents as acute onset hip pain or limp in a well-appearing child. Usually the child is afebrile, or has only a mild temperature elevation. Pain ranges from mild to severe and can be localized to the hip, thigh, or knee. On examination, internal rotation or adduction of the affected hip is limited secondary to pain. Duration of symptoms typically last 1–3 weeks, and prolonged symptoms should suggest a diagnosis other than transient synovitis. The differential diagnosis includes septic arthritis, osteomyelitis, psoas muscle abscess, rheumatic fever, trauma, pauciarticular arthritis, reactive arthritis, malignancy, SCFE, and LCPD.

Laboratory and radiographic studies are done to exclude the aforementioned diagnoses. Radiographs of the hips can be done to exclude SCFE, LCPD, tumor, and osteomyelitis. Ultrasound can be performed to look for the presence of a joint effusion which can be found in as many as 70% of cases. Scintigraphy and computed tomography are less sensitive for the identification of a joint effusion, but may be useful in detecting areas of adjacent osteomyelitis.[23] MRI can be used to differentiate transient synovitis from septic arthritis. Statistically significant MRI findings in transient synovitis include contralateral (asymptomatic) hip effusions and the absence of signal intensity abnormalities of the bone marrow.[24] Ipsilateral effusions and synovial thickening and enhancement are present in both conditions, however.

The white blood cell count (WBC) is usually within normal limits and the erythrocyte sedimentation rate (ESR) may be normal or only slightly elevated. An evidenced-based clinical prediction algorithm was proposed by Kocher *et al.* in 1999 using history of fever, inability to bear weight, complete blood cell count greater than 12,000/mm^3, and ESR greater than 40 mm/h. This study found that if a child with hip pain had all four diagnostic criteria, the probability of septic arthritis was greater than 99% (SOR-B).[25] Conversely, the risk of septic arthritis in the absence of all four criteria was less than 0.2% (Table 7.1). This clinical algorithm was later validated in a subsequent study.[26] In a more recent

TABLE 7.1. Differentiation of septic arthritis from transient synovitis of the hip

Number of positive clinical criteria[a]	Predictive probability of septic arthritis (%)
0	<0.2
1	3.0
2	40
3	93.1
4	99.6

[a]History of fever, non-weight-bearing, ESR>40 mm/h, and WBC>12,000/mm^3
Adapted from Kocher et al. [25]

prospective study of 53 children who underwent hip aspiration for suspected septic arthritis, it was found that fever (oral temperature greater than 38.5) was the best predictor of septic arthritis, followed by an elevated C-reactive protein (CRP), an elevated ESR, refusal to bear weight, and an elevated WBC. A CRP greater than 2.0 mg/dl was found to be a strong independent risk factor and a valuable tool for assessing and diagnosing children suspected of having septic arthritis of the hip (SOR-B).[27]

Treatment
Transient synovitis is a self-limited condition that resolves with rest and supportive therapy. In one study, treatment with ibuprofen was shown to shorten the duration of symptoms (SOR-B).[28] Recurrence of transient synovitis of the hip has been reported to be between 0 and 17% of cases in the literature.[29] The relationship between transient synovitis and LCPD remains speculative. In several series, LCPD or coxa magna followed as many as 30% of cases.[30,31] Some investigators have speculated that the increased intra-articular pressure associated with transient synovitis could potentially lead to the development of LCPD, while others have found no relationship between the two entities other than the similarity in initial clinical presentation.[32] Although most episodes of recurrent transient synovitis have a benign course, some patients with early chronic inflammatory conditions may mimic transient synovitis and further evaluation may be required to rule out these conditions.

SLIPPED CAPITAL FEMORAL EPIPHYSIS

SCFE refers to the posterior and lateral displacement of the proximal femoral epiphysis by mechanical shearing forces with concomitant extension and external rotation of the femoral neck and shaft.[33] This condition represents an orthopedic urgency which requires immediate evaluation and treatment. Although the cause of this disorder remains unknown, it has an increased association with pediatric overweight, puberty, and rapid growth.[34] The preferential site of slippage within the epiphysis appears to be a zone of hypertrophic cartilage cells under the influence of gonadal hormones and growth hormone.[35] SCFE is more likely to occur in older children and adolescents between the ages of 10 and 16 and is more common in males. This condition is bilateral in approximately 20% of patients at the time of presentation and another 20–30% of patients will develop a contralateral SCFE within 12–18 months of the initial slip. Occasionally, this condition is associated with renal failure and endocrinopathies including hypothyroidism and growth hormone deficiency. Therefore, if a child is less than 10 years of age or has a body weight below the 50th percentile presents with a SCFE, evaluation of renal and endocrine function may be warranted.[36]

Classification

Traditionally, the classification of SCFE has been divided into acute, chronic, and acute-on-chronic categories. The differentiation of these three types was temporal; with the symptoms of an acute SCFE lasting less than 3 weeks, a chronic SCFE with symptoms lasting for more than 3 weeks, and a acute-on-chronic SCFE lasting for more than 3 weeks with an exacerbation of symptoms.[37] In many cases, however, this system could be inaccurate because of the inability of parents and children to remember when the onset of symptoms began and because of its poor prediction of prognosis.[38] In 1993, this traditional classification system was abandoned and a new classification system based on stability was adopted in an attempt to impart prognosis.[39] In this new system, a SCFE lesion is classified as stable or unstable. Stability is defined clinically using the ability of the patient to ambulate. A stable SCFE is diagnosed when a child can walk with or without the use of crutches; an unstable SCFE is when the patient cannot walk with or without crutches. The prognosis for a child who has a stable SCFE is very good, with a prevalence of AVN reaching nearly zero.[40] The prognosis of a child with an unstable SCFE is more guarded, however, with the prevalence of AVN ranging from 3 to 84%. Approximately 5% of SCFEs are unstable, and the vast majority of unstable SCFEs are unilateral, with the incidence of bilateral unstable SCFEs being relatively rare (0.25%).[41] The development of AVN in a child with SCFE nearly always results in degenerative hip disease later in life; thus stability imparts prognosis.[42]

Diagnosis

Although SCFE is the most common hip disorder in the adolescent, it is among the most poorly diagnosed of all pediatric orthopedic conditions. It is imperative that this diagnosis be considered in any child aged 10–16 who presents with a limp or pain between the pelvis and tibia.[43] Clinically, the patient may complain of groin, thigh, or knee pain. The referred pain seen in SCFE is secondary to sensory cutaneous nerves that pass close to the hip capsule and innervate the thigh and knee. In fact, in one study, up to 23% of patients who had SCFE presented with a sole complaint of knee pain.[44] A young athlete with a stable SCFE may complain of difficulty with athletic activities and may walk with a limp or an external rotation gait. When there is a complaint of discomfort, it is often vague in nature and is worsened with physical activity. Children with an unstable SCFE present with extreme hip and thigh pain and often have a history of a mild trauma such as tripping on a curb or a fall during a sporting event.

On physical examination, patients with SCFE usually have an asymmetrical outward foot progression angle on the involved side as well as limited internal rotation. In addition, the patient may have obligatory outward rotation of the hip with flexion to allow for clearance of the femoral neck, which would impinge on the anterior acetabulum with flexion in a neutral position. In the case of an unstable SCFE, the patient may lie perfectly still with the hip in a position of flexion, abduction, and external rotation; any attempts to move the hip actively or passively are likely to be met with resistance and significant discomfort. The affected limb may be shortened.

Anteroposterior (AP) radiography of the pelvis is the standard first-line imaging, preferably taken with the patient standing if age and function allow. Radiographs confirm the diagnosis, with the lateral view being most sensitive for detecting early slips with minimal displacement. On the AP view, a line drawn along the superior femoral neck (Klein's line) should intersect some portion of the femoral head (Fig. 7.3). Once the unstable SCFE has been diagnosed on the AP radiograph, a true or cross-table radiograph should be taken. In an unstable SCFE, a frog-leg lateral radiograph should not be attempted because of the significant pain and risk of further iatrogenic slipping that it could potentially cause. At the early preslip stages, other subtle signs on radiographs include asymmetric physeal widening or blurring (the so-called 'blanch sign' of Steel). Alternatively, when SCFE is not evident on standard radiographs, a high-resolution bone scan may demonstrate increased uptake at the superior aspect of the femoral neck and MRI will demonstrate physeal widening on T-1-weighted images. In addition, ultrasound has been shown to reveal an effusion and a step between the epiphyseal and metaphyseal contour.[45]

Treatment

The treatment of unstable SCFE is controversial and the best method for surgical correction is widely debated in the literature. A number of potential risk factors for AVN have been reported, including the use of multiple pins, pin position and penetration, complete or partial reduction, and the stability and severity of the slip. A recent survey of the Pediatric Orthopedic Society of North America found that 57% of responders reported using a single threaded screw for fixation of an unstable SCFE, while 40.3%

7. HIP AND PELVIS INJURIES IN CHILDHOOD AND ADOLESCENCE

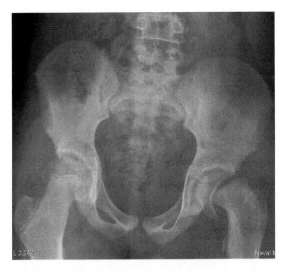

FIGURE 7.3. AP radiograph of the pelvis demonstrating a slipped capital femoral epiphysis (SCFE) on the left (Courtesy of Dr Michael Gibson, National Naval Medical Center).

recommended three threaded screws.[46] The overall goals of surgical treatment are to (1) prevent further slippage until physeal closure, (2) avoid complications, most notably AVN, and (3) maintain adequate hip function. Contralateral radiographs should be obtained in the preoperative period in order to identify an SCFE on the opposite side. Increased physeal stress is placed on the contralateral side after operative treatment of an unstable SCFE, which can lead to progression of the undiagnosed SCFE or transformation of a stable contralateral SCFE to an unstable one.

Prophylactic fixation of the contralateral hip in children who have a unilateral SCFE remains controversial in North America but is more widely accepted in Europe. This option should be strongly considered in children with underlying endocrinopathies and renal failure, as these children have a much higher incidence of bilateral disease (SOR-C). However, if all children with unilateral unstable SCFE underwent prophylactic contralateral fixation, 65–80% of them would have unnecessary surgery, making it difficult to recommend routine prophylactic fixation (SOR-B).[47]

Postoperatively, the child is allowed to get up with crutches once comfortable, and non-weight-bearing is maintained until early evidence of callus formation is seen along the posterior–inferior metaphysis.

Once there is the evidence of bone healing, gradual progression to weight-bearing is allowed (usually between 8 and 12 weeks) and progression to full weight-bearing is usually accomplished by 3–4 months after fixation. Close follow-up is mandatory to observe for the potential development of AVN, which typically occurs within the first 12 months after surgery.

APOPHYSEAL INJURIES OF THE YOUNG ATHLETE

Apophyses are secondary ossification centers that serve as origin and insertion sites of muscles and tendons in the developing skeleton. Whereas muscular strains are common in the adult athlete, apophysitis and apophyseal injuries including avulsion fractures are more common in the athlete who is skeletally immature.[48] This is true because the physis represents the weakest link in the muscle/tendon/bone connection. These conditions usually affect young athletes during the adolescent growth spurt when rapid bone growth exceeds soft tissue development and flexibility. Historically, males are affected up to 9 times more often than females, but now with increased participation of females in athletics at younger ages, this ratio is likely to diminish.[49] While apophysitis is likely caused by repetitive apophyseal microtrauma from activities such as running, apophyseal avulsion fractures usually result from a forceful eccentric muscle contraction that acutely disrupts the apophyseal bony integrity.[50]

Although the true incidence of apophyseal injuries is unknown, 14–40% of pediatric athletes involved in strenuous activity will sustain a pelvic apophyseal avulsion fracture. Ninety percent of these injuries occur in boys between the ages of 14 and 17. One study of 203 acute pelvic apophyseal avulsion fractures in adolescents found that 53% occurred at the ischial tuberosity, 22% at the anterior inferior iliac spine (AIIS), 19% at the anterior superior iliac spine (ASIS), 3% at the superior corner of the pubic symphysis, and 1.5% at the iliac crest.[51] The most commonly involved sports included soccer, gymnastics, fencing, and track and field events.

The ischial tuberosity serves as the site of origin for the medial and lateral hamstrings and is the most common site of apophyseal avulsion injuries in young athletes (Fig. 7.4a).[52] The classic mechanism that has been described is a forceful eccentric hamstring contraction with the hip flexed and the knee extended, as seen in kicking or hurdling.[53] The iliac crest serves as the attachment site for the internal oblique, transversus abdominis, and gluteus medius muscles. Excessive force from arm motion across the trunk while running can cause iliac crest apophysitis. Iliac crest avulsion fractures, however, are uncommon and rarely displace

7. HIP AND PELVIS INJURIES IN CHILDHOOD AND ADOLESCENCE 163

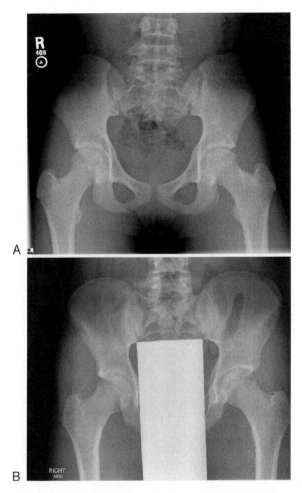

FIGURE 7.4. AP radiographs of the pelvis demonstrating various apophyseal avulsion fractures. (**A**) Right-sided ischial tuberosity avulsion. (**B**) Left-sided iliac crest avulsion. (**C**) Left-sided anterior superior iliac spine (ASIS) avulsion. (**D**) Left-sided lesser trochanter avulsion (Courtesy of Dr Michael Gibson, National Naval Medical Center).

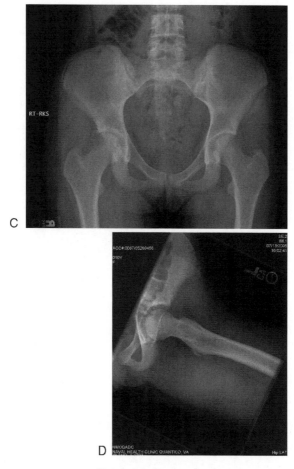

FIGURE 7.4 Continued.

(Fig. 7.4b).[54,55] The ASIS and AIIS serve as attachment sites for the sartorius and biceps femoris muscles, respectively, and can avulse as a result of running and hurdling (Fig. 7.4c).[56] Finally, the iliopsoas muscle inserts on the lesser trochanter, and avulsion injuries have been described in sprinters and jumpers during vigorous hip flexion (Fig. 7.4d). Table 7.2 summarizes characteristics of commonly injured pelvic epiphyses.

TABLE 7.2. Characteristics of common pelvic apophyseal injuries

Apophysis	Age of appearance[52]	Age of fusion[52]	Muscle group	Physical examination[57]	Implicated sports[51,55]
Ischial tuberosity	15–17 years	19–25 years	Hamstrings	Pain with resisted knee flexion or passive hamstring stretch	Gymnastics, soccer, fencing, tennis, track and field
ASIS	13–15 years	21–25 years	Sartorius	Pain with hip flexion/adduction	Soccer, track and field, gymnastics, tennis, fencing, basketball
AIIS	13–15 years	16–18 years	Rectus femoris	Pain with resisted hip flexion with knee extended	Soccer, track and field, tennis, gymnastics, wrestling, fencing
Lesser trochanter	8–12 years	16–18 years	Iliopsoas	Pain with resisted hip flexion with knee flexed	Football, basketball, running
Iliac crest	13–15 years	15–17 years	Gluteus mendius Internal oblique Transversus abdominis	Pain with trunk flexion/rotation/side bend	Soccer, gymnastics, tennis

DIAGNOSIS

Injuries to the pelvic apophyses can be diagnosed by taking a proper history and performing an appropriate physical examination. While apophysitis usually presents as a gradually worsening hip or pelvic pain in an active adolescent athlete, an apophyseal avulsion fracture presents with acute onset of pain, swelling, and a limp. Affected runners may recall a palpable or audible "pop" at the time of injury.[58] The athlete with an apophyseal injury will typically hold his or her pelvis in a position of comfort, minimizing forces placed on the affected muscle and may walk with a limp. Physical examination may reveal tenderness to palpation, swelling, and ecchymosis over the affected apophysis. Resistance testing will exacerbate the patient's pain, and the range of motion is typically limited.[59] Rarely, an avulsion fragment may be palpated.

An AP radiograph of the pelvis should be the first imaging study ordered for patients with a suspected apophyseal avulsion. These avulsion injuries may not be radiographically evident on plain films if the apophysis has not ossified, and additional imaging may be needed for confirmation. Although MRI can reveal these injuries, sonography is advantageous because of its faster examination time and decreased cost.[60] When evaluating for apophyseal injuries with ultrasound, four criteria can be used for diagnosis: (1) a hypoechoic zone in the region of the apophysis representing edema or hemorrhage, (2) widening of the normally hypoechogenic physis, (3) tilting and dislocation of the physis, and (4) hyperemia on Doppler.[61] Finally, if avulsion fracture is clinically suspected and not apparent on radiographs or ultrasound, MRI can be used to confirm this diagnosis.[62] With mild or partial avulsions, elevated signal levels at the muscular origin may be seen on fluid-sensitive sequences. With complete avulsion, fluid signal is found to separate the muscle from the underlying bone, and myotendinous retraction may be identified.[63]

Apophysitis or chronic avulsive injuries may present as areas of bony rarefaction (moth-eaten appearance) or bony lysis on radiographs. Such destructive bony patterns, especially in the absence of obvious pelvic injury, must be differentiated from conditions such as osteomyelitis or Ewing's sarcoma.[64] Finally, nearly one-third of patients in one series of pelvic avulsive injuries had evidence of more than one avulsive site.[65]

Treatment

All cases of apophysitis and the vast majority of pelvic apophyseal avulsion fractures can be treated without surgical intervention. Metzmaker and Pappas have described a five-step rehabilitation program for apophyseal avulsion injuries (SOR-C). The goal of the first step is to rest the injury by relieving the tension on the injured muscle. Bed rest or the use of crutch ambulation with the hips and knees in a position of flexion (in the case of sartorius, rectus, and iliopsoas avulsions) may be necessary to achieve adequate rest, along with ice and anti-inflammatory medications. In the second stage of rehabilitation, which begins once the acute pain has subsided, range of motion exercises are started followed by a progressive strengthening regimen. Limited return to sports can be started once 50% of the anticipated strength has returned. Once the full range of motion and strength has returned, patients may resume their sport without limitations.[66] The risk of re-injury is high if the athlete returns to play before full healing has taken place. Return to sports can usually be anticipated in 4–12 weeks. Rarely, significant displacement of the avulsion fragment can lead to fibrous union and chronic pain and disability; in these instances, surgical excision should be considered (SOR-C).[57] The one exception to conservative management for avulsion fractures may be hamstring avulsions from the ischial tuberosity that are displaced more than 2 cm (SOR-C). In these cases, fibrous nonunion may occur and cause prolonged disability.

References

1. Murray T, Cooperman D, Thompson G, Ballock R. Closed reduction for treatment of developmental dysplasia of the hip in children. Am J Orthop 2007; 36: 82–4.
2. Storer S, Skaggs D. Developmental dysplasia of the hip. Am Fam Physician 2006; 74: 1310–1316.
3. Kamath S, Mehdi A, Wilson N, Duncan R. The lack of evidence of effect of selective ultrasound screening on the incidence of late developmental dysplasia of the hip in the Greater Glasgow Region. J Pediatr Orthop B 2007; 16: 189–191.
4. Desprechins B, Ernst C, De Mey J. Screening for developmental dysplasia of the hip. JBR-BTR. 2007; 90(1):4–5.
5. Lipton GE, Guille JT, Altiok H, et al. A reappraisal of the Ortolani examination in children with developmental dysplasia of the hip. J Pediatr Orthop 2007; 27(1):27–31.
6. Lee M, Eberson C. Growth and development of the child's hip. Orthop Clin N Am 2006; 37: 119–132.
7. Kocher M, Tucker R. Pediatric athlete hip disorders. Clin Sports Med 2006; 25: 241–253.
8. Mehta J, Conybeare M, Hinves B, Winter J. Protein C levels in patients with Legg-Calve-Perthes disease: is it is true deficiency? J Pediatr Orthop 2006; 26(2):200–203.
9. Pearson R, Berkowitz C, Ho S, Heinzman D. Legg-Calve-Perthes Disease. First Consult. MDConsult.com. Last updated April 18, 2007.

10. Canale, S. Osteochondrosis or epiphysitis and other miscellaneous affections. In: Canale S, ed. Campbell's Operative Orthopedics. Philadelphia: Mosby; 2003: 1488–1490.
11. Frick S. Evaluation of the child who has hip pain. Orthop Clin N Am 2006; 37: 133–140.
12. Hubbard A. Imaging pediatric hip disorders. Rad Clin N Am 2001; 39: 721–735.
13. Millis M, Kocher M. Hip, Pelvis, Femur: Pediatric Aspects. In: Koval K, ed. Orthopaedic Knowledge Update 7. Chicago: American Academy of Orthopedic Surgeons; 2002: 387–394.
14. Lee S, Vaidya S, Song H, et al. Bone Age Delay Patters in Legg-Calve-Perthes Disease: an Analysis using the Tanner and Whitehouse 3 Method. J Pediatr Orthop 2007; 27: 198–203.
15. Kim W, Hiroshima K, Imaged T. Multicenter Study for Legg-Calve-Perthes Disease in Japan. J Orthop Sci 2006; 11: 333–341.
16. Brech G, Guarnieiro R. Evaluation of physiotherapy in the treatment of Legg-Calve-Perthes Disease. Clinics 2006; 61: 521–528.
17. Haueisen D, Weiner D, Weiner S. The characterization of "transient synovitis of the hip" in children. J Pediatr Orthop 1986; 6: 11–17.
18. Illingworth C. The limping children with no fracture, sprain, or obvious cause. Clin Pediatr 1978; 17: 139.
19. Landin L, Danielsson L, Wattsgard C. Transient synovitis of the hip: its incidence, epidemiology, and relation to Perthes' disease. J Bone Joint Surg (Br) 1987; 69: 238.
20. Gutierrez K. Transient synovitis. In: Long S, ed. Long: Principles and Practice of Pediatric Infectious Diseases, 2nd ed. Philadelphia: Churchill Livingstone; 2003: 484–485.
21. Tolat V, Carty H, Klenerman L, Hart C. Evidence for a viral etiology of transient synovitis of the hip. Clin Pediatr 1993; 75: 973.
22. Bickerstaff D, Neal L, Brennan P, Bell M. An investigation into the etiology of irritable hip. Clin Pediatr 1991; 30: 353.
23. Kothari N, Pelchovitz D, Meyer J. Imaging of musculoskeletal infections. Radiol Clin North Am 2001; 39: 653–671.
24. Yang W, Im S, Lim G, et al. MR imaging of transient synovitis: differentiation from septic arthritis. Pediatr Radiol 2006; 36: 1154–1158.
25. Kocher M, Zurakowski D, Kasser J. Differentiating between septic arthritis and transient synovitis of the hip in children: an evidenced-based clinical prediction algorithm. J Bone Joint Surg 1999; 81: 1662–1670.
26. Kocher M, Zurakowski D, Kasser J. Validations of a clinical prediction rule for the differentiation between septic arthritis and transient synovitis of the hip in children. J Bone Joint Surg 2004; 86: 1629–1635.
27. Caird M, Flynn J, Leung L, et al. Factors distinguishing septic arthritis from transient arthritis of the hip in children: a prospective study. J Bone Joint Surg 2006; 88: 1251–1257.
28. Kermond S, Fink M, Kerr G, et al. A randomized clinical trial: Should the child with transient synovitis of the hip be treated with nonsteroidal anti-inflammatory drugs? Ann Emerg Med 2002; 3:294–299.

29. Uziel Y, Butbul-Aviel Y, Barash J, et al. Recurrent transient synovitis of the hip in childhood. Longterm outcome among 39 patients. J Rheumatol 2006; 33:810–811.
30. Kallio P. Cox magna following transient synovitis of the hip. Clin Orthop Relat Res 1988; 228: 49–56.
31. Kallio P, Ryoppy S, Kunnamo I. Transient synovitis and Perthes' disease. Is there an etiology connection? J Bone Joint Surg 1986; 68: 808–811.
32. Sharwood P. The irritable hip syndrome in children: Long term follow up. Acta Orthop Scand 1981; 52: 633–638.
33. Kocher M, Tucker R. Pediatric athlete hip disorders. Clin Sports Med 2006; 25: 241–253.
34. Hassink, S. Problems in childhood obesity. Prim Care 2003; 30: 357–374.
35. Kempers M, Noordam C, Rouwe C, Otten B. Can GnRH-agonist treatment cause slipped capital femoral epiphysis? J Pediatr Endocrnol Metab 2001; 14: 729–734.
36. Loder R, Greenfield M. Clinical characteristics of children with atypical and idiopathic slipped capital femoral epiphysis: description of the age-weight test and implications for further diagnostic evaluation. J Pediatr Orthop 2001; 21:481–487.
37. Asdalen R, Weiner D, Hoyt W. Acute slipped capital femoral epiphysis. J Bone Joint Surg 1974; 56A: 473–487.
38. Loder R. Controversies in slipped capital femoral epiphysis. Orthop Clin N Am 2006; 37: 211–221.
39. Loder R, Richards B, Shapiro P. Acute slipped capital femoral epiphysis: the importance of physeal stability. J Bone Joint Surg 1993; 75A: 1134–1140.
40. Rattey T, Piehl F, Wright J. Acute slipped capital femoral epiphysis. Review of outcomes and rates of avascular necrosis. J Bone Joint Surg (AM) 1996; 78(A): 398–402.
41. Peterson M, Weiner D, Green N. Acute slipped capital femoral epiphysis: the value and safety of urgent manipulative reduction. J Pediatr Orthop 1997; 17: 648–654.
42. Krahn T, Canale S, Beaty J. Long term follow up of patients with avascular necrosis after treatment of slipped capital femoral epiphysis. J Pediatr Orthop 1993; 13: 154–158.
43. Millis M, Kocher M. Hip and pelvic injuries in the young athlete. In: DeLee J, Drez D, eds. DeLee and Drez's Orthopaedic Sports Medicine: Principles and Practice. Philadelphia: Saunders; 2003: 1466–1468.
44. Matava J, Patton C, Luhmann S. Knee pain as the initial symptom of slipped capital femoral epiphysis: an analysis of initial presentation and treatment. J Pediatr Orthop 1999; 19: 455–460.
45. Bellah R. Ultrasound in pediatric musculoskeletal disease techniques and applications. Rad Clin North Am 2001; 39: 597–61.
46. Millis M, Kocher M. Hip, pelvis, femur: pediatric aspects. In: Koval K, ed. Orthopedic Knowledge Update 7. Chicago: American Academy of Orthopedic Surgeons; 2002: 387–394.

47. Castro F, Bennett J, Doulens K. Epidemiological perspective on prophylactic pinning in patients with unilateral slipped capital femoral epiphysis. J Pediatr Orthop 2000; 20: 745–748.
48. Morelli V, Weaver V. Groin injuries and groin pain in athletes: Part 1. Prim Care 2005; 32: 163–183.
49. Paluska S. An overview of hip injuries in running. Sports Med 2005; 35: 991–1014.
50. Boyd K, Peirce N, Batt M. Common hip injuries in sport. Sports Med 2001; 24: 273–288.
51. Rossi F, Dragoni S. Acute avulsion fractures of the pelvis in adolescent competitive athletes: prevalence, location, and sports distribution of 203 cases. Skeletal Radiol 2001; 30: 127–131.
52. Paletta G, Andrish J. Injuries about the hip and pelvis in the young athlete. Clin Sports Med 1995; 14: 591–628.
53. Scopp J, Moorman C. The assessment of athletic hip injury. Clin Sports Med 2001; 20: 647–659.
54. Aksoy B, Ozturk K, Ensenyel C. Avulsion of the iliac crest apophysis. Clin Sports Med 1998; 19: 76–78.
55. Metzmaker J, Pappas A. Avulsion fractures of the pelvis. Am J Sports Med 1985; 13: 349–358.
56. Bencardino J, Palmer W. Imaging of hip disorders in athletes. Radiol Clin North Am 2002; 40: 267–287.
57. Anderson S. Sports injuries. Dis Mon 2005; 51: 438–442.
58. Browning K, Donley B. Evaluation and management of common running injuries. Clev Clin J Med 2000; 67: 511–520.
59. Anderson K, Strickland S, Warren R. Hip and groin injuries in athletes. Am J Sports Med 2001; 29: 521–533.
60. Blankenbaker D, De Smet A. The role of ultrasound in the evaluation of sports injuries of the lower extremities. Clin Sports Med 2006; 25: 867–897.
61. Pisacano R, Miller T. Comparing sonography with MR imaging of apophyseal injuries of the pelvis in four boys. Am J Roentgenol 2003; 181: 223–230.
62. Armfield D, Hyun-Min Kim D, Towers J, et al. Sports related muscle injury in the lower extremity. Clin Sports Med 2006; 25: 803–842.
63. Newmann J, Newberg A. MRI of the painful hip in athletes. Clin Sports Med 2006; 25: 613–633.
64. El-Khoury G, Daniel W, Kathol M. Acute and chronic avulsive injuries. Radiol Clin N Am 1997; 35: 747–766.
65. Sundar M, Carty H. Avulsion fractures of the pelvis in children: A report of 32 fractures and their outcome. Skeletal Radiol 1994; 23: 85–90.
66. Waters P, Millis M. Hip and pelvis injuries in the young athlete. Clin Sports Med 1988; 7: 513–526.

Chapter 8
Specific Considerations in Geriatric Athletes

Rochelle M. Nolte

KEY POINTS

- Osteoporosis affects more than 10 million people in the United States, with an estimated 1.5 million osteoporotic fractures annually costing approximately $17 billion annually.
- Risk factors for osteoporosis include physical inactivity, low body weight, low dietary intake of calcium and vitamin D, excessive alcohol use, smoking, certain medications or medical conditions, late menarche and early menopause, personal history of low-trauma fractures, family history of osteoporosis or low-trauma fractures, white or Asian race, and female sex.
- Hip fractures lead to death within 1 year in 20% of cases. One-third of patients with hip fracture require nursing home placement, and fewer than one-third regain their prefracture level of physical function.
- Screening and preventive measures are still not regularly being recommended and implemented in primary care despite current clinical knowledge about osteoporosis and hip fractures.
- Exercise programs for geriatric athletes should include lower body weight-bearing, balance, and flexibility in order to maintain or improve function of the hip and pelvis and to prevent falls and hip fractures.

CASE VIGNETTE

MH is a 72-year-old white woman master swimmer who presents to your office 6 weeks following surgery for a hip fracture. She sustained an intertrochanteric hip fracture after falling on a wet tile floor.

She had surgery on that day with the placement of a compression hip screw with side plate. She was out of bed the day after surgery and underwent 6 weeks of outpatient physical therapy without problems or complications and has been released into your care. Following discharge from the hospital, she had an environmental assessment of her home for fall risks, and she has made all the recommended changes. She has not been going out as much as she used to as she is afraid of falling again and the possibility of "ending up in the nursing home." However, she was very active prior to her fall and she would like to start exercising again.

Her history reveals that she is 20 years postmenopausal and has never taken any hormone replacement therapy or other medications or supplements regularly. She has always been healthy and has been a swimmer since she was a young child. She has had two prior fractures: a fractured ankle in her 40s when she stepped off a curb and turned her ankle, and a fractured wrist in her 50s when she tripped on some steps and caught herself with an outstretched hand. She eats what she considers a healthy diet and averages one serving of dairy every day. She has never been a smoker and she has 1–2 glasses of red wine with dinner every night as she has heard it is good for cholesterol. Family history: her mother had severe kyphosis and at the age of 80 suffered a hip fracture and was admitted to a nursing home and died within 1 year. She has two grown children who are healthy.

On physical exam: She is 63 in. tall, but states she has always been 64 in. She weighs 124 pounds with a body-mass index (BMI) of 22. She is fair-skinned with blue eyes and white hair. She has slightly rounded shoulders and a slightly protuberant abdomen. She walks unassisted without a limp, but with a slow gait. She uses her arms to assist her when rising from a chair. Her surgical site is well healed and her hips have adequate range of motion to permit her to get on and off the examination table without difficulty. However, she is very cautious when moving to take off her shoes. The remainder of her physical exam is unremarkable.

AGE-RELATED PHYSIOLOGICAL CHANGES

Bone
Bone is a dynamic tissue that is constantly remodeling itself. In the adult skeleton, there is an equilibrium between bone formation by osteoblasts and bone resorption by osteoclasts. Normally, during childhood bone formation outpaces bone resorption, resulting in increasing bone density until approximately age 18

when 90% of bone mass is achieved. Over the next decade, the rate of bone deposition begins to level off. At the end of this plateau, there begins a period of net bone loss of about 0.3–0.5% per year.[1] Women typically undergo an accelerated phase of bone loss that starts up to 2–3 years prior to cessation of menses and continues for up to 7 years.[1,2] During this time, women typically lose bone at the rate of about 3–5% per year.[1]

This gradual loss of bone can lead to osteoporosis, defined as "a skeletal disorder characterized by compromised bone strength predisposing to an increased risk of fracture."[3] Currently, it is estimated that there are 10 million people in the United States with osteoporosis and that there are over 1.5 million osteoporotic fractures annually.[3] The decrease in quantity and quality of bone associated with osteoporosis leads to an increased risk of fracture, especially of the hip and spine. Given the insidious onset, the diagnosis of osteoporosis is frequently overlooked until a fracture has occurred and, in some cases, the diagnosis can be overlooked even after a fracture has taken place. Even with substantial evidence that a prior fracture predicts a subsequent fracture, less than 30% of postmenopausal women and less than 10% of men with prior fracture are treated.[4]

There are many known risk factors for osteoporosis. Intrinsic risk factors include being female, advanced age, low peak bone mass, low body weight, white or Asian race, past history of low-trauma fracture, family history of low-trauma fracture or osteoporosis, and low levels of circulating estrogens.[2,3,5] Extrinsic factors include cigarette smoking, excessive alcohol intake, low levels of calcium intake, low levels of vitamin D intake, and physical inactivity.[2,3,5] Age is one of the most important risk factors for women and is one of the criteria used to determine who should be screened by further imaging. Compared to women aged 50–54, women aged 65–69 had a 5.9-fold higher chance of having osteoporosis and women aged 75–79 had a 14.3-fold higher chance of having osteoporosis.[6]

In addition to the above risk factors, some medications are associated with reduced bone mass in adults as listed in Table 8.1. Some underlying medical conditions such as gastrointestinal diseases (e.g., malabsorption syndromes and inflammatory bowel disease), hematologic disorders (e.g., thalassemia and pernicious anemia), and hypogonadal states can also contribute to osteoporosis.[3]

One example of a screening questionnaire that can be used to assess risk and as an instrument to facilitate discussion with women about osteoporosis is the FRACTURE Index shown in Table 8.2.

TABLE 8.1. Drugs that may lead to decreased bone mass

- Aluminum
- Anticonvulsants (phenobarbital, phenytoin, valproate)
- Cytotoxic drugs
- Ethanol (excess use)
- Glucocorticoids
- Gonadotropin-releasing hormone agonists
- Heparin (long-term use)
- Immunosuppressants
- Lithium
- Progesterone (parenteral, long-acting)
- Thyroxine (supraphysiologic doses)
- Tamoxifen (premenopausal use)

TABLE 8.2. Fracture index questions and scoring

	Point value
1. What is your current age?	
Less than 65	0
65–69	1
70–74	2
75–79	3
80–84	4
85 or older	5
2. Have you broken any bones after age 50?	
Yes	1
No/don't know	0
3. Has your mother had a hip fracture after age 50?	
Yes	1
No/don't know	0
4. Do you weigh 125 pounds or less?	
Yes	1
No	0
5. Are you currently a smoker?	
Yes	1
No	0
6. Do you usually need to use your arms to assist yourself in standing up from a chair?	
Yes	2
No/don't know	0
If you have a current bone density (BMD) assessment, then answer next question.	
7. BMD results: Total hip T-score:	
T-score > −1	0
T-score between −1 and −2	2
T-score between −2 and −2.5	3
T-score < −2.5	4

Continued

TABLE 8.2. *Continued*

Without BMD, using a score of 4 as a cutpoint results in a sensitivity of 66.0% and specificity of 66.3% with a positive predictive value of 5.6 for hip fracture in the next 5 years. With BMD, using a score of 6 as a cutpoint results in a sensitivity of 78.6% and specificity of 61.7% with a positive predictive value of 5.8. Using a higher cutpoint in either model increases the specificity, but is accompanied by a sharp decline in sensitivity. The reverse is true if a lower cutpoint is used.
Source: Black et al.[7]

This questionnaire was developed by the Study of Osteoporotic Fracture Research Group on the basis of the major established risk factors for osteoporosis.[7] The FRACTURE Index was developed by a prospective study of healthy white women over the age of 65 in the United States. The index was designed to be used either with or without knowing the patient's bone mineral density (BMD). While the BMD slightly increases the sensitivity of the index, even without the BMD the index is strongly predictive of the risk of hip fracture in the next 5 years.[7] (SOR-A)

OSTEOPOROSIS EVALUATION

A thorough history is the most important part of the evaluation for osteoporosis. Review of the previously mentioned risk factors and possibly using one of the available risk assessment tools such as the FRACTURE Index mentioned above will be helpful in identifying at risk patients.

A physical exam, looking for risk factors for falling, such as decreased mobility or strength (e.g., unable to rise from a chair without using hands), decreased proprioception, decreased visual acuity, signs of osteoporosis (i.e., evidence of vertebral compression fractures with loss of height, kyphosis, and overly protuberant abdomen) should be done. The physical exam should also rule out signs of other possible causes of metabolic disease (i.e., cushingoid features, goiter, jaundice, etc).

The information gathered from the history and physical will help identify patients for whom further diagnostic imaging is indicated.

The United States Preventative Services Task Force (USPSTF) recommends BMD testing for all women aged 65 or older and for younger postmenopausal women who have one or more risk factors for osteoporosis.[6] (SOR-B) Dual energy X-ray absorptiometry (DEXA) is currently considered the gold standard for measuring BMD.[1,3] The radiation level associated with DEXA is low and the precision is high compared to other currently available techniques for measuring BMD.[8] The areal unit of measurement is grams per square centimeter (g/cm^2), although it is usually reported as a T-score, which is a standard deviation without units of measurement. The World Health Organization (WHO) has defined osteoporosis on the basis of BMD of the proximal femur as measured by DEXA.[7] BMD that is greater than 2.5 standard deviations below the mean for a young, white, healthy female is defined as osteoporosis. BMD 1.0–2.5 standard deviations below the mean is defined as osteopenia. The T-score has been applied to define diagnostic thresholds at other skeletal sites and for different technologies. However, difficulties with standardization and accuracy of measurement with the different technologies have given rise to some controversy about the diagnostic criterion of osteoporosis.[8] In addition, the original T-score was developed for use in postmenopausal white women, and how well it applies to men, younger women, and people of different ethnic backgrounds is not completely clear.[8]

DEXA measurement of the hip is the gold standard for predicting the future risk of hip fracture. Other methods used to measure BMD include quantitative computed tomography (QCT), quantitative ultrasound (QUS), and peripheral DEXA.[1,8] However, DEXA of the hip is the best predictor of future hip fracture and peripheral DEXA has not been shown to be predictive of hip fracture.[5,8]

Once the diagnosis of osteoporosis has been made, there are a number of pharmacological and nonpharmacological treatments available. Some of the treatments are also used for the prevention of osteoporosis in high-risk individuals. Some of the nonpharmacological interventions for treatment and prevention of osteoporosis are listed in Table 8.3.

TABLE 8.3. Nonpharmacologic interventions that may help prevent osteoporosis-related fractures

- Diet with adequate calories, protein, and nutrients
- Weight-bearing exercise
- Strength-training exercise
- Balance-training exercise
- Tobacco cessation
- Reducing excessive alcohol intake
- Vision correction
- Assessment of any medical conditions that may decrease bone density or increase the risk for falls
- Assessment of any medications that may decrease bone density or increase the risk for falls
- Elimination of tripping hazards in the home, work, and social environments

Pharmacological treatments used to prevent and treat osteoporosis include antiresorptive drugs such as the bisphosphonates (alendronate, risedronate, ibandronate), calcitonin, estrogen, and selective estrogen receptor modulators (SERMs), such as raloxifene. The bisphosphonates reduce bone turnover and subsequently prevent bone loss. Calcitonin inhibits osteoclasts, and previous studies have shown a decrease in the incidence of vertebral fractures as well as an analgesic effect when administered after acute vertebral fractures,[1,2] but there is no significant information on the effect of calcitonin on early menopausal BMD. Estrogen also inhibits bone resorption, increases total hip BMD, and reduces the risk of fracture at the hip, spine, and wrist, but data from the Women's Health Initiative led to the discontinuation of the estrogen plus progestin arm of the trial in 2002 secondary to an increased risk of breast cancer and cardiovascular outcomes over controls. The estrogen-alone trial was stopped in 2004 because of an increased risk of stroke.[2] Raloxifene is able to exert estrogen-like effects on the skeleton, although not as effectively as estrogen or the bisphosphonates.[2] Calcium and vitamin D supplementation is also important therapy and can be prescribed for prevention of osteoporosis, and should be prescribed for any patients taking bisphosphonates for prevention or treatment of osteoporosis.

The fundamental goal of managing patients at high risk for osteoporosis is to prevent fractures and loss of function, and also to prevent or decrease pain.[1] While there is evidence of increased bone density and decreased risk of fracture with pharmacologic intervention, there are still remaining questions about the effectiveness of interventions in asymptomatic populations.[2,9]

While there is general consensus that women over the age of 65 should have a BMD test, for women under age 65, BMD testing is generally reserved for those considered to be "at risk" for osteoporosis.[2,9] What defines "at risk" is not universally agreed upon, and any data on using medications to prevent bone loss in perimenopausal women with normal BMD are extremely limited. Also, the risk factors, testing, and treatment of osteoporosis in populations other than postmenopausal white women need to be further investigated.

MUSCLE

It is well established that muscular strength declines with age.[10] A gradual decline in muscle mass and strength begins in the fourth decade of life. In fact, between the ages of 30 and 80, the percentage of body weight composed of muscle mass may decline by 30–40%.[11,12] Muscle tissue comprises 40–45% of total body tissue.

Muscle synthesis and maintenance account for 20% of daily resting energy expenditure. Of total body protein turnover, 25% occurs in muscle.[13] Sarcopenia is characterized by muscle loss, muscle weakness, and increased fatigability, but the exact mechanism of disease is yet to be estabilished.[13] There are very little epidemiological data about the relationship between sarcopenia and various adverse outcomes.

It has been recommended that sarcopenia be defined as "lean body mass more than two standard deviations below the young normal mean."[14] Using this definition, the New Mexico Elder Health Survey estimated the prevalence of sarcopenia at 22% in white men and 31% in white women aged 60 years or older.[14] This study found that sarcopenia was associated with a fourfold increase in the risk of disability in at least three of the instrumental activities of daily living (ADL), a 2–3-fold increase in the risk of having a balance disorder, some increase in the risk of a gait abnormality, and about a twofold greater likelihood of having to use a cane or walker.[14] Similar data were found with an elderly population in Rochester, MN, with an incidence of sarcopenia of 25% in men and 52% in women.[14]

In a study of pre and postmenopausal women, there was a correlation between osteopenia or osteoporosis and sarcopenia. In premenopausal women, it was found that there was a 12.5% prevalence of sarcopenia in the osteopenic population and a prevalence of 0.8% in the population with normal BMD.[15] In postmenopausal women, the prevalence of sarcopenia was 16.1% in those with normal BMD, 25% in those with osteopenia, and 50% in those with osteoporosis.[15]

While the best method to prevent and treat sarcopenia is yet to be established, physical activity and resistance exercise stimulate muscle protein synthesis. Current evidence supports resistance exercise to prevent sarcopenia and to increase muscle strength in those with sarcopenia.[11,13] (SOR-C)

CARTILAGE, LIGAMENTS, AND TENDONS

Aging leads to a decrease in the quantity and quality of synovial fluid and a decrease in cartilage proteoglycan content.[16] This leads to decreased water content and elasticity of the cartilage in weight-bearing joints, including the hip.[16,17]

Elasticity of the connective tissue of ligaments and tendons declines with age most likely secondary to changes in collagen, elastin, and water content. This can lead to aging collagen being more subject to overload failure as well as leading to increased stress and force across the joint because of decreased flexibility and decreased range of motion.[16,17] Tendon diameter decreases with age and the tendons become stiffer with a lower failure threshold compared to younger individuals.[16]

BALANCE

Balance can be defined as the ability of an individual to maintain his or her center of gravity within specific boundries.[18] Balance may be either static or dynamic.[18,19] The visual, vestibular, and proprioceptive systems are all important in maintaining balance, and all can suffer degenerative changes with aging. One of the most serious outcomes of poor balance in the elderly is falls.

The accumulative exposure of degenerative, infective, and injurious processes to the sensory, motor, and adaptive systems, combined with slowed protective reflexes, leads to a decreased ability to withstand unexpected perturbations with advancing age.[18–20]

At least 18% of the community-dwelling population over the age of 70 has substantial visual impairment from conditions such as cataracts, glaucoma, or macular degeneration.[20] Three case–control studies demonstrated a significant increase in falls and hip fractures among both men and women with impaired vision.[20]

Aging has a significant effect on the vestibular system, with an estimated neuronal loss of 3% per decade after age 40.[18]

Age-associated changes in postural control, muscle strength, and step height can impair a person's ability to avoid a fall after an unexpected trip or while reaching or bending. These changes can be due to arthritis or decreased range of motion secondary to loss of elasticity in muscle, tendon, or ligaments.

The most common causes of falls in older person are listed in Table 8.4. The most common risk factors for falls are listed in Table 8.5.

About one out of three community-dwelling people over the age of 65 sustain a fall each year.[20] About 1% of those who fall sustain a hip fracture, which carries a 1-year mortality rate of 20–30%.[20] Among community-dwelling people who fall and sustain a hip fracture, between 25% and 75% never recover their prefracture level of function.[20]

EXERCISE TO PREVENT INJURY

Weight-Bearing Exercise

A Cochrane review of 18 randomized controlled trials showed that walking is effective in increasing the density of the bone mass in the spine and the hip.[9] Aerobics and weight-bearing and weight-resistance exercises were also found to be effective; however, the

TABLE 8.4. Causes of falls in older persons: summary of 12 large studies

Cause	Mean (%)[a]	Range[b]
Accident and environment related	31	1–53
Gait and balance disorders or weakness	17	4–39
Dizziness and vertigo	13	0–30
Drop attack	9	0–52
Confusion	5	0–14
Postural hypotension	3	0–24
Visual disorder	2	0–5
Syncope	0.3	0–3
Other specified causes[c]	15	2–39
Unknown	5	0–21

[a]Mean percent calculated from the 3,628 reported falls.
[b]Ranges indicate the percentage reported in each of the 12 studies.
[c]This category includes arthritis, acute illness, drugs, alcohol, pain, epilepsy, and falling from bed.
Source: Rubenstein and Josephson[20]

TABLE 8.5. Risk factors for falls: analysis of 16 studies

Risk factor	Mean RR–OR[a]
Lower extremity weakness	4.4
History of falls	3.0
Gait deficit	2.9
Balance deficit	2.9
Use assistive device	2.6
Visual deficit	2.5
Arthritis	2.4
Impaired ADL	2.3
Depression	2.2
Cognitive impairment	1.8
Age >80 years	1.7

[a]Relative risk ratio (RR) calculated for prospective studies. Odds ratio (OR) calculated for retrospective studies.
Source: Rubenstein and Josephson[20]

review gave no specific information about the amount of walking or exercise needed.

Physical activity provides a positive stimulus for bone formation, but only at the sites of the skeleton that are physically stressed. For example, upper body weight training will not increase bone mass at the hip. Also, the physical activity needs to be continued, as bone mass will return to its previous level if activity returns to the previous level. With a complete lack of activity, such as with immobility or bedrest, bone loss occurs.

For bone gain to occur, the stimulus must be greater than what the bone usually experiences, and physical activities that include a variety of loading patterns such as strength training or aerobics classes may promote increased bone mass more than activities that involve normal or regular loading patterns.[5]

Weight training is also an effective way to approach age-related sarcopenia. Many studies have confirmed an increase in muscle strength and muscle mass with weight training, and current evidence provides support for resistance training as a primary intervention to prevent sarcopenia and to arrest its progression in the elderly.[11,13]

Numerous studies involving both men and women over a wide range of ages (40–90) have shown that strength training aids in increasing muscle strength and muscle hypertrophy as well increasing bone strength and reducing injuries.[21]

Flexibility Exercise

Research regarding flexibility exercises in the elderly is limited. It is generally accepted, however, that flexibility training can optimize joint range of motion and musculoskeletal function, and thus reduce injury potential and enhance functional capability.[17]

Balance Exercise

Numerous studies have shown that exercise can improve fall risks such as poor balance, gait impairment, and muscle weakness.[20] Effective exercise programs include Tai Chi, which consists of slow, rhythmic movements that require trunk rotation, dynamic weight shifting, and coordination between upper and lower extremity movements, and other programs that focus on muscle and balance training.[9] Balance training often includes a range of static and dynamic exercises such as standing on one foot, tandem standing, ball games, moving to music, and functional exercises that involve bending, reaching, and transferring weight.[20]

EXERCISE AFTER HIP SURGERY

Senior citizens are the fastest growing segment of the American population, with 35 million people over the age of 65 in 2000.[22] The majority of total hip arthroplasties (THA) done for end-stage osteoarthritis and the majority of open reduction internal fixation (ORIF) surgeries for hip fractures are done in this population.

Hip fractures are one of the most devastating injuries an elderly individual can suffer. While hip fractures in younger patients are usually due to high-impact trauma, hip fractures in the geriatric population usually result from a fall from a standing height.

This level of force is not usually enough to fracture a bone of normal density, but can be enough to cause a fracture in osteoporotic bone, especially if a person's ability to reach out and cushion the fall is compromised by slowed reflexes, arthritis, or any other condition that limits their movement.

Women account for 80% of all hip fractures, and the incidence of hip fractures increases dramatically with age, from 2 fractures per 100,000 among white women under age 35 to over 3,000 per 100,000 among white women 85 years and older.[5]

Hip fractures are repaired surgically in the majority of cases. Either ORIF or THA may be done depending on the exact location and extent of the fracture, the expectation for level of activity after surgery, and any underlying pre-existing pathology of the hip joint. THA is also done for patients with end-stage osteoarthritis and has been shown to greatly improve mobility and quality of life.[22]

Exercise following hip surgery should be encouraged, but should also be done in a safe environment. Supervised physical therapy is appropriate until a patient is able to ambulate and transfer safely either with or without an assistive device. Any rehabilitation or exercise program should address any underlying muscular weakness or limited mobility that the patient may have had prior to the surgery. The exercise program should also include some weight-bearing exercise to prevent continued bone loss from disuse. Exercises that promote balance and proprioception should also be incorporated to decrease the chances for future falls and further injury. Any exercise program should also enhance the psychological well-being of the patient by helping them overcome any possible fear they may have of falling or further injuring their hip. It should also include activities that they enjoy and assist them in returning to their prior level of social functioning.

For the first 6–8 weeks after THA, patients may have to observe precautions to avoid dislocating the hip, but should participate in a physical therapy program to increase their strength and improve their gait to the point that they can ambulate without an assistive device. After the first 6–8 weeks, patients may begin to resume some recreational activities.

There is concern that after THA excessive load-bearing will increase the amount of wear on the joint, increasing the chances of early loosening and failure. This has led most surgeons to conservatively recommend low-impact activities such as swimming, cycling, and walking, and discourage high-impact activities such as football, handball, basketball, soccer, or hockey.[23] However, there are not many prospective randomized studies on athletic activities after THA in the current literature and not much evidence and information available to assist in counseling patients on sporting activities following THA.

There has been some evidence that more active patients were at an increased risk for revision surgery, but any harmful effects of sports participation were not noticed until 10 years postoperatively.[23] It is not recommended that patients try to pick up any new activities after their THA that may be technically difficult to learn, as the incidence of injury goes up with inexperience. However, for patients who are experienced in some activities and would like to do them occasionally for recreation such as dancing or skating, there is no general consensus that these activities must be avoided. However, it is recommended that any exercise that is done several times each week to maintain aerobic fitness be a low-impact activity such as swimming or cycling rather than jogging or high-impact aerobics to avoid excessive wear on the hip joint.[22–24] For a list of the consensus recommendations for activity after THA, see Table 8.6.

TABLE 8.6. Consensus recommendations for activity after total hip arthroplasty (1999 Hip Society Survey)

Recommended/allowed
- Stationary bicycling
- Croquet
- Ballroom dancing
- Golf
- Horseshoes
- Shooting
- Shuffleboard
- Swimming
- Doubles tennis
- Walking

Allowed with experience
- Low-impact aerobics
- Road bicycling
- Bowling
- Canoeing
- Hiking
- Horseback riding
- Cross-country skiing

Not recommended
- High-impact aerobics
- Baseball/softball
- Basketball
- Football
- Gymnastics
- Handball

Continued

TABLE 8.6. *Continued*

- Hockey
- Jogging
- Lacrosse
- Racquetball
- Squash
- Rock climbing
- Soccer
- Singles tennis
- Volleyball

No conclusion

- Jazz dancing
- Square dancing
- Fencing
- Ice skating
- Roller/inline skating
- Rowing
- Speed walking
- Downhill skiing
- Stationary skiing
- Weight lifting
- Weight machines

Source: Kuster[23]

CASE FOLLOW-UP

MH has suffered a low-trauma hip fracture secondary to underlying osteoporosis. Her history has significant risk factors such as her family history of her mother sustaining a hip fracture, and her personal history of two prior low-trauma fractures. Her alcohol use is relatively high and may put her at further risk as does her lack of use of any osteoporosis prevention medications or supplements. Her loss of height with kyphosis on physical exam is probably secondary to asymptomatic vertebral compression fractures she has already sustained. She also has other risk factors evident on her physical exam such as her low BMI and her relative muscle weakness (needing to use her hands to rise from a chair).

The initial appointment is spent answering her questions about osteoporosis, addressing her fears about the possibility of another hip fracture, discussing measures to prevent falls, and recommending testing and treatment.

She does not like to take pills, but is agreeable to an over-the-counter chewable calcium supplement with vitamin D and is willing to take an oral bisphosphonate she has heard about that only has to be taken once each month. She is also agreeable to decreasing her wine to only one glass with dinner on the weekends.

She will schedule her baseline DEXA scan to be completed before her next appointment with you.

She wants to resume swimming at this time and she is encouraged to do so. Given her underlying osteoporosis and relative muscle weakness, adding more weight-bearing activity such as walking is also recommended. She states she is hesitant to start a walking program as she is nervous about falling again, but she is willing participate in a resistance exercise program and take Tai Chi classes at the local community center in order to build her strength and stability. She will follow up in 1 month to review the results of her DEXA scan and for a functional assessment of her gait, core stability, balance, proprioception, and vision. She will also be assessed to see if her fear of falling has resolved enough to permit her to start a walking program and to resume her previous level of social function.

References

1. Simon LS. Osteoporosis. Clin GeriatrMed 2005; 21: 603–629.
2. Delaney MF. Strategies for the prevention and treatment of osteoporosis during early postmenopause. Am J Obstet Gynecol 2006; 194: S12–S23.
3. Lane NE; Epidemiology, etiology, and diagnosis of osteoporosis. Am J Obstet Gynecol 2006; 194: S3–S11.
4. Center JR, Bliuc D, Nguyen TV, Eisman JA. Risk of Subsequent Fracture After Low-Trauma Fracture in Men and Women" JAMA 2007; 297: 387–394.
5. United States Department of Health and Human Services. Bone Health and Osteoporosis: A Report of the Surgeon General. Rockville, MD: US Department of Health and Human Services, Office of the Surgeon General; 2004.
6. United States Preventive Services Task Force. Recommendations and Rationale: Screening for Osteoporosis in Postmenopausal Women. Ann Intern Med 2002; 137: 526–528.
7. Black DM, Steinbuch M, Palermo L, et al. An Assessment Tool for Predicting Fracture Risk in Postmenopausal Women. Osteoporos Int 2001; 12: 519–528.
8. Link TM, Majumdar S. Osteoporosis Imaging. Radiol Clin North Am 2003; 41: 813–839.
9. Johnell O, Hertzman P. What evidence is there for the prevention and screening of osteoporosis? WHO Regional Office for Europe (Health Evidence Network report). 2006. At: http://www.euro.who.int/document/e88668.pdf. Accessed 5 December 2008.
10. Bemben MG. Age-Related Alterations in Muscular Endurance. Sports Med 1998. 25 (4): 259–269.
11. Nair KS. Aging muscle. Am J Clin Nutr 2005; 81: 953–963.
12. Epperly TD, Newman S. The older athlete. In: Birrer RB, O'Connor FG, eds. Sports Medicine for the Primary Care Physician, 3rd ed. Boca Raton, FL: CRC Press; 2004.

13. Nair KS. Age-Related Changes in Muscle. Mayo Clin Proc 2000; 75: S14–S218.
14. Melton LJ, Khosla S, Riggs BL. Epidemiology of Sarcopenia. Mayo Clin Proc 2000; 75: S10–S13.
15. Walsh MC, Hunter GR, Livingstone MB. Sarcopenia in premenopausal and postmenopausal women with osteopenia, osteoporosis, and normal bone mineral density. Osteoporos Int 2006; 17: 61–67.
16. Singh H. Senescent Changes in the Human Musculoskeletal System. In: Speer KP, ed. Injury Prevention and Rehabilitation for Active Older Adults. Champaign, IL: Human Kinetics; 2005:3–17.
17. Micheo W, Soto-Quijano DA, Rivera-Tavares C, et al. The geriatric runner. In: O'Connor FG, Wilder RP. Textbook of Running Medicine. New York: McGraw-Hill; 2001.
18. Matsumura BA, Ambrose AF. Balance in the Elderly. Clin Geriatric Med 2006; 22: 395–412.
19. Allum JH, Carpenter MG, Honegger F, et al. Age-dependent variations in the directional sensitivity of balance corrections and compensatory arm movements in man. J Physiol 2002; 524: 642–663.
20. Rubenstein LZ, Josephson KR. Falls and Their Prevention in Elderly People: What Does the Evidence Show? Med Clin North Am 2006; 90: 807–824.
21. Escamilla RF. Exercise Testing and Prescription. In: Speer KP, ed. Injury Prevention and Rehabilitation for Active Older Adults. Human Kinetics: Champaign, IL: 2005: 19–48.
22. St Clair SF, Higuera C, Krebs V, et al. Hip and Knee Arthroplasty in the Geriatric Population. Clin Geriatric Med 2006; 22: 515–533.
23. Kuster MS. Exercise Recommendations After Total Joint Replacement: A Review of the Current Literature and Proposal of Scientifically Based Guidelines. Sports Med 2002; 32 (7): 433–445.
24. Chatterji U, Ashworth MJ, Lewis PL, Dobson PJ. Effect of Total Hip Arthroplasty on Recreational and Sporting Activity. ANZ J Surg 2004; 74: 446–449.

Chapter 9
Hip and Pelvis Injuries in Special Populations

Dorianne R. Feldman, Marlís González-Fernández, Aarti A. Singla, Brian J. Krabak, and Sandeep Singh

CLINICAL PEARLS

- Heterotopic ossification is a common complication in disabled populations that can significantly affect hip range of motion, cause pain, and limit functional mobility.
- The most common musculoskeletal injuries among amputee athletes are sprains and strains to the lumbar spine and sacroiliac joint on the uninvolved side.
- Athletes with cerebral palsy typically experience lower extremity injuries that involve the patellofemoral joint which are due to muscle spasms of the surrounding muscles.
- Wheelchair athletes are at a greater risk of long bone fractures due to osteoporosis.
- Disabled athletes require sport- and disability-specific equipment to minimize injury.

CASE STUDY

FM is a 33-year-old South Asian male with a history of a traumatic C5–6 complete spinal cord injury (SCI) who presents with right hip pain and swelling. At the age of 19, FM sustained a C5 posterior vertebral fracture.

For the last 10 years, he has been actively involved in wheelchair athletics such as swimming, skiing, rugby, and wheelchair racing. The patient has complained of right hip pain and mild swelling for approximately 3 years. He then began noticing increased difficulty with hip flexion. The pain worsened and limited hip range of motion, interfering with transfers, bed mobility, and wheelchair positioning. He began requiring more assistance with all functional mobility skills and activities of daily living, significantly affecting his quality of life and prompting him to seek medical care.

FM complained of pain in the anterior–lateral region of the right hip. Musculoskeletal examination was consistent with C6 quadriplegia. Both lower extremities were insensate and atonic. There was significant atrophy throughout the trunk and bilateral lower extremities. Right hip examination demonstrated warmth to palpation. There was no erythema. Passive range of motion was significantly limited in external rotation, internal rotation, and flexion. Radiographs of the right hip revealed extrinsic bone formation lateral to the subcapital femoral region, most evident on anterior–posterior view (Fig. 9.1).

The differential diagnosis for right hip pain is extensive in both able-bodied and disabled athletes. In the absence of obvious trauma, the differential diagnosis is narrower and includes conditions such as osteoporotic fractures, osteoarthritis, septic arthritis, heterotopic ossification, and hip dislocation. In this case, the most likely is heterotopic ossification. Heterotopic ossification is common in SCI, particularly in athletes. Radiography was diagnostic, demonstrating abnormal periarticular bone deposition. Ectopic bone formation is responsible for the limitations in range of motion and pain. In this chapter, we focus our discussion on the most common causes of hip and pelvis dysfunction in the disabled athlete population.

INTRODUCTION

For centuries, able-bodied individuals have engaged in athletic competitions. However, it has only been since the middle of the twentieth century that individuals with physical impairments have been able to participate in competitive sporting events. As a result, functional impairment is no longer a barrier to participation in athletics, and interest in accommodating the needs of those with disabilities continues to grow.

The psychological and physical benefits of exercise are numerous and include improved self-concept, psychosocial attitude, social awareness, social reintegration, perception of well-being, and health (SOR-A).[1,2] Studies show that exercise can significantly increase psychological well-being in wheelchair athletes (SOR-B).[1] Disabled individuals who participate in athletic activities demonstrate better cardiopulmonary endurance, exercise tolerance,

9. HIP AND PELVIS INJURIES IN SPECIAL POPULATIONS   189

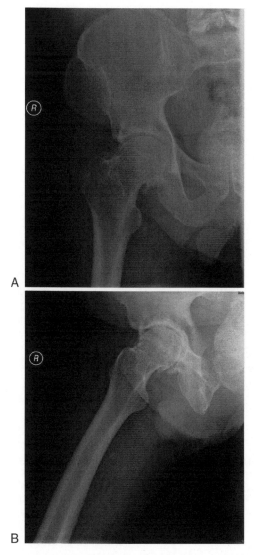

FIGURE 9.1. Heterotopic ossification of the right hip. An irregular linear lucency is seen in the subcapital region. (**A**) AP view of the right hip (**B**) Lateral view of right hip.

mobility, balance, cardiovascular health, and less obesity when compared to those who do not participate (SOR-B).[3] Engaging in sports may also improve bone mineral density (especially for those who are at a wheelchair mobility level) (SOR-B).[4] Proprioceptive-related activities have been associated with improved amputee weight-bearing and gait (SOR-B).[5]

It is well known that physical fitness levels are decreased for individuals with disabilities compared to their able-bodied counterparts.[2] Involvement in sports can significantly improve quality of life and life expectancy, which consequently decreases hospital admissions and medical complications (SOR-B).[6] Individuals who are disabled but active have fewer cardiac risk factors including a better lipid profile (SOR-A).[7,8]

Studies have shown that the injury rate and type of injuries are similar for both disabled and able-bodied athletes (SOR-B).[9] According to injury data,[10] the most common injuries in parathletes (1976 forward) are sprains, strains, abrasions, contusions, fractures, and dislocations. Location of injury is sport- and disability-related (Fig. 9.2). Lower extremity injuries occur more frequently in ambulatory athletes (visually impaired, amputee, cerebral palsy), while upper extremity injuries are more common in wheelchair athletes. Most injuries required less than 7 days without participation in the sport (SOR-B).[10]

Athletes are categorized using the Functional Classification System (FCS) (Table 9.1) for competition purposes. The FCS groups athletes according to their performance and is used as a tool to re-evaluate performance throughout an athlete's career. The FCS is impairment-based, whereas the system for able-bodied athletes is sport-specific. It differentiates between athletes with and without assistive devices and provides a framework for equitable competition among athletes with diverse disabilities. All assistive devices, prosthetics, or other adaptive equipment must be examined to ensure fair competition. For example, an above-knee-amputee skier with either knee disarticulation or hip disarticulation must use a three-track system (ski with two outriggers).[12] We will discuss the challenges these athletes have using the following FCS categories: wheelchair, amputee, and cerebral palsy.

In addition to the FCS, a sports-medical assessment protocol is available. It incorporates cardiovascular and musculoskeletal evaluations geared toward identifying medical problems or impairments and defining therapeutic goals for training programs.

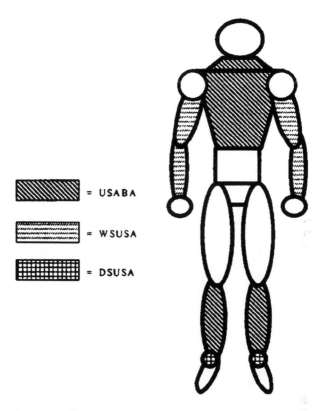

FIGURE 9.2. Predominant unique body region of soft tissue injury for the United States Association of Blind Athletes (USABA), Wheelchair Sports USA (WUSA) athletes, and Disabled Sports USA (DSUSA) athletes. Reprinted from Nyland J, Snouse SL, Anderson M, et al. Soft tissue injuries to USA paralympians at the 1996 summer games. Arch Phys Med Rehabil 2000; 81:368-373. With permission from Elsevier.

TABLE 9.1. Functional classification system categories and classes

Visually impaired (athletics)

T10	No light perception; unable to recognize hand shapes
T11	2/60 and/or visual field of <5_
F11	
T12	2/60–6/60 and visual field of >5_ and <20_
F12	

Continued

TABLE 9.1. *Continued*

Amputee

T42	Single above the knee; combined lower and upper limb amputations; minimum disability
T43	Double below the knee; combined lower and upper limb amputations; normal function in throwing arm
T44	Single below the knee; combined lower and upper limb amputations; moderate reduced function in one or both limbs
T45	Double above the elbow; double below the knee
T46	Single above the elbow; single below the elbow; upper-limb function in throwing arm
F40	Double above the knee; combined lower- and upper-limb amputations; severe problems when walking
F41	Standing athletes with no more than 70 points in the lower limbs
F42	Single above the knee; combined lower- and upper-limb amputations; normal function in throwing arm
F43	Double below the knee; combined lower- and upper-limb amputations; normal function in throwing arm
F44	Single below the knee; combined lower- and upper-limb amputations; normal function in throwing arm
F45	Double above the elbow; double below the elbow
F46	Single above the elbow; single below the elbow; upper-limb function in throwing arm

Cerebral palsy

T30	Severe to moderate involvement; uses one or two arms to push wheelchair; control is poor; affects both arms and legs
T31	Severe to moderate involvement; foot-propelled wheelchair push; affects both arms and legs
T32	Limited control of movements; some throwing motion
F32	Full upper strength in upper extremity; propels wheelchair independently; affects both arms and legs or same-side arm and leg
T33	Good functional strength with minimal limitation or control problems in upper limbs and trunk; affects lower legs
F33	
T34	May use assistive devices; slight loss of balance; affects lower legs or both legs and one arm
F34	
T35	Walks or runs without assistive devices; balance and fine motor control problems
F35	
T36	Good functional ability in dominant side of body; affects arm and leg on same side of body
F36	
T37	Minimal involvement; could be present in lower legs, arm, and leg on same side of body, one leg, or demonstrate problems with balance
F37	

Continued

Table 9.1. *Continued*

Wheelchair

T50	Uses palms to push wheelchair; may have shoulder weakness
T51	Pushing power comes from elbow extension
T52	Normal upper-limb function; no active trunk
T53	Backward movement of trunk; uses trunk to steer; double above-the-knee amputations
F50	No grip with nonthrowing arm; may have shoulder weakness
F51	Difficulty gripping with nonthrowing arm
F52	Nearly normal grip with nonthrowing arm
F53	No sitting balance
F54	Fair to good sitting balance
F55	Good balance and movements backward and forward; good trunk rotation
F56	Good movements backward and forward, usually to one side (side-to-side movements)
F57	Standard muscle chart of all limbs must not exceed 70 points

Functional (swimming)

S1	Unable to catch water; restricted range of motion; no trunk control; leg drag; assisted water start
S2	Unable to catch water; restricted range of motion; no trunk control; slight leg propulsion; unassisted water start
S3	Wrist control limited; limited arm propulsion; minimal trunk control; hips below water; water start
S4	Wrist control; arms not fully fluent; minimal trunk control; hips below water; better body position
S5	Full propulsion in catch phrase; limited arm movement; trunk function; leg propulsion; sit or stand starts
S6	Catch phrase present; arm movement efficient; trunk control; leg propulsion; push start, sit or stand
S7	Good hands; good arms; good trunk; hips level; stand or sit dive start
S8	Hand propulsion; arm cycle good; trunk good; hips and legs level; use of start blocks
S9	Full hand propulsion; full arm propulsion; full trunk control; propulsive kick; dive start from blocks
S10	Full hand and arm propulsion; full arm propulsion; full trunk control; strong leg kick; dive start and propulsion in turns

Visually impaired (cycling, goalball, judo, and swimming)

B1	No light perception; unable to recognize hand shapes
B2	Visual acuity of 2/60 with <5_ field of vision
B3	Visual acuity of 2/60–6/60 and field of vision 5–20_

From Patel DR and Greydanus DE.[11] With permission from Elsevier

HISTORY OF DISABLED ATHLETICS

Sir Ludwig Guttmann, a German-born refugee from Nazi occupation, is credited with originating and popularizing organized sports for the disabled. As director of the SCI unit at the Stokes-Mandeville Hospital in London, Guttmann established a comprehensive rehabilitation program for paralyzed patients and incorporated athletics. In 1948, Guttmann organized a sports competition for World War II veterans with SCI. All the participants were wheelchair athletes. What began as recreational rehabilitation is considered to be the origin of athletic competition for individuals with disability. Four years later, Guttmann's event was transformed into an international competition when a Dutch exserviceman joined the games. The Paralympics were born.[12]

The Paralympics, which began, in Rome, as an event consisting of 400 athletes from 23 different countries, today attracts close to 4,000 participants.[6] As the number of disabled individuals participating in sports continues to grow, it is important that physicians are able to meet the needs of this population.

THE AMPUTEE ATHLETE

The most common musculoskeletal injuries among amputee athletes are sprains and strains to the lumbar spine and sacroiliac joint on the uninvolved side. These injuries are attributed to the mechanical stress of the ground reaction forces during running or ambulation and the asymmetric biomechanical force transmission patterns of the involved and noninvolved sides. In addition, prosthetic alignment (increased hip flexion and ankle plantar flexion) contributes to lumbar spine and pelvic injuries, by causing increased lumbar lordosis (SOR-B).[13] It is important for the sports physician to understand the impact of prostheses and other adaptive equipment on the biomechanics of the specific sport.

Overview

The amputee athlete has a variety of options for adaptive equipment. The new, lightweight, more durable, and better engineered adaptive devices have enabled amputee athletes to attain a better gait pattern (SOR-B).[1] As a result, these athletes can engage in almost any sporting activity. As noted above, it is important that the physician understand (1) the types of amputation, (2) the various adaptive equipment options, (3) biomechanical considerations, and (4) how these factors impact athletic injuries.

Regardless of the level of amputation, there is an automatic change in biomechanics both with and without the use of a prosthesis. The higher the level of amputation, the greater the biomechanical considerations: more energy is required to complete basic functional activities, weight-bearing demands on the residual limb are increased, and the center of gravity is altered, compromising stability and increasing the likelihood of falls (SOR-C). As a result, balance-dependent tasks are more challenging for these individuals.[11]

Lower-extremity amputee athletes use prosthetics that are adapted for their specific sport. All sports prostheses must be able to withstand the demand placed on them by the athlete. Specific prosthetic components are used for activities such as sprinting, endurance, and jumping. Carbon composite and energy storing feet, as well as hydraulic, multiaxial, and computerized knee systems improve gait, athletic prowess, and agility (SOR-C).[12] A shock-absorbing mechanism is desirable for endurance activities (SOR-C).[12] Because shock-absorbing devices are heavier, they may reduce speed, and therefore sprinters prefer lighter prosthetic components (SOR-C).[12] Carbon fiber components, particularly feet, have flexible shanks allowing them to deform on loading and recoil at toe-off, increasing energy return (SOR-C).[14]

Of note, the residual limb is vulnerable to blistering and swelling at pressure-sensitive areas (fibular head, distal tibia, and femoral condyles for transtibial amputees, and ischium for transfemoral amputees) (SOR-C).[1] In athletes with transfemoral amputations, ischial bursitis can occur as a result of weight-bearing patterns and prosthetic socket design. For the same reason, the greater trochanter and femur can also be affected.[1] An improperly fitting prosthesis can further aggravate the situation (SOR-C).[13] Socket irritation can cause prepatellar, infrapatellar, or pretibial bursitis in athletes with transtibial amputations (SOR-C).[11] Amputee athletes can develop residual limb fractures above the prosthesis.[11]

Hyperextension frequently precipitates quadriceps tendon injuries. The quadriceps muscle is subjected to extreme forces during sudden extension movements: acceleration, deceleration, landing, and jumping.[12] The repetitive stress of these forces causes micro-tears at or near the attachment point of the quadriceps tendon to the superior aspect of the patella.[12] Most of the time, these injuries are minimal and do not limit competition. When the symptoms persist or progress, pain will intensify and performance will suffer. Chronic tendinopathy may develop, which could ultimately result in a complete rupture of the quadriceps tendon (SOR-C).[12] Injuries to the uninvolved limb may include plantar fascitis, achilles tendonitis, and stress fractures.[13]

Running

Injuries can affect both the involved and uninvolved extremity. Lower extremity injuries are more common in ambulatory athletes and typically occur during running activities.[10] While engineering has improved knee mechanisms and energy-storing feet designs, the abnormal ground reaction force effect on the residual limb remains a concern. In able-bodied individuals, the ankle is the primary shock absorber and also dampens the rotatory effects of the distal leg and knee.[1] Prosthetic devices attempt to imitate these protective mechanisms, but may still endanger the residual limb. Environmental surfaces, irregular terrain, and malaligned prostheses alter biomechanical forces, affecting balance and increasing the risk for falls.[1] It should be noted that amputee athletes who compete without a prosthesis have an increased risk of injury of the uninvolved limb (SOR-C).[1]

For running, it is necessary to have sufficient lower extremity muscle strength, power, and motor coordination (SOR-C). Similar to normal gait, the running cycle consists of two phases: stance and swing. As speed increases, the amount of time spent in stance decreases. Because runners with transtibial amputations must use an artificial foot and ankle, their performance is dependent on prosthetic design, regardless of prosthetic choice (SOR-C).[14] Running with a transtibial prosthesis increases knee extension time during stance on the involved limb (SOR-B).[14] This alteration in biomechanics can affect resilience and premature fatigue may develop.[1]

Czerniecki et al.[15] found that individuals with transtibial amputations rely heavily on the hip extensors of the affected limb during running for energy production and shock absorption (SOR-B). In a follow-up study comparing able-bodied runners to runners with unilateral transtibial amputations, inherent adaptations in swing phase mechanics were seen. These findings suggest that the uninvolved lower extremity and trunk compensate for the decreased force generation of the stance phase prosthetic limb (SOR-B).[16] Many believe that this energy transformation provides some compensation. Other biomechanical differences in amputee runners include asymmetry of component ankle, knee, and hip forces, all of which increase the risk of injury.

For athletes with transfemoral amputations, running is more challenging because prosthetic choice necessitates a knee component (SOR-C). Gait dynamics change: duration of swing phase increases on the affected side, and toe clearance on the unaffected side is accomplished by hip elevation combined with weight shifting toward the affected side.[12] Computer-enhanced knee components facilitate forward movement of the distal elements approximating normal cadence.[12] This type of prosthesis is a common choice for track athletes because it facilitates swing phase control (Fig. 9.3) (SOR-C).[12] However, gait deviations may still occur. These may include excessive vaulting (rising on the toe of the uninvolved side to assist with forward movement of the prosthesis, minimal knee flexion required), abnormal trunk movement and control, nonreciprocal or symmetric arm movement, and

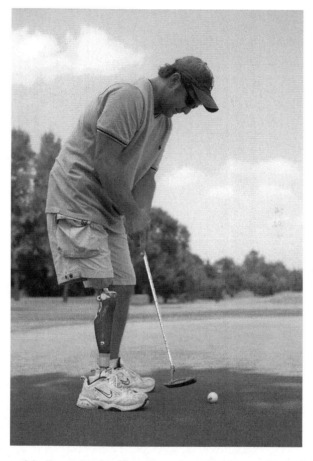

FIGURE 9.3. Recreational golfer with computerized knee unit prosthesis (C-Leg). Courtesy of Otto Bock.

decreased pelvic rotation. Training and modification of prosthetic knee component may alleviate these problems (SOR-B).[1,12]

Skiing

Specialized adaptive equipment is available for amputees who want to ski. For some amputees a three-track system is required: skis attached to two crutches with a third ski on the uninvolved side (Fig. 9.4). Other adaptations include a multiaxial ankle or an ankle fixed in 15–25° of dorsiflexion for athletes with transtibial

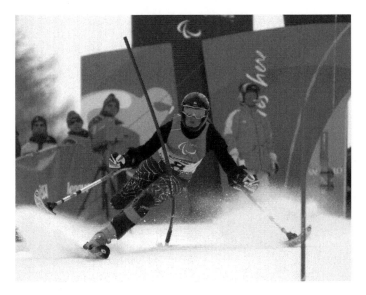

FIGURE 9.4. Paralympic skier using a three-track system: skis are attached to two crutches, with a third ski on the uninvolved side. Courtesy U.S. Paralympic Committee.

amputations, and a mono-ski with a bucket seating device for athletes with bilateral transfemoral amputations or hip disarticulation (SOR-B).[1]

Data from the 2002 Winter Paralympic Games indicate that alpine skiers were more frequently injured than sledge hockey or Nordic skiers (64% vs. 31% vs. 8%; respectively); 38% of alpine skiers had lower extremity injuries; Nordic skiing injuries were located exclusively in the upper extremity, and sledge hockey injuries were more common in the upper extremity (50%) than in the lower extremity (33%).[17] No link has been found between gender and the incidence of ski injuries.[17]

Water Sports

Amputee scuba divers use water-safe prostheses, which are designed to prevent buoyancy. Elastomeric coverings also are available to protect traditional prostheses from limited water exposure. High-level amputees can also swim without a prosthesis (SOR-B).[1] This is important because conventional prosthetic devices are not permitted at governed, international swimming events (although fin attachments are acceptable) (SOR-C).[1]

In any case, training to prevent lateral drifting and trunk dysfunction is recommended (SOR B).[1]

Cycling

Specialized terminal devices enable many amputee athletes to compete in cycling events. As in able-body cycling, binding systems that attach the prosthesis and the contralateral cycling shoe to the pedals are available. It may be necessary to adapt the seat width to optimize balance.[1] Toe clips might be contraindicated if the unaffected foot needs to become free to prevent falls. Some high-level amputees can cycle without a prosthesis using only their intact limb.[1]

Prosthetics for other sports can be tailored to the individual and the specific sport (SOR-C) (Fig. 9.5).[12]

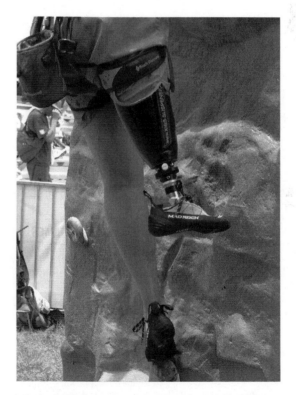

FIGURE 9.5. Rock climber using custom prosthesis with KISS suspension. Courtesy of KISS technologies, LLC.

THE ATHLETE WITH CEREBRAL PALSY

Spasticity, athetosis, and ataxia are classic features of cerebral palsy (CP). Other manifestations include reduced flexibility of muscles and tendons and decreased strength (extensors weaker than flexors). Also, joint contracture can develop if these conditions worsen.

The ratio of ambulatory to nonambulatory athletes with CP is about 50:50. Nonambulatory athletes participate in wheelchair sports.[11] Ambulatory ability determines whether an athlete who has CP is at risk for upper (43%) or lower extremity injuries (44%). In contrast, wheelchair-dependent athletes generally sustain upper extremity injuries (65%).[10] Ferrara and colleagues[18] conducted a retrospective cross-sectional survey of disabled athlete injuries and found that the incidence of injuries to athletes with CP was as follows: 21% knee, 17% shoulder, 15% leg/ankle, and 14% hand/finger. For the purposes of this text, we will concentrate on lower extremity injuries.

Increased muscle tone (spasticity) is the major predisposing factor for athletic injuries in this population.[12] Spasticity can interfere with a person's ability to operate a manual wheelchair, ambulate, fit into clothing properly, or perform transfers and activities of daily living. Other sequelae include contractures, skin breakdown, and pain. The frequent involuntary muscle activity exhibited by this population raises safety issues that are important considerations when organizing competitions and designing training programs. These issues include falling out of the wheelchair, gait dysfunction with forward movement, and loss of balance/postural control.

Athletes with CP typically experience lower extremity injuries that involve the patellofemoral joint and are due to muscle spasms of the surrounding muscles. Classically, there is shortening and tightening of the quadriceps and hamstring muscles, which increase the tension across the joint. Athletes with CP can also have deformities of the ankle and foot (such as equinovarus, equinus, and valgus deformities), which increase the risk for subsequent injuries and pain. Often, athletic involvement is interrupted and orthopedic intervention is needed (SOR-C).[11] Ankle instability, calluses, pressure sores, and metatarsal pain are commonly seen.[11,12]

There is also a tendency for overuse syndromes including muscle strains and chronic knee pain. As stated earlier, there is an increased risk for patellofemoral dysfunction as well as chondromalacia patella.[12] Patella alta (high-riding patella) can be a consequence of decreased quadriceps and hamstring flexibility.[12] Developmental hip abnormalities (coxa valga, acetabular dysplasia, and hip subluxation) may also occur.[11,12] These conditions are more common in the pediatric CP population. Tight hip flexors and extensors can exacerbate lumbar lordosis, chronic back pain, and spondylolytic changes.[11]

For functional and athletic purposes, spasticity must be controlled (SOR-C). Strategies for management include pharmacologic treatment with antispasmodics, positioning, bracing, or physical therapy (SOR-C). Bracing is helpful for tone reduction and ambulation (SOR-C). Pain is usually treated with anti-inflammatory and antispasmodic medications depending on the etiology (SOR-C). Once tone is reduced, stretching is important in preventing contractures and maintaining flexibility. This must be done in a slow, sustained manner to avoid stretch reflex induction.[11] Strengthening programs must also consider the effect of muscle tone in an effort to prevent further muscle imbalance (SOR-B).[11]

THE WHEELCHAIR ATHLETE

Individuals with SCI, CP, amputations, and spina bifida engage in wheelchair athletics. The incidence of lower extremity injuries (specifically the hip and pelvis) is rare because the upper limb is used for transfers and mobility. Despite the limited number of lower extremity injuries, the sports physician should be aware of some specific injuries (Fig. 9.6).

Among those with SCI, osteoporosis is common, increasing the risk of fracture. The distribution of bone demineralization differs in the spinal-cord-injured population where it is predominantly located in the lower extremities and is attributed to disuse.[19] Goktepe and colleagues[4] found reduced trochanter and femoral neck bone density in athletes and individuals with SCI. Bone loss occurs within the first 3 months after the onset of injury.[20]

According to Zehnder et al.,[21] the incidence of known fracture in complete paraplegic males is 2.2% per year. The average time to onset of documented fracture was approximately 9 years. Fracture incidence for males with complete paraplegia increases from 1% within the first year to 5% per year after 20 years.[21] The rate of complications such as osteomyelitis, pressure sores, or contractures can reach 20–40%.[22] Patients can present with symptoms mimicking a viral illness like fever and general malaise.[20] Pain is less commonly identified because of the lack of sensation.[20] Physical examination may reveal swelling and ecchymosis.

Conservative treatment is usually recommended for nondisplaced fractures. A soft well-padded splint is generally prescribed, in the early stages, for functional mobility (SOR-C).[20] Sitting should be started soon after injury, since it is important to help prevent deformities (SOR-C).[20]

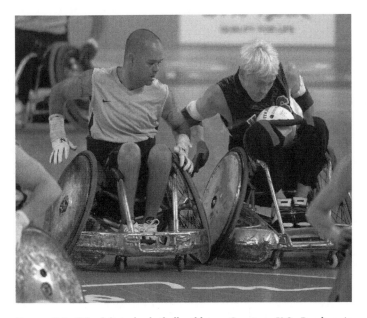

FIGURE 9.6. Wheelchair basketball athletes. Courtesy U.S. Paralympic Committee.

Another complication in the SCI population is heterotopic ossification (HO): formation of bone in ectopic sites. This can be devastating with severe activity limitations in 8–10%.[23] The reported incidence of HO in paraplegic patients is close to 30%.[24] HO typically develops within the first 2 months after SCI,[25] and most frequently occurs at the hips.[26] Other possible sites include the knees, shoulders, and elbows.[26] The etiology of heterotopic ossification is unknown, although risk factors include complete SCI, older age at time of injury, spasticity, pressure ulcers, and other injuries.[26,27] HO can continue for more than 6 months, at which time the bone matures.

Symptoms include local swelling with progression to diffuse edema, limited range of motion, and an elevated serum alkaline phosphatase which usually returns to normal or near-normal levels with maturation (SOR-B).[26,28] There is a low incidence of permanent disability from HO.[26] Radiographic evaluation is helpful in the mature phase, while bone scan can identify HO at earlier stages of development (SOR-B)[26] (see Fig. 9.1).

Treatment focuses on halting progression of ossification and maintaining range of motion and function. Etidronate, a bisphosphonate, is the first-line treatment to prevent further ossification (SOR-B).[23,26] Gentle range-of-motion exercises and radiation therapy are also part of the treatment algorithm. Although radiation therapy is effective, it is not used as frequently (SOR-C).[27,29]

Surgical resection is considered when there is severe restriction of joint range of motion and after maturation has occurred (SOR-B).[26] HO can recur after surgical resection. To prevent recurrence of HO postoperatively, etidronate, anti-inflammatory agents, radiation therapy, and range-of-motion exercises are incorporated in the treatment plan (SOR-B).[26,27]

SUMMARY

With the rapidly growing number of disabled athletes, it is important that the physician fully understand the medical, functional, psychological, and social needs of this population.

Despite the risk for musculoskeletal athletic injuries, there is evidence that supports participation in sporting activities for the disabled population. Athletic involvement has been associated with numerous systemic and mental health benefits that are far more important than the risk of injury.

In our case, FM developed right hip heterotopic ossification, a common and often debilitating complication of SCI. FM was treated with etidronate, a bisphosphonate, and gentle range-of-motion exercises. The goal of this intervention was to reduce ectopic bone formation and preserve hip mobility. After treatment, FM returned to all previous sporting activities.

References

1. Bergeron JW. Athletes with disabilities. Phys Med Rehabil Clin N Am 1999; 10:213,28, viii.
2. Lai AM, Stanish WD, Stanish HI. The young athlete with physical challenges. Clin Sports Med 2000; 19:793–819.
3. Curtis KA, McClanahan S, Hall KM, et al. Health, vocational, and functional status in spinal cord injured athletes and nonathletes. Arch Phys Med Rehabil 1986; 67:862–865.
4. Goktepe AS, Yilmaz B, Alaca R, et al. Bone density loss after spinal cord injury: elite paraplegic basketball players vs. paraplegic sedentary persons. Am J Phys Med Rehabil 2004; 83:279–283.
5. Yigiter K, Sener G, Erbahceci F, et al. A comparison of traditional prosthetic training versus proprioceptive neuromuscular facilitation resistive gait training with trans-femoral amputees. Prosthet Orthot Int 2002; 26:213–217.
6. Groah SL, Lanig IS. Neuromusculoskeletal syndromes in wheelchair athletes. Semin Neurol 2000; 20:201–208.

7. Dearwater SR, LaPorte RE, Robertson RJ, et al. Activity in the spinal cord-injured patient: an epidemiologic analysis of metabolic parameters. Med Sci Sports Exerc 1986; 18:541–544.
8. Brenes G, Dearwater S, Shapera R, et al. High density lipoprotein cholesterol concentrations in physically active and sedentary spinal cord injured patients. Arch Phys Med Rehabil 1986; 67:445–450.
9. Dec KL, Sparrow KJ, McKeag DB. The physically-challenged athlete: medical issues and assessment. Sports Med 2000; 29:245–258.
10. Ferrara MS, Peterson CL. Injuries to athletes with disabilities: identifying injury patterns. Sports Med 2000; 30:137–143.
11. Patel DR, Greydanus DE. The pediatric athlete with disabilities. Pediatr Clin North Am 2002; 49:803–827.
12. Gottschalk F. The Orthopedically Disabled Athlete. In: Stevenson A, ed. DeLee and Drez's Orthopedic Sports Medicine. 3rd ed. Philadelphia, PA: Saunders; 2003.
13. Klenck C, Gebke K. Practical management: common medical problems in disabled athletes. Clin J Sport Med 2007; 17:55–60.
14. Buckley JG. Biomechanical adaptations of transtibial amputee sprinting in athletes using dedicated prostheses. Clin Biomech (Bristol, Avon) 2000; 15:352–358.
15. Czerniecki JM, Gitter A, Munro C. Joint moment and muscle power output characteristics of below knee amputees during running: the influence of energy storing prosthetic feet. J Biomech 1991; 24:63–75.
16. Czerniecki JM, Gitter AJ, Beck JC. Energy transfer mechanisms as a compensatory strategy in below knee amputee runners. J Biomech 1996; 29:717–722.
17. Webborn N, Willick S, Reeser JC. Injuries among disabled athletes during the 2002 Winter Paralympic Games. Med Sci Sports Exerc 2006; 38:811–815.
18. Ferrara MS, Buckley WE, McCann BC, et al. The injury experience of the competitive athlete with a disability: prevention implications. Med Sci Sports Exerc 1992; 24:184–188.
19. Jiang SD, Dai LY, Jiang LS. Osteoporosis after spinal cord injury. Osteoporos Int 2006; 17:180–192.
20. Freehafer AA. Limb fractures in patients with spinal cord injury. Arch Phys Med Rehabil 1995; 76:823–827.
21. Zehnder Y, Luthi M, Michel D, et al. Long-term changes in bone metabolism, bone mineral density, quantitative ultrasound parameters, and fracture incidence after spinal cord injury: a cross-sectional observational study in 100 paraplegic men. Osteoporos Int 2004; 15:180–189.
22. Chen SC, Lai CH, Chan WP, et al. Increases in bone mineral density after functional electrical stimulation cycling exercises in spinal cord injured patients. Disabil Rehabil 2005; 27:1337–1341.
23. Subbarao JV, Garrison SJ. Heterotopic ossification: diagnosis and management, current concepts and controversies. J Spinal Cord Med 1999; 22:273–283.
24. Meiners T, Abel R, Bohm V, Gerner HJ. Resection of heterotopic ossification of the hip in spinal cord injured patients. Spinal Cord 1997; 35:443–445.

25. Banovac K, Williams JM, Patrick LD, Haniff YM. Prevention of heterotopic ossification after spinal cord injury with indomethacin. Spinal Cord 2001; 39:370–374.
26. Kirshblum SC, Priebe MM, Ho CH, et al. Spinal cord injury medicine. 3. Rehabilitation phase after acute spinal cord injury. Arch Phys Med Rehabil 2007; 88:S62–S70.
27. Jamil F, Subbarao JV, Banaovac K, et al. Management of immature heterotopic ossification (HO) of the hip. Spinal Cord 2002; 40:388–395.
28. Singh RS, Craig MC, Katholi CR, et al. The predictive value of creatine phosphokinase and alkaline phosphatase in identification of heterotopic ossification in patients after spinal cord injury. Arch Phys Med Rehabil 2003; 84:1584–1588.
29. Sautter-Bihl ML, Liebermeister E, Nanassy A. Radiotherapy as a local treatment option for heterotopic ossifications in patients with spinal cord injury. Spinal Cord 2000; 38:33–36.

Chapter 10
Functional Therapeutic and Core Strengthening

Gerard A. Malanga and Steve M. Aydin

CLINICAL PEARLS

- Core strengthening is a major part of training programs in athletes as well as patients.
- The kinetic chain theory is a major component of understanding how the core connects and influences movements in the rest of the body.
- Core training program participation should be done with proper evaluation of balance, strength, flexibility, and corrections of difference for optimal benefit.
- Neural systems and proprioceptive feedback play a major role when developing and training the core musculature.
- The long-term benefits of maintaining a strong and endured core have shown to provide optimal athletic functions in sports and decreased dysfunction in patients with low-back pain.

CLINICAL VIGNETTE

A 22-year-old male, who is an avid runner, presents with a 1-year history of low-back, left buttock, and lateral thigh pain. The pain began insidiously and has gotten progressively worse with time and activity. On presentation, the magnetic resonance imaging (MRI) of the patient's lumbar spine demonstrated only a disk bulge at L5/S1, whereas X-rays and MRI of the hip were entirely normal. A bone scan and electrodiagnostic studies were also normal. An injection was administered after a diagnosis of greater trochanteric bursitis, with only transient benefit. A diagnosis of sacroiliac (SI) joint dysfunction was determined as well, which was treated with ultrasound, manipulation, and a fluoroscopically guided injection to the left SI joint, with minimal benefit. Another physician diagnosed him with piriformis syndrome, which was treated with a trigger point injection and then Botox injection, without lasting benefit.

His past medical history was otherwise unremarkable. The athlete occasionally uses nonsteroidal anti-inflammatory drugs, such as ibuprofen, with minimal benefit. He continues to run 23 miles per day, although with the continued symptoms of pain in the left lower back, buttock, and lateral thigh.

On physical examination, he is thin and is a healthy appearing male. The lumbar spine has a mild decrease in lordosis with full pain-free flexion and extension with a mild decrease in segmental motion on the left. His neurological exam is unremarkable. Straight leg raise was negative bilaterally, but a mildly positive Patrick's test was demonstrated on the left. On flexibility testing, he had mildly tight hamstrings and very tight quadriceps muscles, left greater than right. He tested bilaterally positive on Ober's test for iliotibial band tightness, left worse than right. Gait was visually observed and was noted to have increased pronation of the foot on the left greater than right. The leg length, measured by resetting the pelvis and observing the ankles and anterior superior iliac spine levels, showed the left leg to be shorter than the right one.

With functional testing of the patient, the lateral and prone bridges all demonstrated weakness of core muscles with the loss of lumbar support by the patient. Muscle testing of the hip abductors on the left revealed relative weakness.

The patient was evaluated to enter into a comprehensive core strengthening program to improve core strength and improve pain and function.

INTRODUCTION

Core strengthening is now recognized as an integral part of rehabilitation in athletes and an important part of their training programs. The core acts as the stabilizer of the spine and trunk, the generator of power when initiating movement of the limbs, and a point of transition of forces from the lower limbs to the upper limbs, and vice versa, via the abdomen and spine.

When this system becomes altered by injury, the smooth transition of forces that are generated by the limbs and trunk, i.e., the kinetic chain of motion, becomes disrupted. The kinetic chain theory stresses the importance of the core strength.[1]

In this chapter, we will review the anatomy of the core, the properties of the core, and the contribution on the kinetic chain,

10. FUNCTIONAL THERAPEUTIC AND CORE STRENGTHENING

evaluating the strength and endurance of the core and training for the core at different levels.

ANATOMY

The core is often described as a box: a matrix of bones, ligaments, muscles, and nerves in a three-dimensional arrangement. This arrangement of anatomy is what makes the core so functional in providing stability to the spine and in energy transfers. To understand the makeup of the core muscles, it can be imagined as a cube, a three-dimensional layering of tissue, which allows motion in multiple planes.

The core is composed of a floor, a ceiling, front, back, and sides, as shown in Fig. 10.1. The superior aspect or ceiling of the core is made by the diaphragm. The floor is composed of the pelvic floor. The anterior portion of the core is made up by the abdominal muscles, while the posterior aspect is composed of the paraspinals and thoracolumbar fascia. The lateral potions are composed of the lateral hip girdle musculature, and external/internal obliques.[2,3]

The arrangement of the muscles and tissue of the core is done in a layerlike fashion. These are the inner, middle, and outer layers of the core. The outer layer is made up of the power muscles. The middle layer is made up of the abdominal and back-stabilizing muscles. And finally, the inner most layer is comprised of the intersegmental muscle and proprioceptive structures, such as the multifidi and nerves[4] (Fig. 10.2).

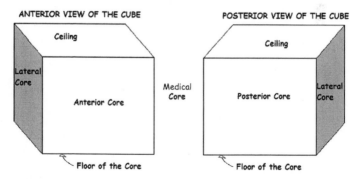

FIGURE 10.1. The core is often thought of as a box; however, it is a three-dimensional structure and resembles a cube or sphere. Viewing it as a cube, with each side contributing a function, while overlapping with one another (like in a sphere), helps in understanding its function and purpose.

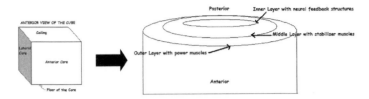

FIGURE 10.2. The core is arranged in a spherical manner with a complex arrangement of tissues. The three layers that make it up are the outer, middle, and inner. Each one contributes a specific function to the core's action. The outer layer functions in the way of producing muscular power. The middle layer uses its muscles and tissues to stabilize the core. And the inner layer functions in providing neural feedback to the body.

TABLE 10.1. The different muscle layers for the anterior, posterior core, lateral borders, floor, and ceiling

Anterior core muscles	*Lateral core muscles*
Rectus abdominus	Gluteus maximus
Transverse abdominus	Gluteus minimus
External obliques	Gluteus medius
Internal obliques	Transverse abdominus
Posterior core muscles	External obliques
Erector spinae group	Internal obliques
Iliopsoas	*Floor and ceiling muscles of the core*
Quadratus lumborum	Diaphragm acting as the ceiling
Multifidi	Pelvic diaphragm acting as the floor
Thoracolumbar fascia	

Looking at the core as a cube simplifies its complexity. All the borders described are connected to one another and overlap. They all function together as one unit in body mechanics to allow transition of forces and stability (Fig. 10.2).

The anterior core is made up mainly of the rectus abdominis, transverse abdominis, external oblique, and internal oblique, as well as their apeneroursis (Table 10.1 and Fig. 10.3a). These muscles also act upon the hip and pelvis region. The rectus abdominis originates on the pubis of the pelvis, and inserts onto the cartilage of the xiphiod, fifth, sixth, and seventh ribs. It allows flexion of the lumbar spine, straightens the pelvis, maintains intra-abdominal pressure, and assists in expiration. The transverse abdominis originates on the posterior–lateral portions of the deep thoracolumbar fascia, anterior iliac spine, and iliac crest. It inserts on the inner surface of the 7th to 12th ribs, the rectus sheath, and linea alba. It functions to bend the trunk unilaterally to the same side of contraction, and rotation to the opposite side. With bilateral contraction, it assists in flexion of the trunk and lumbar spine, increase in intra-abdominal pressure, and expiration. The external oblique originates on the surfaces of ribs 5 to 12 and inserts on the iliac crest and anterior rectus sheath. When it contracts unilaterally, it causes bending of the trunk to the ipsilateral side of contraction and rotation to the opposite side. With bilateral activation of the external oblique, flexion of the trunk, increase in intra-abdominal pressure, and straightening of the pelvis occur. The internal oblique allows the same motion and increase in intra-abdominal pressure as the external oblique. It originates from the thoracolumbar fascia, iliac crest, and anterior superior iliac spine and inserts on the lower borders of ribs 10 to 12, the linea alba, and

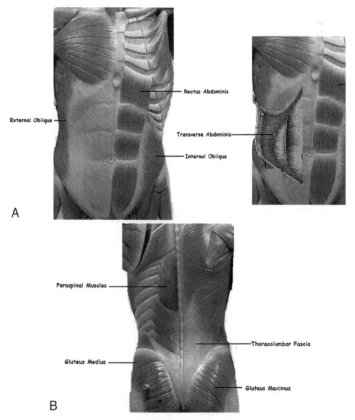

FIGURE 10.3. (**A**) The anterior abdomen and core muscles. (**B**) The posterior aspect of the torso and muscles.

rectus sheath. It is noteworthy that all the origins and insertions have connections to the hip, pelvis, and lumbar spine.[2,3]

The posterior portion of the core consists of the erector spinea, iliopsoas, quatradus lumborum, multifidi muscles, and the thoracolumbar fascia. The erector spinea originate at the sacrum, iliac crest, lumbar spinous process, and lumbar transverse process (Table 10.1 and Fig. 10.3b) and insert onto the 2nd to 12th ribs and thoracic vertebral transverse processes. During bilateral contraction, the erector spinea causes the lumbar spine to extend and bend laterally to the ipsilateral side. The iliopsoas originates on the lateral surfaces of the vertebrae (T12, L14), intervetebral disks, and iliac fossa. It inserts on the lesser trochanter of the femur. The iliopsoas will cause hip flexion and internal rotation at the hip and also tilts the pelvis anteriorly exaggerating lumbar lordosis. Quatratus lumborum originates from the iliac crest and inserts on the 12th rib and L1 to L4 vertebrae. It has three poles: superior, longitudinal, and inferior. The inferior pole is functional in the core musculature, while the superior and middle poles function more with respiration. When the quatratus lumborum unilaterally contracts, it causes the trunk to bend to the ipsilateral side, and when it bilaterally contracts it provides the ability to bear down and increase intra-abdominal pressure.[2] The multifidi originate on the transverse process and then insert superiorly on the spinous process. They function in segmental motion of the lumbar vertebrae and allow extension with bilateral contraction. When they unilaterally contract, they cause flexion, side-bending to the same side, and rotation to the opposite side.[2,3,5,6]

The lateral borders of the core are composed of the gluteal muscles and overlap from the previously discussed muscles; obliques, thoracolumbar fascia, and transverse abdominis. The glueteal muscles consist of the maximus, medius, and minimus (Table 10.1 and Fig. 10.3). The gluteal maximus originates from the dorsal surface of the sacrum and posterior iliac crest, and then inserts on the iliotibial band and gluteal tuberosity of the femur. The motion it primarily contributes to is extension of the hip, with lateral rotation. The gluteus maximus also allows the extension of the trunk from a flexed position. The gluteus medius and minimus both originate from the ilium and insert on the greater trochanter of the femur. The primary motion they allow is hip abduction. The gluteal muscle group as a whole also has an important role in dynamic stabilization of the hip, pelvis, and trunk during motion.[2,3,5]

The thoracolumbar fascia is a retinacular strap that acts as a girdle around the abdomen, consisting of three layers (Fig. 10.3). All three layers – anterior, middle and posterior – function to maintain stability in the spine and trunk while preventing unwanted motion during movements. The anterior and middle potions are those most intimately connected to the iliopsoas, quatratus lumborum, and intrinsic back muscles such as the multifidi. The posterior layer of the thoracolumbar fascia is the most superficial layer. It has a distinct property of covering the back with a tense tissue that is pulled laterally by abdominal muscles. The transverse abdominis has connections to primarily the posterior layer and to the middle layer of the thoracolumbar fascia. This is instrumental in causing a tensing of the fascia, removing the slack, and providing stability (Fig. 10.4).[2,3,5]

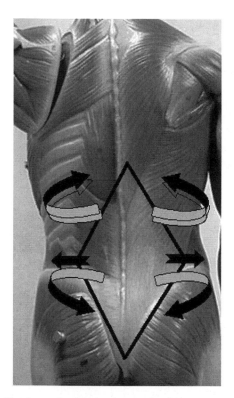

FIGURE 10.4. The thoracolumbar fascia is a crucial component of the core. It is connected to many muscles and, when they contract, it is pulled tight like a girdle and provides stability. The transverse abdominis muscle is one of the major players in pulling the thoracolumbar fascia tight during contraction. The arrows indicate the manner in which the fascia is pulled during a contraction.

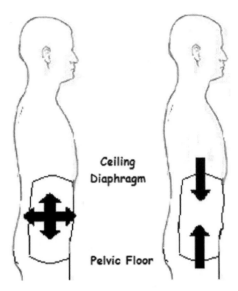

FIGURE 10.5. The pelvic floor and diaphragm are major components in the core and help in providing and maintaining an intra-abdominal pressure during movements. The floor of the core is made up of the pelvic diaphragm muscles. The roof of the core is made up of the diaphragm.

The diaphragm serves as the roof of the core and increases the intra-abdominal pressure by descending. The pelvic floor acts as the base of the core and aids in increasing intra-abdominal pressure by contracting and ascending. The pelvic floor and diaphragm primarily work in co-contraction with the rest of the trunk muscles (Table 10.1 and Fig. 10.5). When a contraction occurs, an increase in abdominal pressure occurs, which, in turn, causes the lumbar spine to stabilize and reduces unwanted movement.[2,3,5–8]

The muscles and tissues described above function by contractions from neuronal firing patterns which result in stabilization, increase in intra-abdominal pressure, and energy transfer. In trying to understand the core, the body's neuron-muscular system has to be looked at as one functioning unit[9] (SOR-C).

MECHANISM OF THE CORE AND THE KINETIC CHAIN

To understand the core and its function, the body should be viewed as having an inherent connection among all the different layers of muscles, fascia, and other connective tissue. The patterns of the muscle contractions allow movement. The motion of an extremity in a plane of space occurs freely at the distal portions from the trunk, while its proximal attachment to the core provides a point of anchor. In most cases, this anchoring is the proximal muscles of the lower or upper extremity anchored to the trunk, or muscles of the trunk attached to the spine. This coupling of musculature of the limbs and trunk allows the body to function as a unit. The resultant motions influence other distal or proximal portions of the body. The motions are generated from forces of contractions within the muscles, which then disperse energy distally and proximally. The spine, hip, pelvis, and trunk are the areas of transition of this energy, force, and motion (Fig. 10.6). Therefore, when a force is generated in the lower extremity, it transmits the force to the trunk, providing stability by securing its position proximally. Furthermore, studies have shown that the generation of force in the extremities is preceded by contraction of the core muscles for stability of the trunk and spine and, as described, the transition of forces from limb to trunk and trunk to limb.[9,10]

The kinetic chain theory, also known as the *link theory*, explains this connection of musculoskeletal motion in the extremities and trunk.

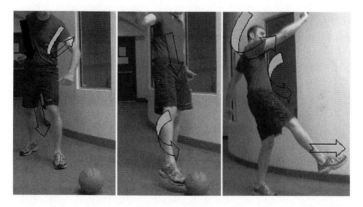

FIGURE 10.6. The kinetic chain theory can often be applied to sports that involve explosive motions. In this example of kicking a soccer ball, the power to kick the ball will often develop in the upper extremities, and transmit downward to the leg during the follow-through. The core contracts prior to all these motions, and stabilizes the body to allow for a fluid transition of the upper body momentum to the lower body. When kicking through the ball, the force generated comes from both the upper body and lower extremity. When the core is functional and intact, the maximal force from these two sources can be achieved.

The definition of the kinetic chain, as described in the literature, is the significant interrelationship of muscle activation and translation of forces within the musculoskeletal system.[11]

The core muscles are thought to be the generators of all initial motion by contracting prior to limb movement, while also allowing forces to transmit from one limb to another by stabilizing the spine and abdomen. This coupling of functions makes the core the center of the kinetic chain. An example of the connections of motion is seen when the end point is the upper limb and the starting point is the lower extremity. In the case of a pitcher throwing a fast ball, the core allows the force to be transmitted from the lower extremity to the upper extremity. When the lower limbs contract in the early part of a pitcher's motion, power is generated in the lower limbs. Prior to start of the pitching stride, the abdominal muscles and back muscles contract, to provide stability. As the pitcher steps forward through his stride, the forces are transferred from the lower limbs though the stabilized core, and up into the upper extremity where the follow-through is made with the upper extremity and the ball is thrown (Fig. 10.7). In an ideal system, there are no weak points of breakdown where the forces can be lost because of instability or weakness. When an interruption in this chain occurs, motion and forces do not transmit correctly and compensation is attempted by other muscle groups; to generate the same amount of power to throw a fast ball in an athlete with a weak core will involve straining of other muscles. As a result, a weak core places a person at greater risk of injury, misalignment, and submaximal performance.[4,9,10,12,13]

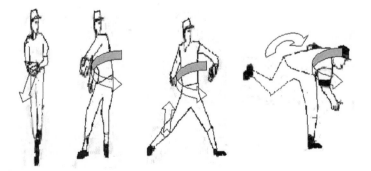

FIGURE 10.7. In the case of a baseball pitcher, the kinetic chain functions similarly to that of a soccer player; however, the forces develop in the lower extremities initially, and then transmits upward to the upper extremities. The core once again contracts, stabilizes, and allows for an efficient throw.

10. FUNCTIONAL THERAPEUTIC AND CORE STRENGTHENING

To understand this, it is important to see how patterns of motion are interrupted in patients with extremity pain and low-back pain. These injuries can result in decreased postural control and proprioception of the core, kinetic chain, and limbs. It has been shown that athletes with lower extremity instability, (i.e., ankle or knee), have a delayed firing pattern of gluteus medius, which functions in hip abduction and posterior-lateral trunk stability, and the anterior abdominal muscles.[13,14] When the core or limbs have a dysfunction present, it is considered an interruption of the kinetic chain. The effect of breakdown in the chain results in abnormal and delayed muscle firing patterns, poor neuronal feedback, and poor proprioception. This, in turn, causes increased instability in the spine and other joints.[4,9,10,14,15]

The core is not only responsible for generating force; it functions to providing stability to the spine and other joints. This is important because joints require control from muscles and proprioceptive feedback from neurons to allow optimal function. The early development of arthritis or joint dysfunction often results from misalignment, unwanted motion, and high shearing tensions. A strong core with sufficient endurance results in spinal stability, and control of motion can be gained[4,9](SOR-B).

The deep muscles of the back, such as the multifidi, are the intersegmental muscles that allow vertebral control, whereas the abdominal muscle, diaphragm, and pelvic floor have the role of increasing intra-abdominal pressure. When the abdominal muscles contract, they increase intra-abdominal pressure, which then causes tension in the spine and thoracolumbar fascia, reducing laxity in the spine.[7,8,16,17] This is analogous to inflating a tire. As air is added to the tire, the walls develop tension, prevent the tire from sagging, and allow it to roll firmly.

There is a built-in neuronal protection system within the core which helps in controlling the patterns of firing muscles in planning a motion and maintains proprioceptive feedback of the body's position. Prior to contraction of limb movement, the core prepares itself for gross motor function of the limb. This is done by the contraction, primarily, of the transverse abdominis muscle and multifidi.[6,11]

The transverse abdominis muscle has been shown to contract prior to the muscles of limb movement. The internal oblique, external oblique, and transverse abdominis all co-contract and increase the intra-abdominal pressure, allowing the tension to increase within the abdomen, tensing the thoracolumbar fascia, and imparting stability onto the lumbar spine.[4] This tension in the trunk also prepares the body for generation of power from the core, which will eventually be translated to a limb. When the core lacks strength or endurance for generating power, it can result in decreased efficiency of motion and power and in injury. The dysfunction present causes an interruption in the contraction pattern of the kinetic chain; the feedback via the nervous system functions inappropriately, resulting in compensatory muscle firing.[12]

For example, when low-back pain is present, the multifidi and transverse abdominis are inhibited. During muscle contraction of the lower extremity, the transverse abdominis is the first to contract in normal individuals. This prevents unwanted trunk movement, and allows the transition of energy/force in the pattern of the kinetic chain, as described previously. With low-back pain, a delayed activation of the transverse abdominis contraction is noted on electromyography evaluation, relative to the limb activation.[18,19]

A strong, balanced, and high endurance core is not only important in the kinetic chain but is also essential in providing stability to the spine, hip, pelvis, and sacrum. When conditioned with strength, and more importantly endurance, the motion in the spine is controlled, and occurs in a fluid manner preventing increased shear. When segmental or micromotion is controlled, it allows more explosive muscle force generation from the core and transmission of forces smoothly from the core to the limbs.

For a more comprehensive discussion of the kinetic chain, refer to Chap. 3 of this text.

ASSESSING THE CORE MUSCULATURE

As previously discussed, the core is the center of the kinetic chain and allows the generation and transmission of forces for optimal movement and function. Many athletes who have been injured or have complaints of low-back pain are likely to have deficiency of their core, which may be a contributing factor. Therefore, the comprehensive evaluation of the athletes should include assessing the strength and endurance of the core[7-9] (SOR-C).

Proper balance is important before initiating a program to strengthen the core. The evaluation includes the assessment of leg lengths, range of motions, flexibility, tight muscles groups, and muscle bulk. When imbalance is present, dysfunction and damage often occur on the weaker side.[7,8,12]

Examination of the lumbar spine, range of motion of the joints, stability and laxity of joint, posture, gait, and flexibility is also an important part of the full assessment of the athlete. When evaluating for balance, range of motion testing, both actively and passively, should be done, comparing sides. This will allow the person to focus on stretching those muscles that are inflexible. The lumbar spine should also be evaluated for range of motion in functional planes of flexion, extension, side-bending, and rotation. Observation and palpation of the spine should be done to assess anatomical alignment and deformity. When the spine is assessed, it should be evaluated in the neutral spine position, which is the position of minimal loading on the spinal joints. The major component being looked at throughout the evaluation is clinical instability, which is defined as the loss of the ability to maintain normal anatomical positions.[20]

When an athlete is being evaluated, the neutral spine should be maintained. The neutral spine is often thought to be the positioning of the lumbar spine to a point of the loss of lordosis, or a flat back. With regard to core strengthening, the neutral spine should be thought of as the point of pain-free position where maximal power can be obtained and balance can be preserved. It should also be understood that this is the position in which training should occur. Furthermore, the maintenance of the neutral spine is important in day-to-day functions. It allows the muscles to train and develop without increasing load, shear, and damage on the spine and other joints. When training is complete, the stabilizers should be strengthened with high endurance and full range, allowing control in all planes which may not occur in the neutral position of the spine. The eventual goal is to improve strength, endurance, balance, and the neuronal output of the trunk and limbs while maintaining a neutral spine position.[4]

Screening examinations can be used to assess joint flexibility, range of motion, and stability (Table 10.2)

TABLE 10.2. Tests for screening stability and flexibility

- Hamstring screens – supine position while raising leg to 90°, while preventing pelvic tilt. Compare to contralateral side.
- Rotation screen – evaluates abdominal and lumbar rotators. Sit in "Indian style" position, with arms over chest, and rotate side to side.
- Hurdle step screen – evaluates hip flexors. Maintain a cross bar behind shoulders, while stepping over a hurdle of about 2 ft high, once leading with the left and then the right.
- Narrow lunge screen – assesses the hamstrings, quadriceps, pelvic muscle, and gluteal groups. Perform by walking a plank, and then alternating squats with the left leading then right, while having a cross bar behind shoulders.
- Deep squat screen – evaluates hip flexors and extensors, the lumbar spine, and abdominal muscles. Done by holding a cross bar above the head, feet in a line, and squatting down then back up, while maintaining static lumbar positioning.

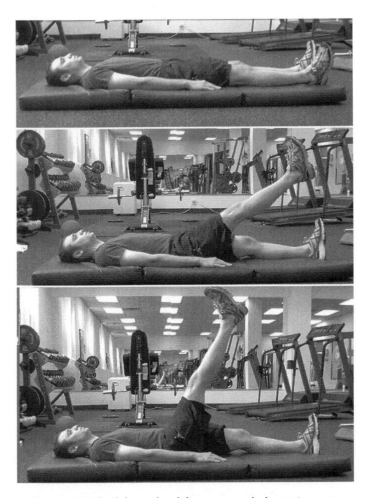

FIGURE 10.8. Flexibility and mobility screens – the hamstrings test.

- The hamstrings can be looked at, with the athlete in the supine position elevating the leg to 80°–90° of flexion at the hip, without introducing pelvic tilt, and comparing bilaterally (Fig. 10.8).
- To evaluate the abdominal and lumbar rotators, a seated-rotation position can be utilized. The athlete sits in the "Indian style" position, arms crossed over chest, and rotates left to right. The rotation is compared side to side looking for asymmetry (Fig. 10.9).

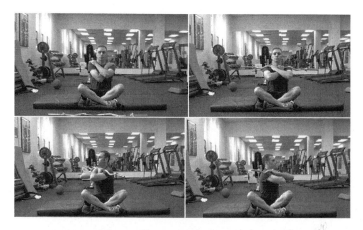

FIGURE 10.9. Flexibility and mobility screens – the rotational test.

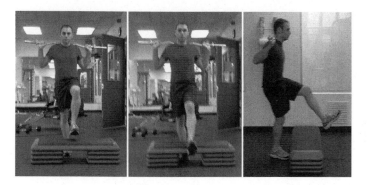

FIGURE 10.10. Flexibility and mobility screens – hurdle step test.

- The hurdle step evaluates the hip flexors and core muscles by maintaining a cross bar behind the shoulders while stepping over a hurdle of about 2 ft high, alternately leading with the left and then the right. Observations of balance control and posture should be noted during the process (Fig. 10.10).
- The narrow lunge is used to assess the hamstrings, quadriceps, pelvic muscle, and gluteal groups. It is performed by walking a plank, and then alternating squats with the left leading the right, while having a cross bar behind the shoulders. Observations to balance control and posture should be noted during the process (Fig. 10.11).

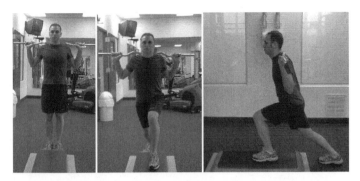

FIGURE 10.11. Flexibility and mobility screens – narrow lunge test.

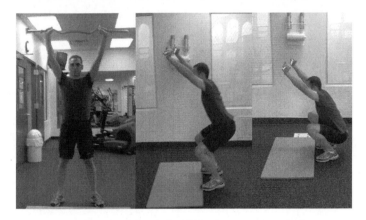

FIGURE 10.12. Flexibility and mobility screens – deep squat test.

- The deep squat is used to evaluate hip flexors and extensors, the lumbar spine, and abdominal muscles. It is done by holding a cross bar above the head, feet in a line, squatting down, and then back up. Evaluators should pay special attention to maintenance of a neutral spine, balance control, and posture[4,7,8,12] (SOR-B) (Fig. 10.12).

After evaluation of balance, the next component to be assessed is endurance. Strength in the absence of endurance of core muscles is insufficient for most sports. This is due to the fact that endurance of muscles in the core allows extended periods of stability. Since the core is recruited prior to most limb movements to brace the body for action, maintaining contraction during the course of the limb movement is done for stability. Various position testing can be done to assess the endurance by seeing how long the

10. FUNCTIONAL THERAPEUTIC AND CORE STRENGTHENING 223

athlete can maintain that position. The four major tests done to evaluate the core's endurance are the prone bridge, lateral bridge, torso flexor, and torso extensor endurance tests[21] (Table 10.3).

The prone bridge is done by having the patient lying prone, with forearms and toes on the floor, assessing the anterior and posterior core muscles (Fig. 10.13). The pelvis should be in a neutral position. Failure of the test is when the pelvis moves from a neutral position and falls into a lordotic position, where the pelvis will rotate anteriorly. If there is a lack of endurance to hold the position, then start with the knees in a bent position, rather than with the knee in extension and resting on the toes, reducing the lever arm. Further assessment of the prone bridge can be done with weights positioned on the back, or the forearms can move more cranially.[4,7,8,12,22]

The lateral bridge assesses the lateral core muscles (Fig. 10.14). The position assesses the abdominal obliques, limiting the psoas participation. Failure occurs when there is a loss of a straight posture and the hip tilts toward the table. An advanced exercise can be done with abducting the upper arm and adding slight rotational movements while holding the position.[12]

Testing the torso flexors can be done by timing how long the patient can hold a position of seated torso flexion (Fig. 10.15). Flex the torso to 60° and the knee/hips flexed to 90°. The toes should be secured under a toe strap or held by the examiner. Failure occurs when the patient's torso falls below 60° of flexion.

TABLE 10.3. Core assessment exercises

- Prone bridge – assesses the anterior and posterior core muscles
- Lateral bridge – assesses the lateral musculature of the core
- Torso flexion – tests the anterior core primarily, and also assesses the posterior core
- Torso extension – mainly tests the posterior core muscles, as well as the anterior core

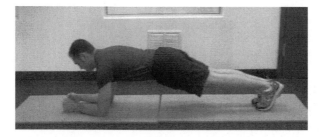

FIGURE 10.13. The prone bridge for core assessment.

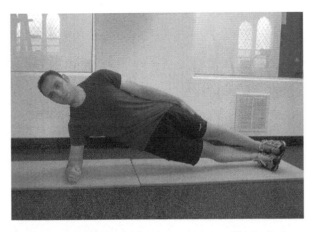

FIGURE 10.14. The lateral bridge for core assessment. This is also known as the *Side Bridge*, which is part of the "Big 3" exercise program.[4]

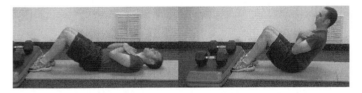

FIGURE 10.15. The torso flexion test for core assessment. The is also known as the *Curl-up*, which is part of the "Big 3" exercise program.[4]

Testing the torso extensors can be done with the athlete in the prone position, while the hip, pelvis, and knees are secured on to a platform or table (Fig. 10.16). The upper body will be held out straight, without the support of the table, at 180°. This demonstrates recruitment of the extensors to a neutral position, while not pass pointing and placing the entire spine into hyperextension. Failure occurs when the 180° posture without the table support is lost and the athlete falls into a flexed position.[12]

The time for maintaining position as described previously should be around 60 s before fatigue is noted and maintenance of the testing posture is lost.[12]

To restore balance, especially in tight muscles groups, the focus should be on restoring the flexibility in the dysfunctional group. This can be done with foam roll exercises, mobility exercises,

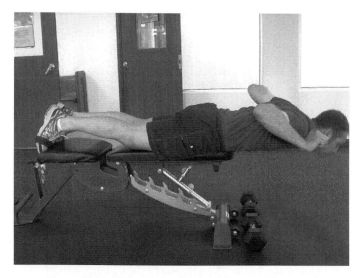

FIGURE 10.16. The torso extension test for core assessment.

contraction–relaxation techniques, active release therapy, and joint mobilization techniques. Each of the positions described has a standardized time to determine whether the muscle group being tested has a functional level of endurance. Reaching those points of time in position with a neutral spine is the goal. The bridge positions along with the torso positions can be the foundation on developing a core strengthening program[4,12] (SOR-B).

By evaluating an individual in all four positions and determining the endurance, one can get a general idea about what shape he or she is in. Once the asymmetries are corrected, the person can enter into a progressive training program, based on his or her capabilities.

EXERCISE PROGRAMS FOR CORE STRENGTHENING AND ENDURANCE

After a person has been assessed and deemed safe to participate in an exercise program, the focus should be on correcting imbalances. The goal of the program is to increase strength, endurance, and neuronal output and to normalize the function of the core. The program should also be individualized for each patient. The goals and level of participation of a patient with low-back pain will differ from those of an athlete training for a sport. At the beginner level, there should be a focus on activating the transverse abdominis and multifidi while maintaining a neutral spine. This involves using techniques of recruiting these muscles into the functions of daily motions. This has been termed development of *core awareness*. A person moves to the intermediate level of training when he or she can maintain a neutral spinal position during simple tasks. At the intermediate level, the goal is to maintain spinal stabilization while increasing challenges to the core musculature. To reach an advanced level of training requires the same ability to maintain spinal control, however, with higher complexities of motions and activities. This includes maintaining trunk control on unsteady surfaces and during plyometric activity[12,21] (Table 10.4).

A general core strengthening program should not begin in the first hour of awakening (**SOR-B**). This is due to the increased hydrostatic pressure in the interverterbral disks.[4] A warm-up can begin with the cat and camel positions. The cat–camel is a range-of-motion exercise that mobilizes the spine by flexion of the spine prior to reaching end point, and then an extension of the spine without reaching end point of motion (Fig. 10.17). This can then be followed by pelvic translation exercises: iliopsoas stretches, piriformis stretches, and hamstring stretches. These will mobilize the point of transition of the kinetic chain and range the joints in

TABLE 10.4. Levels of core strengthening training

- Beginner level – focuses on the transverse abdominis training and recruitment, intrasegmental spinal motion, and training to maintain a neutral spine.
- Intermediate level – at this level the person can maintain a neutral spine during program, and can introduce more core strengthening challenges
- Advance level – maintenance of spinal control, while performing more complex exercises on unstable surfaces, with plyometrics

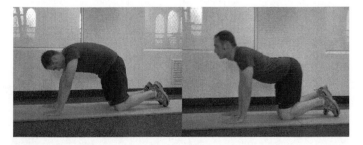

FIGURE 10.17. The Cat–Camel stretch. This exercise is often done at the start of a program to allow for segmental motion in the spine and core.

the pelvis, sacrum, hip, and spine. A short aerobic program can then be incorporated into the core program, during the warm-up portion.[12,21]

The type of training varies from the beginner to the advanced; however, each includes a warm-up stage followed by three stages to be completed during a session (Table 10.5). Stage 1 focuses on motor firing patterns and the muscle motor relearning/plotting patterns for neural feedback. The athlete also focuses on muscle recruitment of specific muscle groups with verbal cuing.[12,21]

Stage 2 stresses stabilization exercises that are done from a beginner to an advanced level. This is known as the "Big 3": curl-ups (Fig. 10.15), side bridge (Fig. 10.14), and bird–dog exercise (Fig. 10.18). Curl-up exercises are done in the supine position, in a neutral spine position, with the knees bent, flexioning at the hips and bringing the contralateral shoulder to the knee. The side bridges are the same as those described when used to assess the core. And the bird–dog position is performed in the same position as the cat–camel, while having one arm and leg outstretched in a reaching position, and one knee flexed and contacting the floor and the other arm supporting the body while contacting the floor. The positions are held for a period of several seconds, maintaining neutral spine, and then alternating with the other leg and arm.[12,21]

TABLE 10.5. Stages of exercise program for all levels

Stage one – focuses on motor patterns, muscle learning patterns, and neural feedback. Cueing for proper technique is done during this portion of the workout

Stage two – works on the exercises done in the program to strengthen. Commonly the "Big 3" exercises are done (see Table 10.6). The Big 3 are used at all levels of training (beginner to advanced) but will have variations in technique

Stage three – addresses the application of the movements and strengthening learned into functional states like walking, running, or daily activities

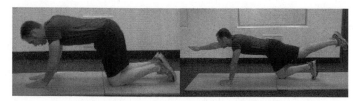

FIGURE 10.18. The Bird–Dog exercise, part of the "Big 3" exercise program.[4]

Stage 3 addresses the functional progression of the exercises and works on exercises which are conducted in standing, walking, and sitting positions. The progression to this stage results in an increase of compressive loads on the lumbar spine.[12,21]

The abdominal exercises in core strengthening programs can be stressful to the lumbar spine if performed incorrectly. This is why the neutral spine must be maintained during early training, to allow the development of control and endurance for future stabilization of the spine (SOR-B). Improper technique will result in loading forces distributed asymmetrically, placing a person at an increased risk for pain and dysfunction at a joint or point of motion.[12,21]

Another focus during core exercising is on co-contraction, specifically the pelvic floor with the transverse abdominis. Diaphragm breathing is also an important part of this system. These allow increasing the intra-abdominal pressure. This results in the box pressure increasing like a balloon, stretching and tightening the muscles that are part of the core.[12,21]

The "Big 3" exercises are curl-ups (for the rectus abdominis), side bridge exercise (for the obliques), and leg/arm extensions (for the back extensors) (Table 10.6). The rectus abdominis is the most active during the initial elevation of the head, neck, and shoulders, while maintaining neutral position of the spine. Side bridge exercises are for the obliques, transverse abdominis, latissimus, and quadratus lumborum. The third exercise is leg and arm extension, which is done in a hands-and-knees position, eventually leading to the bird–dog exercise for the back extensors.[12,21]

The basic exercise strengthening program starts on a flat surface, with eventual progression to positions in functional positions. The participant moves from a stable ground environment to a progressively less stable environment while increasing the complexity of movements.[7-10,12,21]

Achieving functional participation involves getting to a program of exercises in all planes: sagittal plane, frontal plane, transverse/rotational plane. There is also the need to incorporate strengthening, endurance, balance, and proprioceptive training

TABLE 10.6. The "Big 3" exercises

- Curl-ups – strengthens the rectus abdominis and anterior core muscles
- Side bridges – strengthens the internal/external obliques, transverse abdominis, quatratus lumborum, and the lateral core
- Bird–dogs – strengthens the back extensors, transverse abdominis, and posterior core muscles

into the programs. It has been shown that muscle fatigue is coupled with proprioceptive impairment. Using a balance board in the program allows the development of neuronal feedback for improved proprioceptive function. This helps with learning quick unconscious motions, sharpens the body's reaction to postural shifts in its center of gravity, and helps with joint stabilization during motion.[7,8]

Ultimately, the athlete progresses to a program with plyometrics. Plyometrics is an explosive use of energy through the kinetic chain. This is where a strong and balanced core with endurance is most important. Patterns should eventually be established for postural awareness and control to engram motor programming that is automatically patterned in the motor cortex, so that conscious effort is not necessary. Once engram motor programming is established, the athlete no longer has to think about drawing in and co-contracting various muscle groups, as they fire automatically during activities.[7–10,12,21]

ROLE OF CORE STRENGTHENING AND SPECIFIC MUSCLE GROUPS

Core strength plays a significant role in allowing activities of ambulation, limb motions, and athletic motions. When there is a breakdown in the kinetic chain, for example, when the center of the chain is weak, there is the potential for injury to occur.

Core and hip extensors, primarily the gluteus maximus, play a major role in stabilizing the pelvis during trunk rotation, or when the center of gravity is grossly shifted. When there is asymmetry in hip muscle strength or inflexibility is present, the athlete is at risk for increased incidence of injury. When poor endurance is present, there is often delayed firing in the hip extensors and abductors, which has been theorized to have an increased report of lower extremity injury and low-back pain. This can be attributed to the interruption of neuronal firing patterns, which in turn results in poor muscular control.[10]

The hip abductors function in midstance to stabilize the pelvis, preventing downward inclination (Trendelenburg sign) during single leg stance (gluteus medius/minimus). When hip abduction weakness occurs, there is an increase in lateral trunk stabilizer firing. Furthermore, when there is an anterior cruciate ligament (ACL) dysfunction or ankle instability, the firing patterns of the hip and core muscle become disrupted in their neuronal contraction patterns, as shown in studies. In response to an ACL injury or knee instability, the hip flexors and knee extensors do not function at optimal contraction. This reduces the stress on the ACL and knee joint.

This results in poor firing patterns on the ipsilateral side and a disruption in the kinetic chain.[15] With regard to ankle injuries, it has been shown that a pattern of increased firing of the hip muscles is noted on the ipsilateral side of the ankle injury. Early recruitment of hip muscles, coupled with ankle instability, also results in a poor conduction of muscle firing and disrupts the kinetic chain.[14] In cases where distal extremity dysfunction develops, there is a greater risk for developing proximal injury due to compensatory mechanisms. A core strengthening program prevents injury by improving dynamic control of the core and stabilization of motion of the limbs through different planes.[7]

In treating patients and athletes with chronic low-back pain, the program should focus on increasing the ability to stabilize the spine, reaching a level in the program where the patient can function without limitation from pain. Patients with low-back pain have been shown to develop an abnormal pattern of muscle contraction. The multifidi and transverse abdominis have been shown not to function correctly when low-back pain is present. During muscle contraction during anterior loading, the transverse abdominis is activated, first preventing unwanted trunk movement and then allowing the transition of energy and forces in a normal pattern of the kinetic chain. However, patients with low-back pain have demonstrated delayed activation of the transverse abdominis relative to the limbs.[6–8,12,23]

Core strengthening for low-back pain needs a focus on the muscles associated with twisting motion and repetitive flexion/extension motions. People with poor musculature control of the trunk and hips are often at greater risk for developing low-back pain due to abnormal or unstable transferences of forces when motion is occurring. Correction of this can help with improving function, allowing more stability for prevention of injury, and improving quality of life by decreasing pain.[6,23]

There is also a major role for core strengthening in athletes and the general public in promoting good health and preventing injuries. It has been a part of strengthening programs in athletes for years. Athletes generally progress through the first two stages over a period of time and eventually reach the third stage. The third stage then focuses on exercises for core strengthening in multiple planes on uneven/unstable surfaces, progressing to plyometrics. In athletes, greater explosive power is generated from the muscles and in multiple planes. Power may explode through one limb and needs to transfer motion through the core to other extremities. A conditioned core will allow the athlete to function at a superior level in balance, neuronal control, endurance, and strength.

This will result in the optimal amount of force throughout the kinetic chain while having a protective affect from future injury.[1,9]

CONCLUSION

In summary, the competitive athletic training program has become molded to have elements of a core strengthening program in it. As in the clinical vignette, it is evident that the athlete has deficiencies in his core, which have resulted in pain and a decreased level in participation. On follow-up, after entering into a core training program which was advanced to a plyometric level, he was pain-free, more conditioned, and participating at a higher level than he was previously to examination.

References

1. Nadler SF. Visual vignette: injury in a throwing athlete: understanding the kinetic chain. Am J Phys Med Rehabil 2004; 83(1):79.
2. Schuenke M, et al. Thieme atlas of anatomy, general anatomy and musculoskeletal system. New York: Thieme, 2006.
3. Netter, FH. Atlas of human anatomy, second edition. Canada: Icon Learning Systems LLC, 2001.
4. Akuthota V, Nadler SF. Core strengthening. Arch Phys Med Rehabil 2004; 85:S86–S92.
5. Norris CM. Abdominal muscle training in sport. Br J Sp Med 1993; 27(1): 19–27.
6. Callaghan JP, Patla AE, McGill SM. Low back three-dimensional joint forces, kinematics, and kinetics during walking. Clin Biomech 1999; 14:203–216.
7. Barr KP, Griggs M, Cadby T. Lumbar stabilization: core concepts and current literature, part 1. Am J Phys Med Rehabil 2005; 84:473–480.
8. Barr KP, Griggs M, Cadby T. Lumbar stabilization: a review of core concepts and current literature, part 2. Am J Med Rehabil 2007; 86: 72–80.
9. Nadler SF, Malanga GA, DePrince M, et al. The relationship between lower extremity injury, low back pain, and hip muscle strength in male and female college athletes. Clin J Sport Med 2000; 80:89–97.
10. Nadler SF, Malanga GA, Feinberg JH, et al. Relationship between hip muscle imbalance and occurrence of low back pain in collegiate athletes: a prospective study. Am J Phys Med Rehabil 2001; 80: 572–577.
11. Nadler SF, Malanga GA, Bartoli LA, et al. Hip muscle imbalance and low back pain in athletes: influence of core strengthening. Med Sci Sports Exerc 2002; 34:9–16.
12. Bliss LS, Teeple P. Core stability: the centerpiece of any training program. Curr Sports Med Rep 2005;4:179–183.
13. Keankaampaa M, Taimela S, Laaksonen D, et al. Back and hip extensor fatigability in chronic low back pain patients and controls. Arch Phys Med Rehabil 1998; 79:412–417.

14. Beckman SM, Buchanan TS. Ankle inversion injury and hypermobility: effect on hip and ankle muscle electromyography onset latency. Arch Phys Med Rehabil 1995; 76:1138–1143.
15. DeVita P, Hunter PB, Skelly WA. Effects of a functional knee brace on the biomechanics of running. Med Sci Sports Exerc 1992; 24:797–806.
16. Vleeming A, Pool-Goudzwaad AL, Stoeckart R, et al. The posterior layer of the thoracolumbar fascia: its function in load transfer from spine to legs. Spine 1995; 20:753–758.
17. Solomonow M, Zhou B, Harris M, et al. The ligamento-muscular stabilizing system of the spine. Spine 1998; 23:2552–2562.
18. Juker D, McGill S, Kropf P, Steffen T. Quantitative intramuscular myoelectric activity of lumbar portions of psoas and the abdominal wall during a wide variety of tasks. Med Sci Sports Exerc 1998; 30:301–310.
19. Hodges PW, Richardson CA. Delayed postural contraction of transversus abdominis in low back pain associated with movement of the lower limb. J Spinal Disord 1998; 11:46–56.
20. Panjabi M. The stabilizing system of the spine: I. function, dysfunction, adaptation and enhancement. J Spinal Disord 1992; 5:383–389.
21. Fredericson M. A Systematic approach to core strengthening for improved athletic improvement. Lecture handout, 2007.
22. Gilchrist RV, Frey ME, Nadler SF. Muscular control of the lumbar spine. Pain Physician 2003; 6:361–368.
23. Saal JA. Dynamic muscular stabilization in the nonoperative treatment of lumbar pain syndromes. Orthop Rev 1990; 19(8):691–700.

Chapter 11
Manual Medicine of the Hip and Pelvis

Charles W. Webb and Jayson Cannon

> *The important of injuries to the hip is too much overlooked. To the Sports Physician it should be a subject of the deepest throught.*
>
> A.T. Still

CLINICAL PEARLS

- Do not forget to treat sacroiliac joint and the lumbar spine. The supine direct articulatory technique for the lumbar spine is a quick, easy, and very low risk treatment.
- The six muscle groups of the pelvis are the adductors, abductors, external rotators, internal rotators, extensors, and flexors. Always look for a restriction of motion as a potential cause for the discomfort.
- Somatic dysfunction is impaired or altered the function of related components of the somatic (body framework) system: skeletal, arthrodial, and myofascial structures; and related vascular, lymphatic, and neural elements.
- Somatic dysfunction is found in areas where TART exists. (TART: tissue texture changes, asymmetry, restriction in motion, and tenderness)
- The minor motions, not the major motions, usually become restricted when somatic dysfunction occurs.

CASE

A 25-year-old married woman, a recreational runner presents herself to the office with the chief complaint of right hip pain. The pain has been present for 3 weeks, worse during her last run after

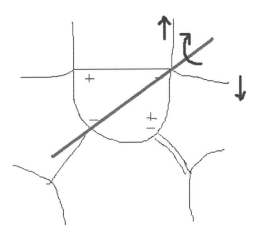

FIGURE 11.1. Graphic depiction of the case pelvic findings.

slipping off a curb awkwardly. The pain gets worse with activity and lightens during rest. She is currently training for a marathon. Her last menstrual period was within the last month. She is not pregnant and she uses oral contraception regularly. She is not taking any other medications other than an occasional acetaminophen or ibuprofen for headaches and menstrual pain. Her past medical and surgical histories are negative, and she has never been pregnant. She has no known allergies. She denies tobacco use of any kind, nor any illicit drugs. She admits to having an occasional glass of wine, and she drinks coffee in the mornings.

Physical examination reveals stable vital signs. She has a positive Ober's test on the right. Her popliteal angle is 140° bilaterally. She has a positive modified Thomas test on the right as well as a positive standing and seated flexion test on the right. She has mild tenderness over her right greater trochanter as well as the right sacroiliac (SI) joint. Her sacral sulcus is deep on the left, and the inferior lateral angle (ILA) of the sacrum is shallow on the right. She has good motion of the sacral base on the left, with none on the right and minimal motion of the right ILA. She has decreased internal and external rotation of the hip on the right compared to the left. Patrick/FABER test is negative. Her piriformis muscle is tight on the right with several noted tender points on both the right piriformis and psoas (Fig. 11.1).

X-rays of the hip and pelvis are negative for evidence of fracture, arthritis, and other boney abnormalities.

INTRODUCTION

How do you approach this patient and many more that present themselves to the sports clinic with hip pain? This is a very typical patient seen in many sports medicine clinics. They are usually athletes who are training for a specific event and have pushed themselves to the point where even the most benign mechanism of injury is enough to cause them to "fall off the edge" and have an injury that necessitates a significant decrease in training. The first step in evaluating a patient, with this type of presentation is to have a thorough systematic examination process to ensure an accurate pathoanatomic diagnosis. (SOR-C)

Hip pain/pelvis pain in the athlete can be from a multitude of problems. These problems range from simple greater trochanteric bursitis to fracture or abscess in the hip musculature (Table 11.1).[1-8]

The osteopathic and chiropractic philosophy embraces an approach to wellness through knowledge of interrelationships of structure and function, and a search for the cause of the patient's problems. When applied to addressing pain in the hip and pelvis, one must use a global approach to narrow the differential. Foot and lower extremity malalignment, joint restrictions, muscular imbalances, leg length discrepancy, and sport specific mobility abnormalities can all place abnormal loads on the hip and cause pain. Once the provider is confident that the cause of the problem is musculoskeletal, the search for dysfunction begins.[1,6,9]

In order to quickly and accurately diagnose hip dysfunction, the sports provider must understand the muscles and ligaments of the hip and pelvis, the lymphatic drainage patterns of the leg, the nerves of the lumbar and sacral plexi in addition to the sympathetic innervations and associated reflexes.

TABLE 11.1. Differential diagnosis for hip and pelvic pain

Visceral
  Endometriosis
  Pelvic inflammatory disease
  Ovarian cysts
  Pelvic vascular congestion
  Myofascial pain syndrome
  Irritable bowel syndrome
  Nephrolithiasis (bacterial/viral/inflammatory)
  Dysmenorrhea
  Inguinal hernia
  Femoral hernia
Somatic dysfunction
  Rotated inominate

Continued

TABLE 11.1 *Continued*

    Pubic shear
    Sacral shear
    Sacral torsion
    Inominate shear
    Lumbar segmental dysfunction
    Muscle restriction (abductors, adductors, external rotators, internal rotators, flexors, extensors)

Ligament sprains
    Sacrotuberous
    Sacrococcygeal
    Sacrospinous
    Ischiofemoral
    Iliolumbar

Muscle strains and tendonosis
    Piriformis
    Psoas
    Glutei
    Hamstrings
    Quadriceps
    Adductors

Structural
    Iliotibial band syndrome
    Lumbago
    Osteoarthritis
    Stress fracture
    Labral tear
    Synovitis
    Osteitis pubis
    Snapping hip syndrome
    Scoliosis
    Spondylolithesis
    Slipped capital epiphysis
    Congenital short leg
    Congenital asymmetry of the facets
    Inflammatory arthritis
    Apophyseal injury

FUNCTIONAL ANATOMY OF THE HIP AND PELVIS

The hip and pelvis are built for support and motion. Composed of the largest bones and muscles in the body they are the foundation for locomotion. The body's center of gravity is located in the pelvis, just anterior to the second sacral vertebra. Once the provider understands the anatomy of the hip and pelvis, it is easy to understand how dysfunction (decrease in motion) of the hip can produce not only lower extremity pain, but also low back pain, pelvic pain, and changes in the gait cycle that may lead to other pain syndromes.[4,10,11]

Functional anatomy relationships of the hip and pelvis are the key to determining the cause of the dysfunction and correcting it. The inominates articulate with the sacrum via the sacroiliac joints. The pubic symphysis acts as an anterior static bar providing stability to the pelvis during both ambulation and sitting. Tension on the ligaments, which cross the SI joint, can cause dysfunction in the leg. Patients with iliolumbar ligament strains often present thinking they have an inguinal hernia; however, the physical findings are not supportive. Somatic dysfunction of the sacrum, inominates, and lubosacral junction are common causes of hip and pelvic pain in active patients. In about 10% of patients the sciatic nerve divides before entering the gluteal region and the peroneal portion passes through the piriformis muscle; in less than 1% it will pass superior to the piriformis muscles. The piriformis muscle is found in the midpoint of a triangle made between the posterior superior iliac spine (PSIS), the coccyx, and the superior aspect of the greater trochanter (Fig. 11.2). When the composite sciatic nerve is compressed secondary to piriformis spasm, the superficial nerve bundles are mechanically irritated and the resultant pain can radiate down the leg, usually not below the knee. Pain from nerve root pressure usually radiates below the knee.[8,11-13]

The hip is the term for the composite of the inominate bone, the head of the femur, and the acetabular joint. The acetabulum of the inominate is composed of portions of the ilium, ischium, and the pubic bone. The femur travels along three axes in the hip joint. The transverse axis is where flexion (130°) and extension (35°) occur. Abduction (55°) and adduction (35°) occur along the anteroposterior (AP) axis, and internal rotation (35°) and external rotation (45°) occur along he longitudinal axis.

It is the minor motions, not the major motions that usually become restricted when somatic dysfunction occurs, and it is the compensations for these minor motion restrictions that become the issue over a period of time. Posterior and anterior glide of the femoral head in relation to internal and external rotation of the hip are the minor motions. Flexion, extension, abduction, and adduction are considered the major motions of the hip.[12,14-16]

As other chapters of this book focus on various treatments of the pelvis and hip in regards to sports medicine and primary

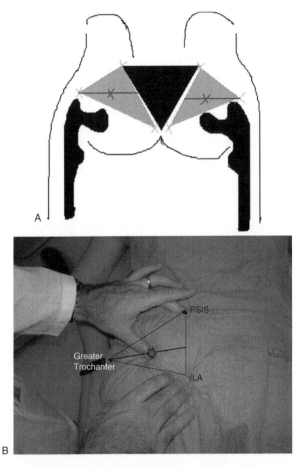

FIGURE 11.2. (**A**) Graphic depiction of the location of the piriformis muscle. (**B**) Location of the piriformis tender points.

care, this chapter will focus on manual medicine techniques. The use of manual therapy is an ancient healing form that has been documented as early as 2,700 B.C.[17] Osteopathic manipulation has been part of the mainstream medical establishment since 1872 when A. T. Still, MD opened the first osteopathic medical school in Kirksville, Missouri. In 1895 the first chiropractic school was opened by David Palmer.

MANIPULATION BASICS

Before we can discuss manual treatments, we must first understand some basics about manipulations. Osteopathic and chiropractic manipulations are forms of manual medicine that stress the need for normal and symmetrical motion in the joints. Osteopathic manipulations are done to enhance or restore motion in a joint. Chiropractic manipulations are done to enhance or restore alignment of the boney structures. By restoring motion to a joint and homeostasis to the tissues we are allowing the body to function in a more optimum state of health or well being. Regardless of the theory utilized, the goals are the same, to quickly return the athlete to the activity of choice safely. The growth of manual medicine has been fueled by patient outcome. The rise of modern-day manipulative medicine by osteopathic physicians, chiropractors, and physical therapists has come behind that of efficacy studies such as the RAND study by Dr. Paul Shekelle, who said: "Spinal Manipulation is the most commonly used conservative treatment for back pain supported by the most research evidence of effectiveness in terms of early results and long term effectiveness."(SOR = B).[18]

There are three general considerations that a provider must understand before deploying manual medicine as a treatment option: (1) One technique may treat more than one type of dysfunction; (2) More than one technique may be required to treat a single type of dysfunction; and (3) All techniques work best when applied to a specific diagnosis. The goals of treatment are to enhance the movement of body fluids, modify somatosomatic, viscerosomatic, and viscerosomatovisceral reflexes, provide maintenance treatment to irreversible conditions (osteoarthritis), and to mobilize articular restrictions.

METHODS OF MANIPULATION

There are three distinct methods of manipulation: direct, indirect, and combined. Direct is when the restrictive barrier is engaged in one or more planes of motion normal to the articulation so that the activating force applied may carry the dysfunctional component through the restrictive barrier. Indirect is when the provider moves the dysfunctional component away from the restrictive barrier (the direction that it wants to go) in one or more planes of motion normal to the articulation. The joint, structure, or tissue is moved to the point of balanced ligamentous tension or ease. Combined is a combination of direct and indirect methods. This method is most useful in treating myofascial tissues.

ACTIVATING FORCES

There are various activating forces that are used in treating somatic dysfunction. Many are beyond the scope of this text. If further reading is desired, please refer to the references at the end of this chapter. The activating forces discussed here will be discussed in detail in the treatment section of this chapter. *Patient cooperation* is an activating force that is required when treating dysfunction with strain/counter strain (treatment of tender points) and when using muscle energy. The patient is instructed to move his/her body in specific directions involving various planes of articulation to aid in the mobilizing of an area of restriction. In muscle energy techniques, the activating force is the *patient's contraction of muscles* in a specific direction against the physician's counterforce. A *physician guiding force* is exerted when the physician positions the patient away from the restrictive barrier to a point of release and then guides the tissue or joint somatic dysfunction through various positions that move with ease until the dysfunctional pathway has been completely retraced. *Springing* is also known as the low velocity moderate amplitude force: the provider makes contact upon the restrictive barrier and with variable degrees of force, springs the structure with intermittent pressures. High velocity low amplitude (HVLA) is used only with direct methods: the restrictive barrier is properly engaged to yield along one of the planes of a joint. A HVLA force is applied to move the joint or tissues through the restrictive barrier. An articulatory procedure is of a low velocity and low to a high amplitude technique where a joint is carried through its full range of motion.[9,14,19–22]

GOALS OF TREATMENT

The primary goal of treatment is to restore function to the tissues. Hypo or hyper mobility of a joint leads to muscle imbalance, altered movement, and eventually pain syndrome. The manual medicine approach is holistic in nature. The few contraindications to manual medicine are listed in Table 11.2.

TABLE 11.2. Contraindications to manipulation

Conditions
Fracture
Acute rheumatoid arthritis
Joint instability
Infection
Malignancy
Advanced neurological deficit/urinary incontinence
Severe osteoporosis

MANUAL MEDICINE TECHNIQUES

There are a plethora of manipulative techniques for the hip and pelvis in both chiropractic and osteopathic literature. Covering all of these techniques is not practical for this text. The techniques presented here are the authors' preferred techniques and the ones that they teach on a regular basis. Considerations for these techniques include the time involved in the clinic to perform, the ease of patient education, and the ease of teaching to other providers. We hope you find these techniques helpful.

Counterstrain[9,15,21]

Psoas

Indications for psoas strain include hip flexor contracture and anterior hip pain. The psoas tender points are routinely found just medial to the anterior superior iliac spine (ASIS), upon palpation. They are treated using a supine counter strain technique (Fig. 11.3.). The provider places his fingers on the tender points and then flexes the hip to fold the psoas around the tender point. This is the point where the pain from the tender point is gone or 80% of the tenderness is gone. Then the provider holds this position for approximately 90 seconds or until the tender point melts away under the provider's fingertips. Then the provider moves the legs back to the neutral position. This must be done passively to avoid re-aggravating the tender point. The premise is that the Golgi tendon apparatus of the muscle fibers are being reset.

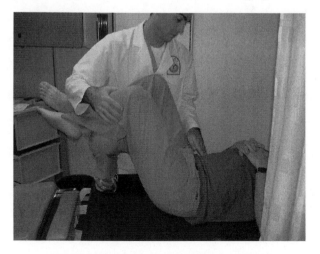

FIGURE 11.3. Treatment of psoas tender points.

Piriformis

Piriformis strains are restricted internal rotation and posterior hip pain. The piriformis tender points are treated in a similar fashion (Fig. 11.4), but the patient is in the prone position and the hip is extended and rotated to find the position of comfort. This is again held until the point melts away, approximately 90 seconds, then the hip is passively moved back to the neutral position.

Muscle Energy Techniques[15,20,22,23]

Anteriorly Rotated Inominate, or the Inferior Pubic Shear

Indications are osteitis pubis, groin strain, low back pain, hip or pelvic pain and restriction in hip extension.

Findings show that the ASIS is inferior, the pubic bone is inferior, and the PSIS is superior on the affected side. There is a positive flexion test on the affected side; the pelvic rock test will also be positive (restricted) on the affected side.

To treat, the patient is asked to lie supine on the table; the provider stabilizes the opposite ASIS with one hand then flexes the knee and the hip. The provider then leans on the patient's knee to flex and abduct the thigh to the barrier (ligamentous tension). The patient is instructed to push against the provider's equally

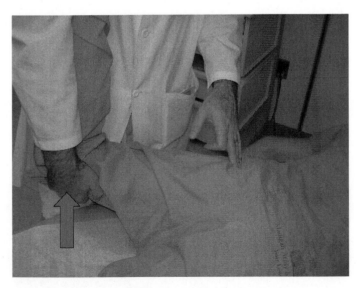

FIGURE 11.4. Treatment of piriformis tender points.

applied force for 3–5 s., then instructed to relax, pause, and asked to loosen up/ take up the slack. This is repeated 3–5 times or until the ASIS/pubes are equal.

Posterior Rotated Inominate, or Superior Pubic Shear

Indications are osteitis pubis, groin strain, low back pain, hip or pelvic pain and restriction in hip flexion.

Findings show the ASIS is superior, the pubic bone is superior, and the PSIS, is inferior on the affected side. There is a positive flexion test on the affected side; the pelvic rock test will also be positive (restricted) on the affected side.

The patient, while supine on the table, moves the affected side to the edge of the table and drops the involved leg off the side of the table. The clinician places one hand on the opposite ASIS to stabilize the pelvis and the other hand on the thigh just above the knee. The clinician extends the affected hip to the barrier (ligamentous tension) and has the patient push up against the counterforce for 3–5 s, pause, and take up the slack to reengage the barrier. This is repeated 3–5 times or until the ASIS/pubes are equal. The pressure needed from the patient is 8–10 pounds of force, so caution them not to throw you across the room.

SI Joint Dysfunction/Pubic Shear

Indications are osteitis pubis, groin strain, low back pain, hip/ pelvic pain, and SI joint pain from sacral dysfunction.

Findings include a positive flexion test on the side with the dysfunction. The pelvic rock test is positive. The pubic symphysis or the SI joint is tender to palpation at the sacral base or the lumbosacral junction.

To treat, the patient is asked to lie supine on the examination table. The knees and the hips are flexed to 90°. The clinician wraps his/her arm around the patient's knees and asks the patient to separate the knees with a strong effort. This will stretch the abductors and cause a loosening of the SI joint. Repeat this 3–5 times. With the patient in the same position, the clinician separates the patient's knees and places his/her forearm between the patient's knees with the hand on the knee and the elbow on the opposite knee. Then the patient is asked to push the knees together with a strong effort. This is an isometric contraction that should be held for 3–5 s and repeated 3–5 times. Then reassess for ASIS/pubes equality.

Restricted Hip Abduction

Indications are osteitis pubis, greater trochanteric bursitis, groin strain, hip pointer (contusion), and snapping hip syndrome (iliotibial band [ITB] tightness).

Findings show decreased range of motion in abduction of the hip compared to the uninvolved side.

For treatment, the patient is asked to lie supine on the examination table with the involved hip near the edge of the table. The provider stands between the patient's legs, lifts the involved leg with the caudal hand, and stabilizes the opposite ASIS with the cephalad hand. The patient adducts the leg against the provider's counterforce for 3–5 s. When the patient relaxes, the provider pauses and then reengages the barrier. Repeat 3–5 times, then reassess for increased symmetrical motion.

Restricted Hip Adduction
Indications are osteitis pubis, greater trochanteric bursitis, hip pointer, andsnapping hip syndrome.

Findings demonstrate a decreased range of motion in adduction of the hip compared to the uninvolved side.

For treatment, the patient is asked to lie supine on the examination table with the feet at the end of the table (Fig. 11.5). The provider lifts the involved leg at the proximal tibia and adducts it to the restrictive barrier. The patient abducts the leg against the provider's counterforce for 3–5 s. When the patient relaxes, the provider pauses then takes up the slack to reengage the barrier. Repeat the process 3–5 times and reassess for improved range of motion in adduction.

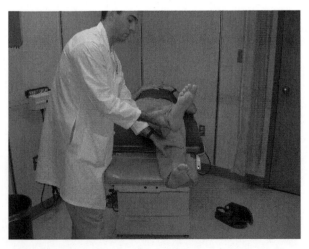

FIGURE 11.5. Treatment for restricted hip adduction.

Restricted Hip Extension
See anterior rotated inominate. The treatment techniques are the same as that for the anterior rotated inominate.

Restricted Hip Flexion
See posterior rotated inominate. The treatment techniques are the same as that for the posterior rotated inominate.

Restriction in Hip External Rotation
Indications include osteitis pubis, hip pointer, snapping hip syndrome, and tight internal rotators.

Findings show a decreased range of motion in external rotation of the hip.

To treat, the patient is asked to lie supine on the examination table with the affected hip flexed to 90° and the knee flexed to 90° (Fig. 11.6). The provider places his/her cephalad hand on the patent's knee and uses the caudad hand to apply force to the ankle, externally rotating the hip to the restrictive barrier. The patient is asked to push against the provider's hand to internally rotate the hip for 3–5 s. and then asked to relax. The provider pauses and takes up the slack to reengage the barrier. Repeat 3–5 times then reassess for improved range of motion.

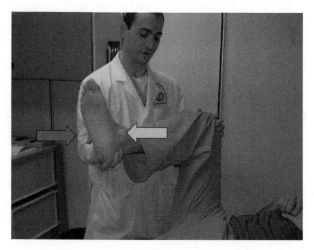

FIGURE 11.6. Treatment for restricted hip external rotation.

Restricted in Internal Rotation

Indications are osteitis pubis, hip pointer, snapping hip syndrome, and tight external rotators (piriformis).

Findings show a decreased range of motion in internal rotation and tight external rotators of the hip.

For treatment, the patient is asked to lie supine on the examination table with the affected hip and knee flexed to 90° (Fig. 11.7). The provider places his/her cephalad hand on the patient's knee and uses the caudad hand to apply force to the ankle, internally rotating the hip to the restrictive barrier. The patient is asked to push against the provider's hand to externally rotate the hip for 3–5 s., and then asked to relax. The provider will pause and then take up the slack to reengage the barrier. Repeat 3–5 times then reassess for improved range of motion.

Sacral Base Anterior

Indications include low back pain, pelvis pain, and hip pain.

On examination, sacral sulci are deep bilaterally, ILAs are level bilaterally, the sacral base will move anteriorly bilaterally, and the sacrotuberous ligaments are tight bilaterally.

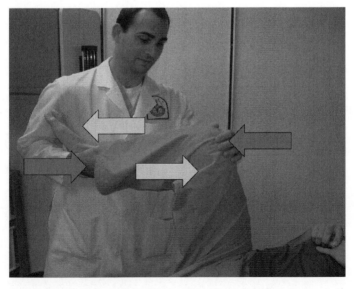

FIGURE 11.7. Treatment for restricted hip internal rotation.

For treatment, the patient is asked to lie supine on the table with both hips and knees flexed to the chest (Fig. 11.8). The provider places his/her hands on the sacral base bilaterally to monitor motion and asks the patient to push against the force for 3–5 s,

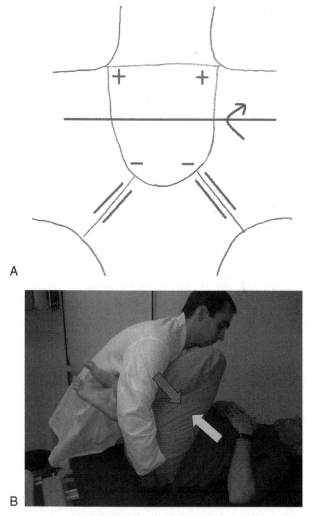

FIGURE 11.8. (**A**) Graphic depiction of exam findings for sacral base anterior treatment for sacral base anterior. (**B**) Treatment for sacral base anterior.

then asked to relax. The provider applies pressure to take up the slack and reengage the barrier. Repeat 3–5 times and then reassess for improved sacral positioning and motion.

Sacral Torsion About the Same Axis
Indications are low back pain, pelvic pain, hip pain, hip pointer, and snapping hip syndrome.

Findings reveal left rotation about a left oblique axis. They will be the opposite for a right-sided rotation on a right axis. Left ILA is posterior and inferior compared to the right. The left **PSIS** will be inferior; the right sacral sulcus will have motion and may be deeper than the left. The segmental examination of the lumbar spine will have an L5 sidebent left rotated right (SlRr) and the left sacrotuberous ligament will be tense with the right being loose.

To treat, the patient is placed prone on the examination table (Fig. 11.9). With the patient relaxed, have the patient move the hips so that the left hip is on the examination table and the knees and hips are flexed to 90°. The provider sits on a stool next to the table, supporting the patient's legs on the provider's thigh. The provider holds the patient's ankles and asks the patient to push them toward the ceiling for 3–5 s and then asked to relax. The provider applies a counterforce, then pauses and takes up the slack to reengage the barrier. The provider's other hand is monitoring the motion of the sacral base and inducing a left rotation of the spinous processes of L4–L5 vertebra. Repeat this process 3–5 times then reevaluate the sacrum for improved motion. This may be done on the right side for a right sacral torsion about a right oblige axis. This technique, when done with the patient supine to start, will treat a right rotation about a left oblique axis (Fig. 11.10).

High Velocity Low Amplitude Techniques[15,20,22,23]

Unilateral Sacral Shear, Superior Inominate Shear
Indications include low back pain, pelvic pain, SI joint pain, hip pain, and superior iliac shear.

On examination, one ILA is markedly inferior and posterior compared to the other. PSIS are usually equal, but may be superior on the affected side. The sacral base on the affected side may be anterior. Flexion and pelvic rock tests will be positive on the affected side.

To treat, the patient is placed supine with a small, rolled-up towel under the affected ILA (Fig. 11.11). From the end of the table, the provider grasps the affected lower extremity with both hands and abducts and internally rotates the hip to a point of the

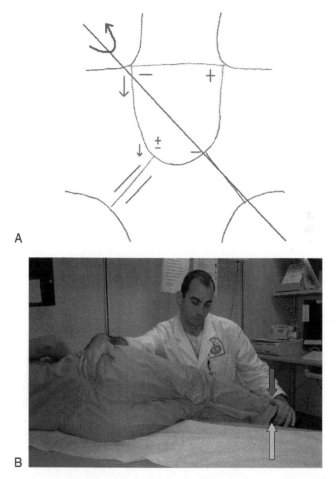

FIGURE 11.9. (**A**) Graphic depiction of exam findings for left sacral rotation about a left oblique axis. (**B**) Treatment of a left on left sacral torsion.

closed packed position. Gentle traction is applied along the long axis of the leg. The patient is asked to take a few deep breaths and exhale fully; at the end of the full exhalation the provider applies a short quick tug on the leg, taking care not to pull on the ankle itself. The leg is then returned to midline on the table and the patient is reexamined.

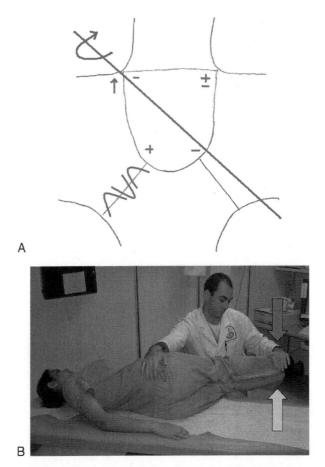

FIGURE 11.10. (**A**) Graphic depiction of exam findings for a right sacral rotation about a left oblique axis. (**B**) Treatment of a right on left sacral torsion.

Right Posterior Innominate
Indications are low back pain and SI dysfunction.

To treat, the patient is asked to lie on his/her side; the lower thigh and leg are straight and the upper thigh and leg are flexed (Fig. 11.12). The pelvis is brought toward edge of the table. The provider is anterior to the patient with the caudad hand making pisiform contact medial and inferior to the PSIS and the cephalad

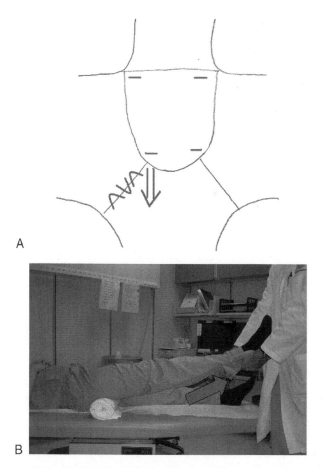

FIGURE 11.11. (**A**) Graphic depiction of exam findings for sacral shear. (**B**) Treatment for a unilateral sacral shear.

hand on the front of the shoulder. The caudad hand drives the PSIS anterior accompanied with a body drop.

Sacral Base Posterior
Indications include low back pain and SI joint pain. This condition is very common in the postpartum period.

On examination, the sacral sulci will be shallow bilaterally; there will be some motion at the ILAs bilaterally but not the sacral

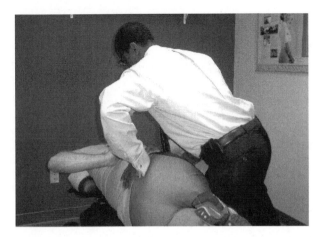

FIGURE 11.12. Treatment for right posterior innominate shear using a high velocity low amplitude (HVLA) technique.

base. The PSISs and ILAs are equal and the sacrotuberous ligaments are relaxed bilaterally.

To treat, the patient is placed prone on the examination table and is asked to rise up on their elbows (Fig. 11.13). The provider places the heel of one hand on the sacral base and the other hand on the lower extremity to stabilize the patient. Pressure is applied to the sacral base to engage the barrier. As the patient exhales a short quick thrust is applied to the sacral base. The sacrum is then rechecked.

Table Assisted Technique

Right Posterior Innominate
Patient is placed prone with the provider standing on either side of the table (Fig. 11.14). The provider's contact hand is on medial inferior aspect of the involved PSIS. The stabilization hand is on the inferior aspect of the ischial tuberosity on the uninvolved side. The thrust or line of correction is posterior to anterior with an inferior-to-superior aspect.

Articulatory Technique for the Lumbar Spine and the SI Joint[15]

Indications are low back pain, SI joint pain, and somatic dysfunction of the lumbar spine or pelvis.

Findings show lumbar segmental dysfunction, sacral rotation about a vertical axis, and a positive pelvic rock test on the involved side.

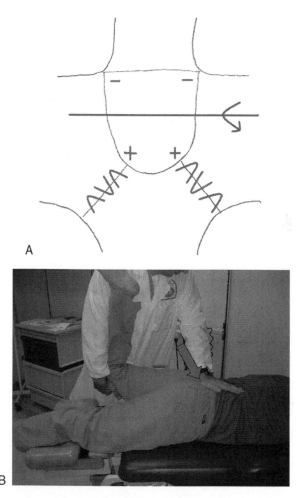

FIGURE 11.13. (**A**) Graphic depiction of exam findings for a sacral base posterior. (**B**) Treatment for a sacral base posterior.

With the patient supine on the table, the provider stands opposite to the side with the dysfunction (Fig. 11.15). The patient is asked to interlock their fingers behind their neck. The provider then will place the cephalad hand through the patient's opposite arm and rest the dorsum of their hand on the patient's sternum. (This technique is best for males; with female patients, place the cephalad hand through the patient's opposite arm and grasp the

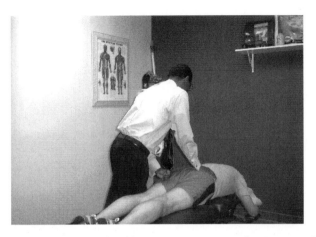

FIGURE 11.14. Treatment for right posterior innominate shear using a table assisted technique.

inferior angle of the scapula.) Place the heel of the caudal hand on the opposite ASIS to stabilize the pelvis. Have the patient take a deep breath. As the patient exhales the provider stands, inducing a stretch of the entire spine from the thoracic region to the SI joint. Popping sounds are commonly heard but should cause no alarm.

Stretching Techniques
Stretching of the hip and pelvis to maintain the motion that is restored via manipulation is imperative for long-term success. Below are the stretches that this author routinely teaches to the patients seen in his clinic. Patients must understand that stretching must become a part of their daily activities. These stretches are to be done in sets of three for 15 s each.[5,6,8,23]

Hamstrings (Semitendinosus, Biceps Femoris, Semimembranosus)
The patient stands with feet together. Keeping both knees fully extended, the patient slowly bends forward at the waist trying to place the palms on the ground. Hold this stretch for 15 s. and repeat three times. Then the patient crosses the right foot over the left foot and repeats, then the left foot over the right foot and repeats (Fig. 11.16).

Iliopsoas
The patient kneels on the right knee with the left foot forward on the floor, turning the right foot out to turn the right hip in

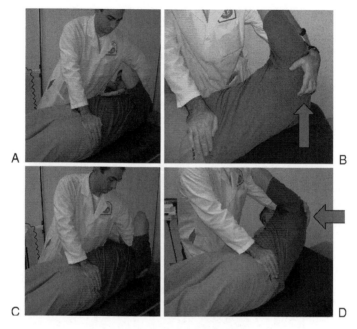

FIGURE 11.15. (**A**) Supine direct articulatory technique.

and leaning forward from the waist while keeping the back straight. The stretch should be felt in the front of the right hip (Fig. 11.17).

Quadriceps Femoris Stretch
The patient stands with the left hand supported on a stationary object to maintain balance. The right hand holds the right ankle. The patient pulls the right leg toward the buttocks keeping both knees together. The stretch is felt in the front of the right thigh. Repeat for the left leg (Fig. 11.18).

Iliotibial Band Stretch
The patient stands perpendicular to and 2–3 feet from a door or wall with the right hand on the wall for support and the right leg behind the left leg. As the provider pushes down on the left hip, a stretch is felt in the lateral right thigh as the patient

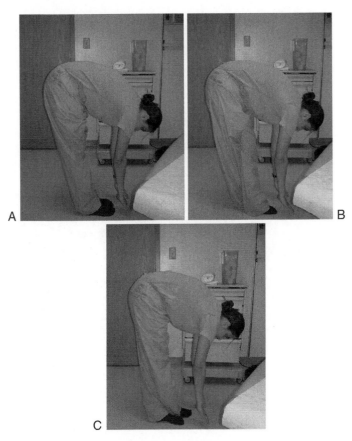

FIGURE 11.16. (**A**) Hamstring stretch (*straight leg hang*). (**B**) Hamstring stretch (*left over right*). (**C**) Hamstring stretch (*right over left*).

pushes the right hip toward the junction of the wall and the floor (Fig. 11.19).

Gluteal Stretch (Figure 4 Stretch)
The patient lies supine on the table. The ipsilateral lower extremity is flexed, abducted, and externally rotated to place the ankle on the opposite thigh just above the knee. The opposite hip is flexed with the knee bent by the patient reaching up and grapping the leg at mid-thigh. The stretch is felt with the patient pulling the leg to their chest (Fig. 11.20).

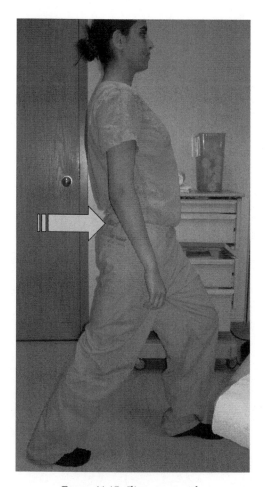

FIGURE 11.17. Iliopsoas stretch.

Piriformis Stretch
This, stretch is similar to the gluteal stretch, but instead of placing the ankle just above the knee, when the legs are crossed, place the knee on just above the opposite knee, and then pull the leg toward the chest.

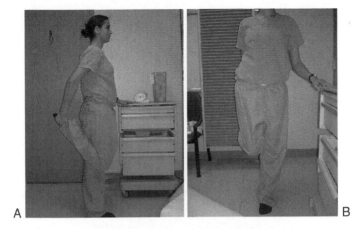

FIGURE 11.18. Quadriceps stretch.

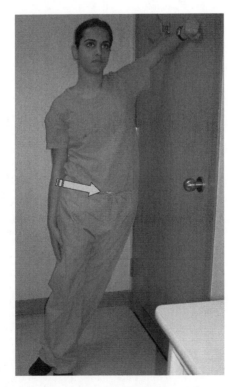

FIGURE 11.19. Iliotibial band stretch.

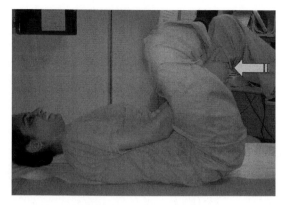

FIGURE 11.20. Gluteal stretch.

Doctor-Assisted Resisted Piriformis Stretch
The patient lies supine on the table. The involved lower extremity is flexed and crossed over the contralateral extremity. The involved side is internally rotated with the doctor resisting the patient's external rotation by standing on the ipsilateral side with his hand resisting external rotation. This stretch should be held for 20 s. and is usually done 2–3 times per leg (Fig. 11.21).

Groin Stretch
With the patient sitting up with feet together and knees bent, separate the knees to feel the stretch in the groin and inner thighs (Fig. 11.22).

SUMMARY

The patient was found to have iliotibial band syndrome, as her pain was exacerbated shortly into her run, then would dissipate shortly after stopping. She had a positive Ober's test and tenderness over the greater trochanter on the right; she also has a right on right sacral torsion. X-rays of the hip and pelvis are negative for evidence of fracture, arthritis, and other bony abnormalities. She was treated with manipulation to include the ones listed above and did very well. She was given a stretching program and to follow up in 3 weeks. Upon returning in 3 weeks she was able to run without difficulty and was able to complete her goal; running the Portland Marathon.

These are but a few of the large variety of manual medicine techniques that have been described in both the chiropractic and osteopathic literature. Manual medicine or manipulative medicine

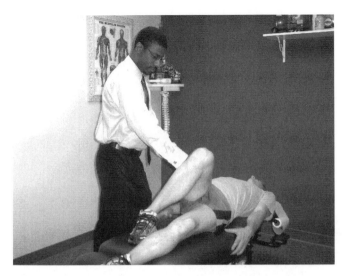

Figure 11.21. Doctor-assisted resisted piriformis stretch.

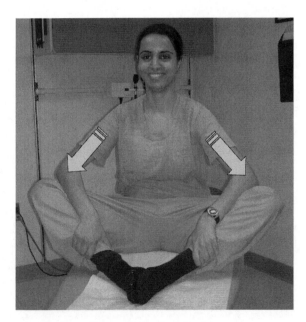

Figure 11.22. Groin stretch.

or adjustments are all plays on a tool that is found in several physicians bags. It is but another method of evaluating and treating the athlete not only in one's clinic but also on the field, court, or track, or anywhere else that athletes find themselves in competition. Manual medicine techniques have been found to be effective in the treatment of a variety of musculoskeletal as well as visceral ailments. So regardless of one's training, be it allopathic, osteopathic or chiropractic, the sports minded provider that practices manual medicine has the ability to lay on hands, help restore motion to an area of the body, improve alignment for optimal performance, and above all do no harm.

References

1. Tettambel MA. An osteopathic approach to treating women with chronic pelvic pain. JAOA 2005; 105: S20–S22.
2. Pedowitz RN. Use of Osteopathic Manipulative Treatment for Iliotibial Band Friction Syndrome. JAOA 2005; 105: 563–567.
3. Patriquin DA. Pain in the lateral hip, inguinal, and anterior thigh regions; differential diagnosis. JAOA 1972; 71: 729.
4. Anderson K, Strickland SM, Warren R. Current Concepts: Hip and Groin Injuries in Athletes. Am J Sports Med 2001; 29: 521–533.
5. Adkins SB, Figler RA. Hip Pain in Athletes. Am Fam Physician 2000; 61: 2109–2118.
6. Morelli V, Smith V. Groin Injuries in Athletes. Am Fam Physician 2001; 64: 1405–1413.
7. O'Kane JW. Anterior Hip Pain. Am Fam Phys 1999; 60(6): 1687–1696.
8. Retzlaff EW, Berry AH, Haight AS, et al. The Piriformis Muscle Syndrome. JAOA 1974; 73: 799–807.
9. Ward RC, ed. Foundations for Osteopathic Medicine. Baltimore: Williams & Wilkins, 1997.
10. Beal MC. The sacroiliac problem: review of anatomy, mechanics, and diagnosis. JAOA 1982; 81: 667.
11. Torry MR, Schenker ML, Martin HD, et al. Neuromuscular Hip Biomechanics and Pathology in the Athlete. Clin Sports Med 2006; 25(2):177–197.
12. Braly BA, Beall DP, Martin HD. Clinical Examination of the Athletic Hip. Clin Sports Med 2006; 25(2):199–210.
13. TePoorten BA. The Piriformis Muscle. JAOA 1969; 69: 150.
14. Kuchera WA, Kuchera ML. Osteopathic Principles in Practice. Kirksville, MO: KCOM Press; 1994.
15. Greenman PE, ed. Principles of Manual Medicine 3rd edition. Philadelphia: Lippincott Williams & Wilkins, 2003.
16. Fuller DB. Osteopathic medical component missed in treating anterior hip pain. JAOA 1997; 97: 514.
17. Gardner S, Mosby JS. Chiropractic Secrets. Philadelphia: Hanley & Belfus; 2000:231.

18. Shekelle, PG, Adams AH, Chassin MR, et al. The Appropriateness of Spinal Manipulation for Low Back Pain. Monograph No. R-4025/2-CCR/FCER. Santa Monica, CA: RAND/UCLA; 1991.
19. Rumney IC. Techniques for determining, and ultimately modifying, areas of restricted motion in the lumbar spine and pelvis. JAOA 1971; 70: 1203.
20. Kimberly PE. Outline of Osteopathic Manipulative Procedures; The Kimberly Manual, Millennium Edition. Marceline, MO: Walsworth Publishing, 2000.
21. DiGiovanna EL, Schiowitz S, ed. An Osteopathic Approach to Diagnosis and Treatment. Philadelphia: JB Lippincott; 1991.
22. Howard WH. Easy OMT. Ashville: C-4 Publishing; 1998.
23. Karageanes SJ, ed. Principles of Manual Sports Medicine. Philadelphia: Lippincott Williams & Wilkins; 2005.

Chapter 12
Taping and Bracing for Pelvic and Hip Injuries

Scott A. Magnes, Lance Ringhausen, and Peter H. Seidenberg

CLINICAL PEARLS

- There is little research available regarding the use of athletic taping and bracing for the hip and pelvis.
- The disadvantages of using athletic tape are the expense, the difficulty of application, and possible skin irritation.
- Tape's effectiveness at decreasing joint motion lessens after 30 min.
- Further research is needed to determine if compression shorts are able to prevent injury or enhance athletic performance.

CASE STUDY

A 20-year-old female collegiate goalie presents herself to the athletic training clinic for the evaluation of right lateral hip pain. The pain started a day earlier when she dove and landed on the lateral aspect of her right hip in order to block a shot. She complains of pain in that area exacerbated by hip abduction.

On examination, there is edema overlying the greater trochanter but no ecchymosis is present. She has full passive range of motion of the hip and resisted abduction increases pain in the area of the greater trochanter. Log roll is negative. Ober test is negative but produces pain in the area of the greater trochanter. There is no pelvic obliquity noted. She is neurovascularly intact.

INTRODUCTION

Taping has been utilized since ancient Roman times and was first introduced to organized sports in the 1890s in college athletics.

Although the ankle is the most common joint taped and the most often studied, athletic taping techniques are used for nearly all body parts, including the shoulder, elbow, wrist, hand, fingers, knee, foot, and hip. To date, research has been focused mainly on taping for the ankle, wrist, hand, and knee joints. Unfortunately, there are very little data regarding the hip and pelvis to guide clinicians in its potential use in these areas.

INDICATIONS FOR TAPING

Athletic taping techniques can be utilized after acute injury, for rehabilitation from injury, for injury prophylaxis, or for functional purposes. In general, taping is performed with the involved joint in a neutral position to limit the range of motion. Compressive taping techniques are used for an acute injury to limit joint motion and control edema. Tape may be applied during return to activity to protect the injured joint from further damage.

EFFICACY OF TAPING

Originally, it was postulated that taping techniques could hold bones rigidly in approximation and, consequently, prevent injury to the associated ligament. However, research has proven that the effect of taping is mostly proprioceptive.[1–7] Radiographic studies showed that the affected bones do not maintain the same relationship in a weight-bearing dynamic position as they do in the non-weight-bearing static position after taping,[8] disproving this theory. Contrary to most athletes' beliefs, tape's effectiveness at restricting joint motion is decreased within 30 minutes of the onset of physical activity.[9,10] These undesirable changes were attributed to perspiration and loosening or stretching of the tape during weight-bearing activities.

DRAWBACKS

Although widely utilized, athletic taping has several obvious drawbacks.[6] For example, a trained individual is required to correctly apply the tape to the affected body part. Also, since the tape cannot be recycled after application, costs may be high. Frequent reapplication of tape can lead to skin irritation.

TYPES OF TAPE

There are many different types of athletic tape. The most commonly used is Zonus. Other commonly used tape types include Elasticon, Elastoplast, Blister Tape, Leukotape, Cover Roll, and Kinesiotex (Kinesiotape). Except Kinesiotex, the tape is generally applied over a foam-like material called underwrap, or prewrap.

The purpose of the prewrap is to protect the skin from the adhesive backing of the tape. In order to provide better adherence, a tacky substance (e.g., Tuf-Skin spray adherent) is often applied to the skin prior to the application of the underwrap.

Kinesiotape was invented by Kenzo Kase, D.C. in Japan. Kase attended chiropractic school in the United States, but practiced in Japan. He invented Kinesiotape in an effort to decrease pain and edema, assist in muscle function, and improve joint function. Kinesiotape was first utilized on Japanese Olympic volleyball players in the 1980s and now is commonly utilized in all professional sports in Japan. It is also very commonly utilized in the nonathletic population in that country. It was first introduced in the United States in 1995.

The theory behind the mechanism of action of Kinesiotape is based on augmenting the body's natural healing processes. The tape is flexible and has physical properties that affect the neurologic, proprioceptive, musculoskeletal, and lymphatic systems. Unlike traditional taping methods that employ compression to control edema, Kinesiotape is applied to the surface of the skin to facilitate lymphatic drainage. It is purported that the elasticity of the tape allows the skin to be gently lifted directly under the tape to facilitate extracellular fluid drainage. Kase and Hashimoto utilized Doppler ultrasound to measure fluid flow in patients with and without circulatory insufficiency. They found that there is an increase in flow after application of Kinesiotape and were unable to demonstrate any adverse effects from its use.[11,12]

Kinesiotape has also been utilized successfully in the treatment of muscle injuries. Its mechanism of action is purported to be much different from that of traditional athletic taping techniques. The tape has an elastic component that will attempt to recoil, once applied. Therefore, application of tape from the origin of the muscle to its distal insertion helps facilitate muscle function. When placed in the opposite direction, Kinesiotape has a tendency to inhibit or decrease muscle activity. This distinction is extremely important clinically, when utilizing Kinesiotape for rehabilitation of any musculoskeletal injury. Studies have been conducted measuring electromyographic muscle activity with the tape applied in each direction confirming that there is more electromyographic activity when the tape is applied in the facilitatory role and less electromyographic activity when it is applied for muscle inhibition.[11,12]

Kinesiotape is manufactured to mimic the thickness, weight, and elasticity of human skin. Kinesiotape has an elastic component that allows it to stretch 30–40% beyond its original length.[13]

The adhesive is heat activated and allows the tape to function for several days without reapplication. It is also water resistant, such that it can be worn in a pool, shower, or bath without coming off. Kinesiotape is designed to "breathe" and also functions to remove sweat from the surface of the skin. It causes fewer skin reactions than conventional tape. The tape contains no latex and is hypoallergenic. It is available in different colors including neutral, blue, and pink. As per Eastern medicine theory, pink absorbs more light and generates a warming effect while blue reflects light and produces a cooling effect.[6] Unlike conventional tape, Kinesiotape can be cut lengthwise without losing any of its unique properties.

TAPING TECHNIQUES

Numerous taping techniques have been purported to be efficacious in the treatment and prevention of injury about the hips and pelvis (Fig. 12.1.). Some examples of injuries/ conditions in which taping/ bracing have been utilized include greater trochanteric bursitis, iliac crest contusion (hip pointer), and osteoarthritis of the hip.

BRACING

Bracing has several advantages over taping. Its use does not require any special expertise and there is no repeated expense as with each reapplication of tape (Fig. 12.2). The effectiveness of bracing compared to taping has been researched by several authors and no significant differences were found in the injured joint. Yet bracing and taping both increased the effectiveness of proprioceptive feedback and when studied were found to have a reduction in muscle action while landing. [2,7,10,14]

Compression Shorts

One common brace utilized in sports for injury prevention and rehabilitation about the hip and pelvis is compression shorts. It has become increasingly popular during the last decade despite little research to support its efficacy. Light compression materials (i.e., Spandex) have not been found to hinder performance.[1,15] While no increase in single maximal jump power was noted, compression shorts did help maintain higher jumping power during repeated vertical jumping exercise.[15]

Performance and proprioception at the hip with the use of elasticized compression shorts that offer considerably more compression and resistance to movement than conventional compression shorts have been studied. Their use did not limit performance on any measures except active range of motion during hip flexion.[16,17]

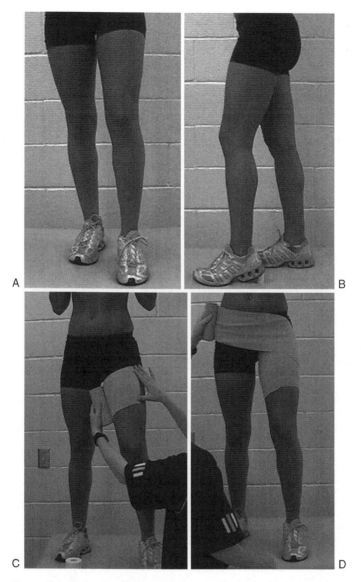

FIGURE 12.1. Hip spica technique. (**A**) Place a 1–2 inch object under the heel to slightly flex the hip. (**B**) Lateral view of 12.1a. (**C**) Using a 6-in., double-length elastic bandage, wrap lateral to medial on the involved side at a slight downward angle. (**D**) Wrap the bandage around the involved side and cross the anterior hip. (**E**) Wrap the bandage around the back of the patient and around the anterior aspect of the involved side. (**F**) Continue across the anterior aspect of the hip.

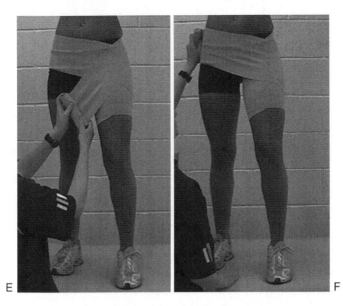

FIGURE 12.1. Continued.

There is scientific evidence that movement of skin overlying activated muscle triggers cutaneous receptors to send proprioceptive information to the brain;[2,9] however, there was no increased proprioception at the hip noted with the use of the compression shorts.[17] Subjective data revealed over 93% of subjects felt the shorts were supportive, although its proper fit was an issue.[17] Doan et al.[16] found countermovement vertical jump height and 60-m. sprint times to be enhanced with the use of neoprene and rubber compression shorts which provided compression similar to those used in the previous study. Further research is needed to delineate if compression shorts offer any enhancement to athletic performance or efficacy in prevention of injury.

CASE CONCLUSION
The patient was diagnosed with traumatic greater trochanteric bursitis. Ice and analgesics were used for pain control. The athlete was advised to wear compression shorts and hip spica taping was performed during practice and competition. This treatment provided her with more confidence in hip movement but did not decrease her pain. Her symptoms completely resolved after 2 weeks.

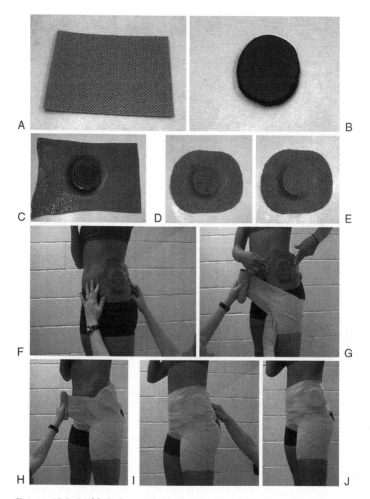

FIGURE 12.2. Molded thermoplastic protection of the hip. (**A**) Select an appropriate thermoplastic material. (**B**) Half-inch high density foam. (**C**) Place the heated thermoplastic material over the foam. (**D**) Cut the thermoplastic material to appropriate size. (**E**) Remove the foam from the thermoplastic material. (**F**) Place the thermoplastic material over the involved side. (**G–I**) Using a hip spica technique, wrap the mold to the patient. (**J**) Secure the elastic bandage with white athletic tape.

References

1. Kraemer WJ, Bush JA, Triplett-McBride NT, et al. Compression garments: Influence on muscle fatigue. J Strength Cond Res 1998; 12:211–215.
2. Simoneau GG, Denger RM, Cramper CA, Kittleson KH. Changes in ankle joint proprioception resulting from strips of athletic tape applied over the skin. J Athl Train 1997; 32:141–147.
3. Carmines DV, Nunley JA, McElhaney JH. Effects of ankle taping on the motion and loading pattern of the foot for walking subjects. J Orthop Res 1988; 6:223–229.
4. Cordova ML, Ingersoll CD, LeBlanc MJ. Influence of ankle support on joint range of motion before and after exercise: a meta-analysis. J Orthop Sports Phys Ther 2000; 30:170–182.
5. Refshauge KM, Kilbreath SL, Raymond J. The effect of recurrent ankle inversion sprain and taping on prorioception at the ankle. Med Sci Sports Exerc 2000; 32:10–15.
6. Kase K. Illustrated Kinesiotaping, 3rd ed. Albuquerque: Universal Printing and Publishing; 1994.
7. Hopper DM, McNair P, Elliott BC. Landing in netball: Effects of taping and bracing the ankle. Br J Sports Med 1999; 33:109–113.
8. Cameron MH. Patellar taping in the treatment of patellofemoral pain. A Prospective randomized study. Am J Sports Med 1997; 25:417.
9. Moberg, E. The role of cutaneous afferents in position sense, kinaesthesia, and motor function of the hand. Brain 1983; 106:1–19.
10. MacKean LC, Bell G, Burnham RS. Prophylactic ankle bracing versus taping: Effects on functional performance in female basketball players. J Orthop Sports Phys Ther1995; 22:77–81.
11. Kinesio-taping Association. Kinesio-taping Perfect manual. Albuquerque: Universal Printing and Publishing; 1998.
12. Karlsson J, Sward L, Adreason GO. The affect of taping on ankle stability. Practical implications. Sports Med 1993; 16:210–215.
13. Burke WS, Bailey C. Believe the hype. Physical therapy products. July/August 2002.
14. McGaw ST, Cerullo JF. Prophylactic ankle stabilizers affect ankle joint kinematics during drop landings. Med Sci Sports Exerc 1999; 31:702–707.
15. Kraemer WJ, Bush JA, Bauer JA, et al. Influence of compression garments on vertical jump performance in NCAA Division I volleyball players. J Strength Cond Res 1006; 10:180–183.
16. Doan BK, Kwon Y-H, Newton RU, et al. Evaluation of a lower-body compression garment. J Sports Sci 2003; 21:601–610.
17. Bernhardt T, Anderson GS. Influence of moderate prophylactic compression on sports performance. J Strength Cond Res 2005; 19(2):292–297.

Chapter 13
Nonsurgical Interventions

Michael D. Osborne and Tariq M. Awan

CLINICAL PEARLS

- Given their relative safety, the ease of use in trained hands, and cost-effectiveness, injection therapies can be beneficial when more conservative treatment measures have failed.
- Injection therapies containing local anesthetics may help confirm a diagnosis, particularly when performed with the precision of image guidance.
- Informed consent should be obtained for all procedures and should include a discussion regarding the indications, anticipated outcome, potential risks and complications, possible side effects, and alternatives to the procedure.
- It is incumbent on the proceduralist to have a thorough understanding of the relevant anatomy, procedural technique, potential risks, and procedural contraindications and to be prepared to manage any unforeseen complications prior to attempting injection therapies.
- Injection therapies are very rarely indicated as first-line treatment.

CASE PRESENTAION

A 24-year-old male recreational basketball player presented himself with right hip and groin pain of 2 months duration. The patient was playing basketball and landed awkwardly on his right leg. He subsequently developed progressive pain with activity, sharp in quality and predominantly over the anterior hip with radiation to the groin. He denied any mechanical catching or locking. He was unable to run or play basketball without discomfort. Pain could be relieved by laying supine with his hip and knee flexed. Mild relief was obtained with nonsteroidal anti-inflammatory drugs (NSAIDs) and physical therapy.

Physical Examination
- Normal appearance, gait, and station.
- Normal strength, reflexes, and full hip range of motion.
- Tenderness over iliopsoas at the pelvic brim, and hip adductors.
- FABER test negative; Stinchfield test positive.
- Passive hip extension, internal rotation, and adduction caused discomfort but did not reproduce the typical pain.
- Modified Thomas test was positive for anterior hip pain.

Differential Diagnosis
- Hip adductor strain
- Iliopsoas bursitis/tendonitis
- Hip labral tear
- Snapping hip syndrome
- Osteitis pubis
- Sports hernia/athletic pubalgia
- Femoral/pelvic stress fracture

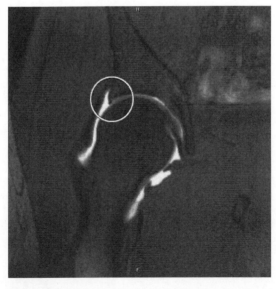

FIGURE 13.1. MRI arthrogram of the hip demonstrating a small superior labral tear.

Imaging
- Plain radiographs were unremarkable.
- Magnetic resonance imaging (MRI) arthrogram demonstrated a small linear extension of contrast beneath the superior acetabular labrum compatible with labral detachment (Fig. 13.1).

INTRODUCTION

The aim of this chapter is to provide an overview of some of the more common injection therapies for sports-related disorders of the hip and pelvis. Additionally, we provide technical instruction that will allow the interested clinician an opportunity to learn basic office-based procedures.

The principal form of injection therapies involves the use of a combined corticosteroid and anesthetic injection into or around a symptomatic musculoskeletal structure. The use of cortisone was first reported in 1949 by a team of physicians at the Mayo Clinic[1] and resulted in a Nobel Prize in 1950. Since 1950, the injection of corticosteroid has been applied to a plethora of musculoskeletal conditions with varied efficacy.

Although corticosteroid injections are an exceedingly common form of treatment applied today, their role in symptomatic management of sports injuries remains a topic of some controversy. Prospective, randomized, controlled studies support their use in disorders such as osteoarthritis of the hip and knee.[2,3] However, one should not automatically conclude that these results can be generalized to all musculoskeletal conditions.

In addition to corticosteroids and local anesthetics, proliferative therapy (prolotherapy) and viscosupplementation (injection of hyaluronic acid compounds) have been investigated as treatments for injured athletes. Preliminary studies have shown effectiveness for select musculoskeletal conditions and provide promise for further randomized, clinical controlled studies.[4-7]

RATIONALE FOR USE

Given their relative safety, ease of use in trained hands, and cost-effectiveness, injection therapies can be a very useful modality when more conservative treatment measures have failed. Prior to performing any type of injection, the clinician must have a thorough understanding of the regional anatomy as well as procedural contraindications and precautions. The proceduralist must also have a thorough understanding of the various injection constituents and their potential side effects.

DIAGNOSTIC INJECTIONS

Injection therapies containing local anesthetics can be helpful in establishing a diagnosis when performed with precision. The rationale is that one can identify a symptomatic nociceptive structure by infiltrating it with a local anesthetic. Examples include intra-articular injections (hip, sacroiliac joint, pubic symphysis), soft tissue injections (bursa and peritenon infiltration), and peripheral nerve blocks (such as lateral femoral cutaneous nerve block).

To reduce the incidence of false positive responses one must use a small enough volume of injectate, such that it will only anesthetize the targeted nociceptive structure. Otherwise, the anesthetic may diffuse to nearby tissues and cause pain relief by inadvertent effect on structures not targeted in the procedure.

Image guidance can be used to significantly increase the accuracy of reaching the desired target tissue and thereby enhance diagnostic accuracy. Image guidance is highly recommended when performing diagnostic injections (SOR-A). Increasingly, ultrasound is being used in office-based sports medicine practices to help guide injection therapies.[8,9] Ultrasound can be particularly helpful when trying to localize peripheral nerves and musculature for diagnostic block.[10] One advantage of ultrasound is that during the injection, additional relevant pathology such as hip joint effusion, bursitis, or tendinopathy may be visualized which may impact what structures are ultimately targeted during the procedure. One potential limitation, however, is the lack of penetration in large patients, which may limit visualization of deeper tissues. Additionally, it takes considerable training and experience with diagnostic ultrasound to use this method of image guidance effectively (written communication, Jay Smith, MD, April 2007).

Fluoroscopy is the standard method of image guidance used in pain clinics, interventional radiology suites, and large sports medicine practices. Accurate placement of the procedural needle can be directly visualized under fluoroscopic guidance. With the injection of a radiopaque contrast media, one can confirm the injection has reached the target tissue. Furthermore, the use of contrast can identify vascular uptake when injections are being performed near blood vessels such as during nerve blocks. This reduces false negative responses (through inadvertent vascular injection) and guards against systemic toxicity when performing large-volume field blocks.

Diagnostic blocks can also be performed with great accuracy using computed tomography (CT) and MRI guidance;[11] however, this is rarely necessary if ultrasound or fluoroscopy are available to the experienced proceduralist (SOR-B).

An additional diagnostic application of injection therapies is aspiration and analysis of joint effusions. Joint fluid analysis can differentiate among various pathophysiologies such as infection, gout, pseudo gout, inflammation, and hemorrhage.

THERAPEUTIC INJECTIONS

The purpose of therapeutic injections is principally to improve pain and allow for restoration of function. The precise effect of each procedure depends on the structure injected and the pharmacologic agent utilized.

PHARMACOLOGICAL AGENTS

Corticosteroids

Corticosteroid preparations are the most commonly utilized injectate because of their effects as potent inhibitors of inflammation. They modify the local inflammatory response through stabilization of lysosomal membranes, inhibition of cellular metabolism (e.g., neutrophil chemotaxis and function), inhibition of polymorphonuclear leukocyte membrane microtubular function, and establishment of decreased local synovial permeability. Corticosteroids can also increase the viscosity of synovial fluid, alter production of hyaluronic acid synthesis, and change synovial fluid leukocyte activity,[12] all of which may improve symptoms secondary to degenerative, inflammatory and overuse syndromes.

Though many different preparations are available for joint and soft tissue injections, corticosteroids differ with respect to potency, solubility, and relative duration of action. The relative potency of individual corticosteroids is compared in Table 13.1. Few studies

TABLE 13.1. Relative potency of corticosteroid preparations

Corticosteroid	Relative anti-inflammatory potencies	Equipotent doses (in mg)
Cortisone	0.8	25
Hydrocortisone	1.0	20
Prednisone	4	5
Methylprednisolone acetate (Depo-Medrol)	5	4
Dexamethasone sodium phosphate (Decadron)	25	0.6
Betamethasone (Celestone Soluspan)	25	0.6

Adapted from: Cardone and Tallia[13]

have investigated the duration of action of corticosteroid agents in joints or soft tissues. In general, the duration of effect is inversely related to the solubility of the therapeutic agent. The less soluble agents remain in the joint or soft tissue longer and provide more prolonged effect. Nevertheless, shorter acting solutions are less irritating to the joint space and less likely to produce a post-injection pain flare. Agents with low solubility should be used primarily for intra-articular therapy and should be avoided in soft tissues due to the increased risk of soft tissue atrophy from prolonged local corticosteroid action.

Hyaluronic Acid

Intra-articular injection of hyaluronic acid is used to treat the pain associated with osteoarthritis of the knee with several randomized controlled studies showing reasonable efficacy.[14] The rationale for the use of hyalurons therapeutically is based on observations that hyaluronic acid is an important component of synovial fluid that acts as a cushion and lubricant for the joint (**SOR-A**). It serves as a major component of the extracellular matrix of the cartilage, helping to enhance the ability of cartilage to resist shear forces and maintain a resiliency to compression.[15] A limited number of studies suggest that injections with hyaluronic acid may also benefit people with osteoarthritis of the hip.[6] However, in the absence of placebo-controlled studies, the efficacy of hyaluronic acid injections or its derivatives in the symptomatic treatment of hip osteoarthritis cannot be determined conclusively.

Anesthetics

Local anesthetics can assist in identification of a symptomatic nociceptive structure by producing a rapid reduction in pain following injection/infiltration. Typically however, when performing intra-articular and soft tissue injections an anesthetic is usually mixed with a corticosteroid. Not only does this provide temporary analgesia and confirm delivery of the medication to the symptomatic structure, it dilutes the crystalline suspension of the corticosteroid and thus provides better diffusion of medication throughout the injected region. An allergic reaction to the amide local anesthetics such as lidocaine and bupivacaine is very rare.

Lidocaine

For most procedures 1% lidocaine is frequently used due to its rapid onset of action. However, because of its short half-life, lidocaine's duration of effect is short (1–2 h).[12] At high concentrations lidocaine (5%) is neurotoxic to local peripheral nerves and thus it can be used as a form of peripheral neurolysis.[16] Systemic toxicity would be rare in a standard sports medicine practice. The toxic effects of local anesthetics are highly dependent on the route of injection and the rapidity of absorption or uptake into the local vasculature.[17] Intra-articular and most soft tissue injections are not heavily vascularized, thus reducing the chance of central toxicity.

Bupivacaine
When longer acting local analgesia is desired, the use of an agent such as bupivicaine is preferable because of its duration of effect of 3–6 h.[18] However, bupivacaine has a longer time to the onset than lidocaine (2–10 min) and thus will not help attenuate the pain of the injection procedure itself. Bupivacaine is typically used in a strength of 0.25% for musculoskeletal injections.

Proliferants

Prolotherapy is the injection of a substance that activates the inflammatory cascade and thus induces fibroblast proliferation. One objective of proliferative therapy is to strengthen incompetent ligaments that exhibit increased laxity.[19] Thus, for example, for a gymnast who has low back pain from a hypermobile sacroiliac joint, a series of prolotherapy treatments over the dorsal sacral ligaments may, over a period of time, strengthen them and thereby reduce motion and thus reduce pain. A second application of prolotherapy is to stimulate the repair of tendons that have undergone chronic degeneration (tendonosis), once again by inciting an inflammatory response which then reactivates the healing process.[19] A number of substances can be used for prolotherapy such as compounds containing phenol, glucose and glycerine. Another commonly used substance is dextrose (10–12% concentration) which is potentially less neurotoxic than phenol preparations. However, part of the pain-relieving effect of compounds containing dilute phenol might also be due to its toxic action on nociceptors.[20]

SAFETY CONSIDERATIONS

The procedures described in this chapter are by-and-large considered minimally invasive. However, this does not mean that they are totally without risk. Informed consent should always be obtained for any procedure irrespective of the relative risks. Discussion with the patient should include the indications, anticipated outcome, potential risks and complications, possible side effects, and alternatives to the procedure. Patients should sign the documentation that informed consent was given and understood. The documentation should be kept as part of the patient's record.

CONTRAINDICATIONS

Contraindications to corticosteroid injections include infection, drug allergy, coagulopathy, and anticoagulated state. It is imperative to assess for any underlying medical contraindications, as well as confirm the patient's allergies and coagulation status, prior to performing any type of procedure.

POTENTIAL COMPLICATIONS

Intra-articular and periarticular steroid injections have been found to be safe and to have low complication rates if performed while taking adequate precautions.[21,22] Potential complications that could result from joint and soft tissue procedures include: post procedural pain flair, subcutaneous fat atrophy, soft tissue calcification, tendon rupture, bleeding, infection, and allergic reaction.[21] These potential complications can be minimized with proper exclusion of patients with known contraindications as well as meticulous attention to injection site preparation and procedural technique.

Injection site preparation is arguably the most important part of the procedure. Skin preparation can be performed with a variety of microbicides including alcohol, clorhexadine and alcohol solutions, or povidone–iodine. One must allow the selected microbicide, time enough to kill the bacteria after application (30–60 s is typically satisfactory, though for optimal bacteriocidal effects povidone–iodine products should be dry). Post-injection infection rates of 1:16,000 to 1–2:150,000 have been cited.[12]

Local reactions at the injection site may include swelling, tenderness, and warmth, all of which can develop a few hours after the injection and may last up to 2 days. A post-injection steroid flare, thought to be a crystal-induced inflammatory response caused by preservatives in the injectate, may occur within the first 24–36 h after injection.[23] This reaction is self-limited and symptomatic patients are instructed to apply ice packs for temporary amelioration. Also, failure to remove residual skin preparation may cause local skin irritation.

Soft tissue (adipose) atrophy and local skin depigmentation are possible with any steroid injection into soft tissue, particularly at superficial sites and bony prominences where the subcutaneous adipose is less thick. Rarely, periarticular and soft tissue calcifications may occur, seemingly most preferentially at sites of multiple injections. The risk of tendon rupture can be reduced by taking great care to avoid intrasubstance injection of steroid into the tendon itself. The peritenon is the target tissue for treatment of tendonitis/tendonosis. To avoid direct needle injury to articular cartilage or local nerves, strict attention should be paid to anatomic landmarks and depth of the injection.

Systemic effects are uncommon but may arise, particularly following injection into highly vascularized tissue (such as a site of prior surgery) or with inadvertent direct vascular injection. The proceduralist must be vigilant to reduce the potential for systemic side effects. Patients should remain in the office for an appropriate period time following their procedure to monitor for adverse reactions. Typically 10 min will suffice with minor procedures. If large volumes of long-acting anesthetics are used, a lengthier period of observation should be instituted. Symptoms of vascular uptake of local anesthetic include lightheadedness, tinnitus, a metallic taste in the mouth, and perioral tingling. Patients who exhibit these symptoms should not be released to home and should be moved to a setting where additional monitoring can be instituted to observe for signs of central nervous system and cardiotoxicity.

Exogenous corticosteroids can have an effect on the endocrine system. Hyperglycemia can certainly occur following corticosteroid injection in patients with diabetes,[23] particularly if they typically exhibit poor glycemic control or require high doses of insulin for management. All diabetics should be counseled regarding this possibility and given instructions for frequent glucose monitoring for the first several days following the injection. Other rare, but reported, complications include adrenal suppression, and abnormal uterine bleeding.[13,24]

ANATOMY

Surface anatomy landmarks that are palpable and help guide injections into the hip and pelvic region include the ilium with its large anterior superior iliac spine (**ASIS**) and posterior superior iliac spine (**PSIS**), the greater trochanter, ischial tuberosity, and the coccyx. Palpable joints include the hip joint, sacroiliac joint, pubic symphysis, and the sacrococcygeal articulation. The sciatic notch is formed by the ilium and the lateral border of the sacrum. The proceduralist should have a detailed understanding of musculoskeletal anatomy, including muscle attachments, bursa, nerves, and blood vessels. Hip and pelvic anatomy with common injection target tissues, are depicted in Fig. 13.2.

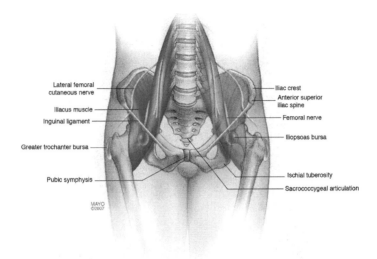

FIGURE 13.2. Anterior view of the pelvis with common injection target tissues identified.

PROCEDURES

Documentation

As previously discussed, the physician should review the rationale for the procedure and obtain written informed consent. In July 2004, the Joint Commission on the Accreditation of Healthcare Organizations (JCAHO) began requiring providers to follow a universal protocol for preventing wrong site, wrong procedure and wrong person surgery. The protocol's three major elements include: (1) initial verification of the intended patient, procedure, and site of the procedure; (2) marking the intended site with a sterile pen, where applicable; and (3) a final "time-out" immediately before beginning the procedure.[25]

Injection Technique Fundamentals

Image Guidance
Determine whether image guidance (if available) will be necessary to appropriately perform the procedure. For injections such as the hip joint, iliopsoas bursa, sacroiliac joint and pubic symphysis, image guidance is recommended.

Positioning
Position the patient in a comfortable manner that will allow easy access to the target anatomy.

Target Selection
Superficial anatomy is palpated and a needle entry point is marked.

Sterile Preparation
The area is generously prepped with a microbicidal agent.

Drapes
Drapes can be used if necessary to maintain a sterile field, however, are not typically necessary for routine soft tissue and joint injections that have been prepped in a wide fashion around the target anatomy.

Universal Precautions
Universal precautions should always be observed.

Gloves
Sterile gloves must be worn if the physician needs to palpate the needle entry site after it has been prepped or to touch the needle. This is often the case with novice proceduralists. For the experienced proceduralist, once the needle entry point is marked and prepped, the injection can typically be performed without touching (contaminating) the needle entry point or needle. Thus nonsterile gloves may be worn.

Skin Wheel
Injections are much more tolerable for the patient if the proceduralist takes time to perform a separate skin wheel with 1% lidocaine at the needle entry point using a 30 gage needle, and infiltrates a little lidocaine along the initial needle trajectory. When performing a skin wheel, infiltrate very slowly; this will minimize the initial burning pain associated with subcutaneous lidocaine. Patients will return for further procedures if they know their physician has excellent technique and causes them minimal pain.

Negative Aspiration
When the needle has reached the target site one should perform a 5 s. aspiration by applying negative pressure on the syringe. This will reduce the risk of inadvertent intravascular injection. The authors recommend using a 10 ml control syringe for this purpose with finger loops that allow a one-handed aspiration.

Injectate Volume

Typically when performing a therapeutic injection, an ample amount of injectate should be used to ensure adequate coverage of the target structure. If the diagnosis is in question and the patient's response to the procedure will influence further treatment, then the smallest possible injectate volume should be used. The volumes indicated in the forthcoming procedure descriptions reflect a standard therapeutic volume rather than a diagnostic volume.

Steroid Dosing

There are little data identifying the "necessary" amount of corticosteroid to administer with various procedures (SOR-C). The precise dose selected may be influenced by a number of factors, including the presence of systemic diseases like diabetes and osteoporosis or the amount of exogenous corticosteroid already administered in the preceding months. The doses listed reflect the authors' preferences and will be listed in milligrams of methylprednisolone. For equal-potency conversion to other corticosteroids, please consult Table 13.1.

Injection Resistance

With intra-articular and soft tissue injections there should be only slight resistance to the flow of medication while compressing the syringe. If resistance is considerable or there is significant pain induced, the needle tip should be repositioned. Usually this signifies injection into the bone, sub-periosteal, or within the substance of a tendon, all of which one wants to avoid! Withdrawing the needle by a millimeter or two will often alleviate the problem.

Microbicide Removal

All residual skin preparation solution should be washed off following the procedure to minimize skin irritation.

Dressing

Hold pressure on the punctured site until all the bleeding has stopped. A simple adhesive bandage will suffice as a dressing in most cases.

Sharps

Dispose of all sharps in properly labeled, puncture-proof containers.

SOFT TISSUE INJECTIONS

Greater Trochanteric Bursa (Fig. 13.3)

Positioning: Lying on one's side with the bottom leg straight and the top leg in partial hip and knee flexion.

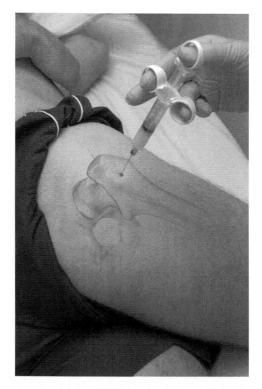

Figure 13.3. Greater trochanteric bursa injection.

Injection landmarks: The greater trochanter is palpable on the lateral aspect of the hip. Select the site of maximal tenderness over the trochanter for the target site.

Injectate composition: 5 ml of 1% lidocaine and 30 mg of methylprednisolone.

Injection technique: Following an appropriate skin wheel, a 5 cm, 25 gage needle is advanced to the bone. Once the bone is contacted, the needle is withdrawn 3–5 mm (to the level of the bursa) and, following negative aspiration, the injection is performed.

Pearls: If the patient has more diffuse pain on palpation of the trochanter, consider placing one-half of the injectate at the site of maximal tenderness and then perform a four quadrant infiltration about the greater trochanter with the remainder of the solution.

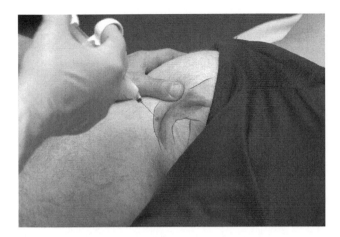

Figure 13.4. Ischial bursa injection.

Ischial Bursa (Fig. 13.4)

Positioning: Prone.

Injection landmarks: The ischium is palpable on the inferior aspect of the buttocks. Select the site of maximal tenderness over the ischium for the target site.

Injectate composition: 4 ml of 1% lidocaine and 20–30 mg of methylprednisolone.

Injection technique: Following an appropriate skin wheel, a 6 cm, 22 gage needle is advanced to the bone. Once ischium is contacted, the needle is withdrawn 3–5 mm (to the level of the bursa) and, following negative aspiration, the injection is performed.

Pearls: If the patient has more diffuse pain on palpation of the ischium, consider placing one-half of the injectate at the site of maximal pain, and then perform a four quadrant infiltration about the remainder of the ischium. For obese patients a longer (9 cm) needle may be required.

Hamstring Origin (Fig. 13.5)

Positioning: Prone.

Injection landmarks: The ischium is palpable on the inferior aspect of the buttocks. Have the patient activate the hamstring muscles to aid palpation of the attachments to the ischium. Select the site of maximal tenderness for the target site.

Injectate composition: 4 ml of 1% lidocaine and 20–30 mg of methylprednisolone.

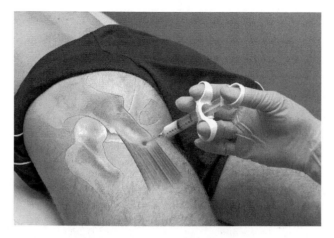

Figure 13.5. Hamstring origin injection.

Injection technique: Following an appropriate skin wheel, a 6 cm, 22 gage needle is advanced to the hamstring tendon origins at their attachments to the ischium. Initially aim for the proximal tendon and "walk" the needle cephalad until the inferior aspect of the ischium is contacted. Once the bone/tendon junction is contacted, the needle is withdrawn 1–2 mm and, following negative aspiration, the injection is performed.

Pearls: There should be minimal resistance to the flow of the injectate. If resistance is high, this may signify that the needle tip is within the substance of the tendon. In this case, the needle should be slowly withdrawn until minimal resistance is encountered. For obese patients, a longer (9 cm) needle may be required.

Iliopsoas Bursa (Fig. 13.6)

Positioning: Supine.

Injection landmarks: Identify and mark the femoral pulse and neurovascular bundle at the level of the inguinal ligament. The needle entry point is 2.5 cm lateral and 2.5 cm inferior.

Injectate composition: 5 ml of 1% lidocaine and 20–30 mg of methylprednisolone.

Injection technique: Following an appropriate skin wheel, a 9 cm, 22 gage needle is advanced via a slightly superior and medial trajectory from the entry point until the bone is contacted. Once the bone is contacted, the needle is withdrawn 3–5 mm (to the level of the bursa) and, following careful negative aspiration, the injection is performed.

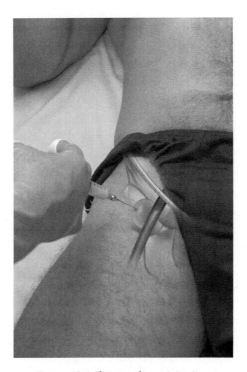

Figure 13.6. Iliopsoas bursa injection.

Pearls: The accuracy of this injection is significantly enhanced by using image guidance such as ultrasound where the iliopsoas tendon and bursa can be visualized and targeted, or fluoroscopy where the lip of the acetabulum or inferomedial femoral neck can be directly targeted.

Hip Adductor Origin (Fig. 13.7)

Positioning: Supine with hip slightly flexed, abducted, and externally rotated.

Injection landmarks: The pubis is easily palpable at the medial aspect of the inguinal crease. Have the patient activate the adductor muscles to aid palpation of the attachments to the inferior pubic ramus. Select the site of maximal tenderness for the target site.

Injectate composition: 4 ml of 1% lidocaine and 20–30 mg of methylprednisolone.

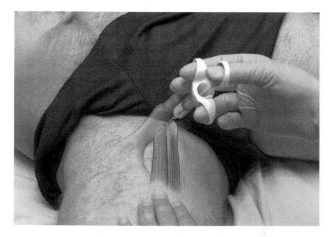

Figure 13.7. Hip adductor origin injection.

Injection technique: Following an appropriate skin wheel, a 6 cm, 22 gage needle is advanced to the adductor tendon origins at their attachments to the inferior pubic ramus. Once the bone/tendon junction is contacted, the needle is withdrawn 1–2 mm and, following negative aspiration, the injection is performed.

Pearls: There should be minimal resistance to the flow of the injectate. If resistance is high this may signify that the needle tip is within the substance of the tendon. In this case the needle should be slowly withdrawn until minimal resistance is encountered.

JOINT INJECTIONS

Sacroiliac (Fig. 13.8)

Positioning: Prone.

Injection landmarks: Identify and mark the PSIS. The needle point is 1 cm medial to the midpoint of the PSIS.

Injectate composition: 5 ml of 1% lidocaine and 30–40 mg of methylprednisolone.

Injection technique: Following an appropriate skin wheel, a 6 cm or 9 cm, 22 gage needle is advanced in an oblique fashion laterally under the PSIS until the bone is contacted. The injectate should be infiltrated in a fan-type distribution along the dorsal aspect of the posterior sacroiliac ligaments. This technique accomplishes a periarticular injection.

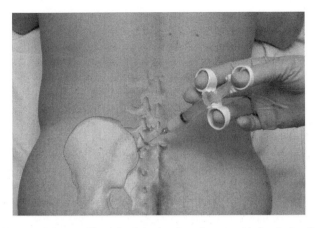

Figure 13.8. Sacroiliac joint injection (non-image guided technique).

Pearls: The accuracy of sacroiliac injections are significantly enhanced by using image guidance such as fluoroscopy (or ultrasound) where the posterior inferior (synovial) aspect of the sacroiliac joint is targeted and the needle can be placed for an intra-articular injection.

Hip (Fig. 13.9)

Positioning: Lateral – symptomatic side up with bottom leg flexed at the hip and knee. The midpoint of the ilium, greater trochanter, and femoral shaft should all line up in the same coronal plane.

Injection landmarks: Palpate and mark the top of the ilium, greater trochanter, and proximal femoral shaft. The needle entry point is 1 cm cephalad to the most proximal portion of the greater trochanter (which may be as much as 5 cm cephalad to the most easily palpable lateral portion of the greater trochanter).

Injectate composition: 5–8 ml of 1% lidocaine and 40 mg of methylprednisolone.

Injection technique: Following an appropriate skin wheel, a 9 cm, 22 gage needle is inserted in the coronal plane of the femoral neck at a 30° (downward) angle. The needle is advanced until the bone is contacted. The injection is made through the capsular attachment to the femoral neck.

Pearls: The accuracy of this injection is significantly enhanced by using image guidance such as fluoroscopy. Under fluoroscopic guidance a more anterior approach is used to directly guide the needle through the hip capsule and into the joint space.

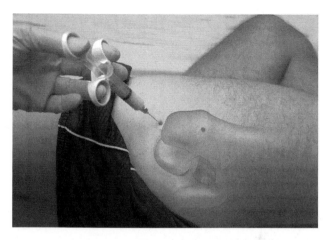

Figure 13.9. Hip joint injection (non-image guided technique).

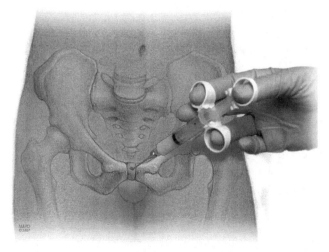

Figure 13.10. Pubic symphysis injection.

Pubic Symphysis (Fig. 13.10)

Positioning: Supine.

Injection landmarks: Identify the pubic tubercles bilaterally and mark the cleft midline between.

Injectate composition: 3 ml of 1% lidocaine and 20 mg of methylprednisolone.

Injection technique: Following an appropriate skin wheel, a 3.75–5 cm, 25 gage needle is advanced to the symphysis. Once the fibrocartilaginous disc is contacted, advance the needle an additional 5 mm into the cleft.

Pearls: The accuracy of this injection is significantly enhanced by using image guidance. Prior to performing a corticosteroid injection into the pubic symphysis, infectious osteitis pubis must be definitively excluded.

Sacrococcygeal (Fig. 13.11)

Positioning: Prone.

Injection landmarks: Identify the sacral cornu bilaterally and mark 1 cm inferior, midline. The articulation of the sacrum and coccyx should be palpable near this position. Adjust the needle entry point accordingly.

Injectate composition: 3 ml of 1% lidocaine and 20 mg of methylprednisolone.

Injection technique: Following an appropriate skin wheel, a 3.75 cm, 25 gage needle is advanced until the bone is contacted. The needle is withdrawn 1–2 mm and, following negative aspiration, the injection is performed.

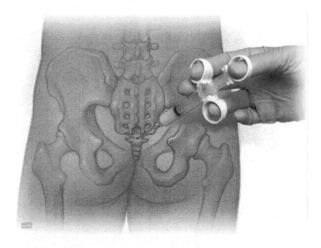

Figure 13.11. Sacrococcygeal injection.

Pearls: Caution should be exercised upon advancing the needle to guard against inadvertent puncture of the rectum by missing the coccyx.

NERVE BLOCKS

Lateral Femoral Cutaneous Nerve (Fig. 13.12)

Positioning: Supine.

Injection landmarks: Identify the ASIS and mark 1 cm medial and inferior as the needle entry point.

Injectate Composition: 6 ml of 1% lidocaine and 20 mg of methylprednisolone.

Injection technique: Following an appropriate skin wheel, a 5 cm, 25 gage needle is advanced slightly superior and laterally, underneath the ASIS until the ilium is contacted. The injection is then performed by infiltrating in a fan type distribution perpen-

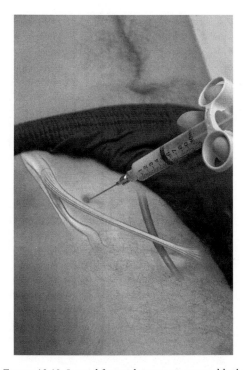

FIGURE 13.12. Lateral femoral cutaneous nerve block.

dicular to the course of the traversing lateral femoral cutaneous nerve.

Pearls: The ilioinguinal and iliohypogastric nerves run in close proximity to this target site and the patient should be forewarned about the possibility of inadvertently anesthetizing these structures.

CASE PRESENTATION WRAP-UP
Fluoroscopically guided intra-articular local anesthetic/corticosteroid injection of the hip did not alleviate his pain (Fig. 13.13.). Fluoroscopically, guided local anesthetic/corticosteroid injection of the iliopsoas bursa did completely relieve his pain (Fig. 13.14). Diagnosis was iliopsoas bursitis.

Treatment consisted of temporary activity modification, scheduled NSAID administration, physical therapy directed at gentle stretching of the iliopsoas, and iliopsoas and hip girdle strengthening.

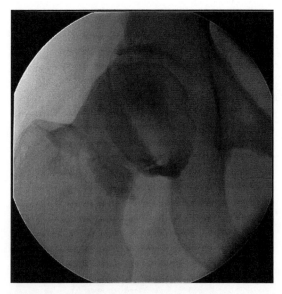

FIGURE 13.13. Fluoroscopically guided intra-articular hip injection with contrast filling diffusely throughout the joint capsule.

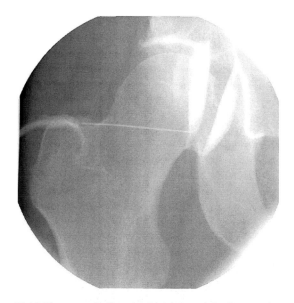

FIGURE 13.14. Fluoroscopically guided injection of the iliopsoas bursa with the iliopsoas tendon traversing the center of the bursa.

On follow-up, the patient was able to gradually return to running and basketball. No subsequent discomfort or dysfunction developed from the labral tear identified on MR arthrogram.

Various hip and pelvis disorders may often present with similar symptoms and examination findings. Diagnostic injections can be an effective tool to help identify the pain generator. In the case presented the iliopsoas bursa injection confirmed the diagnosis, distinguishing it from an incidental non-symptomatic hip labral tear.

References
1. Hench PS, Kendall E, Slocumb CH, Polly HF. The effect of a hormone of the adrenal cortex (17-hydroxy-11dehydrocorticosterone: Compound E) and of pituitary adrenocorticotropic hormone on rheumatoid arthritis. Proc Staff Meet Mayo Clin 1949; 24:181–197.
2. Raynauld JP, Buckland-Wright C, Ward R, et al. Safety and efficacy of long-term intra-articular steroid injections in osteoarthritis of the knee: a randomized, double-blind, placebo-controlled trial. Arthritis Rheum 2003; 48:370–377.

3. Qvistgaard E, Christensen R, Torp-Pedersen S, Bliddal H. Intra-articular treatment of hip osteoarthritis: a randomized trial of hyaluronic acid, corticosteroid, and isotonic saline. Osteoarthritis Cartilage 2006; 14(2):163–170.
4. Rabago D, Best TM, Beamsley M, Patterson J. A systematic review of prolotherapy for chronic musculoskeletal pain. Clin J Sport Med 2005; 15(5):376–380.
5. Topol GA, Reeves KD, Hassanein KM. Efficacy of dextrose prolotherapy in elite male kicking-sport athletes with chronic groin pain. Arch Phys Med Rehabil 2005; 86(4):697–702.
6. Fernandez Lopez JC, Ruano-Ravina A. Efficacy and Safety of Intra-articular Hyaluronic Acid in the Treatment of Osteoarthritis of the Hip: A systematic review. Osteoarthritis Cartilage 2006; 14(12):1306–1311.
7. Kim SR, Stitik TP, Foye PM, et al. Critical review of prolotherapy for osteoarthritis, low back pain, and other musculoskeletal conditions: a physiatric perspective. Am J Phys Med Rehabil 2004; 83(5):379–389.
8. Naredo E, Cabero F, Beneyto P, et al. A randomized comparative study of short term response to blind injection versus sonographic-guided injection of local corticosteroids in patients with painful shoulder. J Rheumatol 2004; 31:308–314.
9. Sofka CM, Adler RS. Ultrasound-guided interventions in the foot and ankle. Semin Musculoskelet Radiol 2002; 6(2):163–168.
10. Smith J, Hurdle MF, Locketz AJ, Wisniewski SJ. Ultrasound-guided piriformis injection: technique description and verification. Arch Phys Med Rehabil 2006; 87(12):1664–1667.
11. Pulisetti D, Ebraheim NA. CT-guided sacroiliac joint injections. J Spinal Disord 1999; 12(4):310–322.
12. Carek PJ. Joint and Soft Tissue Injections in Primary Care. Clin Fam Pract 2005; 7(2); 359–378.
13. Mader R, Lavi I, Luboshitzky R. Evaluation of the pituitary-adrenal axis function following single intra-articular injection of methylprednisolone. Arthritis Rheum 2005; 52(3):924–928.
14. Bellamy N, Campbell J, Robinson V, et al. Viscosupplementation for the treatment of osteoarthritis of the knee. Cochrane Database Syst Rev 2006 Apr 19; (2):CD005321.
15. Kelly MA, Kurzweil PR, Moskowitz RW. Intra-articular hyalurons in knee osteoarthritis: rationale and practical considerations. Am J Orthop 2004; 33:15–22.
16. Choi YK, Liu J. The use of 5% of lidocaine for prolonged analgesia in chronic pain patients: a new technique. Reg Anesth Pain Med 1998; 23(1):96–100.
17. Product Information: Xylocaine injection, lidocaine HCl and epinephrine injection. AstraZeneca Pharmaceuticals, Wilmington, DE, 2001.
18. Product Information: Marcaine injection, bupivacaine HCl injection. Hospira, Inc, Lake Forest, IL, 2004.
19. Hackett GS. Ligament and Tendon Relaxation (Skeletal Disability) Treated by Prolotherapy (Fibro-Osseous Proliferation), 3rd ed. Springfield, IL: Charles C Thomas Publishers; 1958.

20. Saunders S, Longworth S. Injection Techniques in Orthopedics and Sport Medicine, 3rd ed. New York: Elsevier; 2006.
21. Gray RG, Gottlieb NL. Intra-articular corticosteroids: an updated assessment. Clin Orthop 1983; 177:235–263.
22. Kumar N, Newman RJ. Complications of intra- and peri-articular steroid injections. Br J Gen Pract 1999; 49:465–466.
23. Cardone DA, Tallia AF. Joint and soft tissue injection. Am Fam Physician 2002; 66:283–288.
24. Menes JMA, De Wolf AN, Berthoud BJ, Stem HJ. Disturbance of the menstrual pattern after local injection with triamcinolone acetonide. Ann Rheum Dis 1998; 57:500.
25. Universal Protocol for Preventing Wrong Site, Wrong Procedure, Wrong Person Surgery.™ Copyright © 2007 Joint Commission. At: <jointcommission.org/PatientSafety/UniversalProtocol/>. Accessed May 8, 2007.

Chapter 14
Treatment Options for Osteoarthritis of the Hip

Heather M. Gillespie and William W. Dexter

CLINICAL PEARLS

- Strength training and aerobic exercise can reduce pain and improve function and health status in patients with hip osteoarthritis and should be recommended for all patients (SOR = C).
- Acetaminophen is recommended as the first line of pharmacologic therapy in hip osteoarthritis (SOR = C).
- Additional therapeutic options include intra-articular injections, nutritional supplements and alternative therapies.
- Current treatment is focused on symptom control; however, disease-modifying agents are currently in development.
- After all conservative measures are exhausted, pain and function are the primary determinants for surgery (SOR = C).

CASE VINETTE

The Patient is a 40-year-old nurse and aerobics instructor with a history of depression and fibromyalgia who presents herself with hip pain, increasing over a period of 2 years. She describes a dull, achy pain on the lateral hip that radiates to the groin. The pain is worse with activity and limits her range of motion; however, she has been able to remain active with bicycling. On examination, she has a body mass index (BMI) of 24, no tenderness to palpation over the hip, but pain is reproduced with hip internal rotation. She has decreased range of motion in internal rotation of the right hip compared to the left. Radiographs show a mild amount of joint space narrowing and subchondral sclerosis (Fig. 14.1).

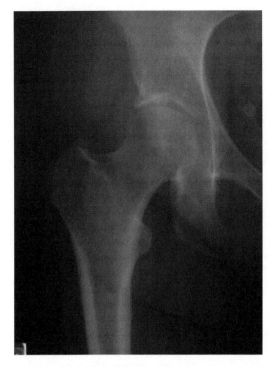

FIGURE 14.1. Right hip osteoarthritis with joint space narrowing and subchondral sclerosis.

EPIDEMIOLOGY

Osteoarthritis is the most common cause of musculoskeletal pain and disability. A progressive and debilitating disease, osteoarthritis affects over 15% of the world's population[1] and is a major cause of morbidity and health care expenditures. As the population continues to age, the cost and consequences from osteoarthritis will continue to grow.

Osteoarthritis, characterized by joint pain and dysfunction, is associated with defective integrity of the articular cartilage and related changes in the underlying bone and joint margins. Currently, there is no known cure for osteoarthritis. New treatments and disease-modifying therapies are currently under investigation, but the etiology of osteoarthritis is still not completely understood. Therapy is aimed at decreasing pain and dysfunction and increasing mobility and overall quality of life.

The hip is the second most common large joint to be affected by osteoarthritis.[2,3] The prevalence of hip osteoarthritis ranges from 3% to 11% in Western populations aged over 35 years,[3] with reported prevalence variation due to differences in radiographic case definitions.[4]

RISK FACTORS

Risk factors associated with osteoarthritis include systemic factors, such as genetics and bone density, as well as biomechanical factors that affect the joints, such as reduced muscle strength. Age, joint location, obesity, joint malalignment, trauma, gender, comorbidities, biochemical changes, and lifestyle have all been associated with the development of osteoarthritis.[1] Age-related changes in cartilage alter the biomechanical characteristics of collagen and proteoglycans. Mechanical wear, chondrocytes, and cytokines, principally interleukin (IL)-1β (beta) and transforming growth factor (TGF)-β (beta), all play roles in the pathogenesis of the disease.[5]

In males, trauma and age are associated with osteoarthritis. A positive association of hip trauma is also found with unilateral but not bilateral hip osteoarthritis. Obesity is associated with bilateral but not unilateral hip osteoarthritis.[6] A recent systematic review that examined the influence of obesity on the development of hip osteoarthritis found only moderate evidence to support the influence of obesity on the development of hip osteoarthritis, primarily due to the lack of high-quality studies.[7]

DIAGNOSIS

The accurate diagnosis of hip osteoarthritis relies on a combination of both clinical and radiographic findings. Radiographic evidence of joint degeneration and characteristic subjective symptoms of pain and disability have been found to be superior to clinical criteria alone.

Physical symptoms include generalized hip pain, pain in the lateral or anterior thigh and groin, and pain with prolonged ambulation. Physical signs include antalgic gait, decreased range of motion, and pain with internal rotation. The pain is often described as deep and achy. In early disease, the pain may be intermittent and mostly with joint use, but as the pain becomes more chronic, patients may also experience pain at night. The joint is often described as "stiff" and patients have difficulty with initiating movements. In advanced disease, crepitus may develop and range of motion may become limited.[8] Radiographic findings in patients with osteoarthritis include cartilage space narrowing, osteophytosis, subchondral cysts, subchondral sclerosis, femoral neck buttressing, and femoral head remodeling (Figs. 14.2–14.5).[5,9] Historically, radiographic evidence of osteophytes, cysts and subchondral sclerosis have been used to diagnose osteoarthritis; however, recent research has focused on joint space width (JSW) as the primary determinant and radiographic criterion for hip osteoarthritis.

Jacobsen et al. found that minimum JSW less than or equal to 2 mm had the closest association with self-reported hip pain in 3,807 subjects whose mean age was 61 years old.[4] In a recent study by Gupta et al., cartilage space narrowing was the most sensitive predictor of hip osteoarthritis.[5] Croft et al. studied 1,315 men aged 60–75 and found minimal joint space to be the best radiographic criterion of hip osteoarthritis to use in epidemiologic studies, at least for men.[10] In 1991, Altman et al. proposed a classification tree of (1) hip pain and osteophytosis or (2) hip pain and cartilage

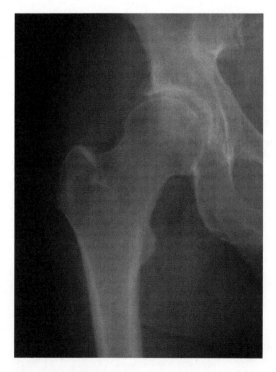

FIGURE 14.2. Hip osteoarthritis with joint space narrowing.

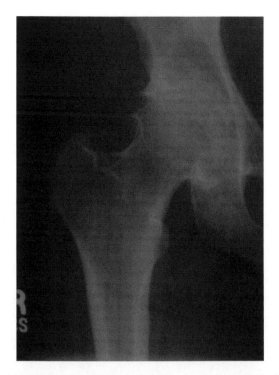

FIGURE 14.3. Hip osteoarthritis with osteophytes and subchondral sclerosis.

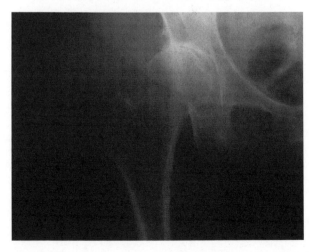

FIGURE 14.4. Severe hip osteoarthritis with loss of joint space and subchondral sclerosis.

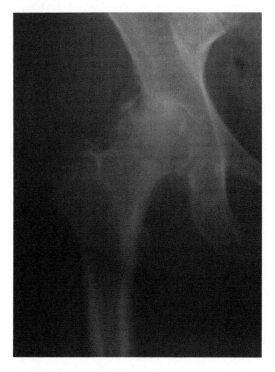

FIGURE 14.5. Severe hip osteoarthritis with subchondral cysts, osteophytes, subchondral sclerosis and joint space loss.

space narrowing with a sedimentation rate less than 22 mm/h. The study demonstrated a sensitivity of 91% and a specificity of 89% for hip osteoarthritis.[11]

NONOPERATIVE MANAGEMENT

Overall, the goals of nonoperative management in osteoarthritis should be to reduce pain and functional impairment, to improve mobility, and perhaps to delay or prevent the need for surgery. Treatments should be chosen to limit the side effects of therapy. Expert opinion supports the statement that optimal management of hip osteoarthritis requires a combination of nonpharmacologic and pharmacologic treatment modalities.[3]

A systematic review of the literature by a multidisciplinary expert group (European League Against Rheumatism) generated recommendations for the treatment of hip osteoarthritis.

This review evaluated the clinical efficacy, cost effectiveness, and strength of ten key recommendations for hip osteoarthritis. In general, evidence specific to hip osteoarthritis is strikingly lacking and most recommendations are based on expert opinion or extrapolated from evidence and studies of knee osteoarthritis.[3]

Treatment of hip osteoarthritis should be tailored to the individual patient taking into account patient comorbidities, current medications, level of pain, disability and handicap, degree of structural damage, and baseline physical activity and functional status (SOR = C).

Nonpharmacologic Therapy

Nonpharmacologic treatment of hip osteoarthritis should include patient education, self-management programs, exercise and physical therapy, lifestyle changes, assistive devices such as a cane, and weight reduction if obese or overweight.

Exercise: General Benefit

Exercise and physical activity have clearly been shown to benefit those with large-joint osteoarthritis.[2,8] Decreased lower extremity strength is associated with increased disability in people with osteoarthritis. Disease-related factors such as impaired muscle function and reduced fitness are amenable to therapeutic exercise. Tak et al. conducted a randomized controlled trial (RCT) in 109 patients, which demonstrated a positive effect on pain and hip function from an 8-week exercise program.[12] Strengthening and aerobic exercise have been shown to reduce pain and improve function and health status in patients with hip osteoarthritis. Expert opinion from a recent systematic review states that improvement in muscle strength and proprioception gained from exercise programs may reduce the progression of hip osteoarthritis. Notably, the effectiveness of exercise is thought to be independent of the presence or severity of radiographic findings.[2]

Exercise: Type

Land-based exercise programs, hydrotherapy, and strength training have all reported positive improvements in functional performance and reduction of pain in osteoarthritis. A systematic review published in 2005 combined research evidence and expert opinion to develop recommendations for exercise in the management of hip osteoarthritis. Due to a paucity of studies, many recommendations are extrapolated from studies in knee osteoarthritis; however, in one RCT of aerobic exercise of hip osteoarthritis, home exercise was found to be as effective as hydrotherapy.[2] Supervised classes appeared to be as beneficial as treatments on a one-to-one basis.[8] Group exercise and home exercise were found to be equally effective while a supervised group format potentially provides a more cost-effective alternative; also, social contact with peers may help to increase adherence.[2,8] While there are no data regarding intensity of exercise in hip osteoarthritis, a Cochrane review examining the effectiveness of therapeutic exercise at different intensities in people with osteoarthritis of the knee found both high-intensity and low-intensity aerobic exercise to be equally effective in improving patient's functional status, gait, pain, and aerobic capacity.[13] Studies have also shown that dropout rates are related to the intensity of the exercise, with higher intensity having a higher rate of withdrawal.[13] It is important to carefully tailor the exercise type and intensity to the individual patient, erring on the side of a low-intensity exercise program with a slow progression to achieve maximum short and long term effects.

Hydrotherapy

If the resources and facilities are available, hydrotherapy (aquatic physical therapy/water-based therapy) can be an ideal setting for people with osteoarthritis. Hydrotherapy should incorporate both aerobic and strength/resistance-based training to achieve full benefit (SOR = C). The buoyancy of the water reduces the load across the joints affected by pain and allows for performance of functional closed-chain exercises that would otherwise be too difficult. The warmth and pressure of the water may aid in pain relief, swelling reduction, and ease of movement. Warm water encourages muscle relaxation and reduces guarding around the joints, which leads to increased range of motion and ultimate functional gains.

In a recent RCT of 71 patients comparing 6 weeks of hydrotherapy versus no treatment, the hydrotherapy group had significantly less pain and improved physical function, strength, and quality of life compared to controls, with benefit sustained 6 weeks after cessation of the program.[14] Foley et al. studied 105 patients randomized to three water- or land-based exercise sessions a week for 6 weeks. Both water and gym exercises were found to improve function, with land-based exercises being better for strength and water-based superior for aerobic conditioning.[15]

Exercise: Adherence and Risk

One of the leading indicators of success and benefit from exercise therapy is patient adherence to the program. The bottom line is that performing exercise is more important than the type performed. Strategies to improve adherence such as long-term monitoring and review, setting specific exercise-related goals that are easy to achieve, frequent encouragement, and inclusion of a spouse or other family member in the exercise should be considered in the exercise prescription.

There is no direct evidence concerning contraindications to exercise therapy for hip osteoarthritis, but an expert group has recommended that there are few contraindications to the prescription of strengthening or aerobic exercise in patients with hip osteoarthritis.[2] Consistent with general patient-centered care, exercise prescription for osteoarthritis should include both aerobic and strength training and be individualized. Age, comorbidities, resources, and overall mobility should all be taken into account to ultimately increase patient adherence and overall success (SOR=C).

Patient Education and Self-Management Programs
Arthritis self help groups that teach patients how to manage their disease have been shown to decrease pain and improve quality of life in patients with osteoarthritis. One RCT for education and hip osteoarthritis suggests that education reduces pain, and systematic reviews for education have demonstrated positive, although nonsignificant, effects for education programs compared to controls.[3] Community organizations as well as the Arthritis Foundation can serve as a resource for education materials.

Self-management programs have been shown to reduce anxiety and improve participants' perceived self-efficacy to manage their symptoms of osteoarthritis. Education that the disease is not relentlessly progressive and self-management tools, such as techniques to deal with problems such as pain, fatigue, frustration, and isolation, can decrease doctor visits. In addition, treating depression in patients with osteoarthritis may help reduce the amount of pain and improve their functional status and quality of life.[16]

Assistive Devices
There is no research evidence for appliances such as canes and insoles[3] in the treatment of hip osteoarthritis, but theoretically they may help to alter joint forces. In general, there are few contraindications if the device is found to be effective for individual patients.

Weight Loss
A positive relationship exists between obesity and hip osteoarthritis. While there is no RCT evidence, some case–control studies demonstrate the benefit of weight loss in reducing pain and disability. Weight loss combined with strength training increases the muscle strength surrounding the joint, which also may attenuate the impact load. In general, interventions that reduce the force across the

compromised hip joint such as weight loss and the use of assistive devices have face validity and expert opinion support (SOR = C).[3]

Pharmacologic Therapy

Pharmacologic therapy in osteoarthritis should be undertaken as a supplement, not a replacement, for nonpharmacologic therapy. Drug therapy has been found to be most potent when combined with nonpharmacologic treatment. The majority of current pharmacologic options in the treatment of osteoarthritis are symptom-modifying therapies; however, structure- and disease-modifying therapies are currently in development. Current symptom-modifying medications include analgesics (acetaminophen, opioids, and tramadol), nonsteroidal anti-inflammatory drugs (NSAIDs), COX-2 inhibitors, corticosteroids, and viscosupplementation.

Acetaminophen

Balancing efficacy and safety, acetaminophen (up to 4 g/day) is the oral analgesic of first choice for mild-moderate pain in osteoarthritis and is the preferred long term analgesic (SOR = C).[3]

Some research has shown acetaminophen to be inferior to NSAIDs in pain relief, but acetaminophen is less toxic and has a favorable safety profile (4 g/day dosing limit).[3] A decision analysis model in 2003 by Kamath et al. comparing acetaminophen to NSAIDs and COX-2 inhibitors, found acetaminophen to be the least toxic and most cost effective therapy.[17] A systematic review of RCTs showed acetaminophen with no higher risk of gastrointestinal (GI) upset than placebo and sparse evidence for renal toxicity.[3] A study in knee osteoarthritis showed acetaminophen to be superior to NSAIDs, NSAIDs plus gastro protective agents, and selective cox-2 inhibitors (coxibs) for the cost of each GI adverse effect avoided.[3]

General precautions in prescribing acetaminophen include hepatic dysfunction, high alcohol intake, and Coumadin use. The concern for hepatotoxicity and alanine transaminase (ALT) elevations in acetaminophen-treated patients with baseline normal liver function was recently systematically reviewed. Low level, transient ALT elevations were shown to usually resolve or decrease with continued therapy and were not accompanied by signs of liver injury. The transient elevations were, therefore, thought to be clinically insignificant, and it was concluded that maximum daily doses of acetaminophen did not cause liver failure or dysfunction and acetaminophen "remains safest oral analgesic available.[18]"

NSAIDs

NSAIDs are widely used to control the pain of osteoarthritis. There is strong evidence that NSAIDs provide significant pain relief for osteoarthritis; however, they are also associated with significant side effects and risks, particularly adverse GI events.[3] GI side effects associated with NSAID use are reported to lead to over $500 million annually in health care costs.[19] There is a 2–4% annual incidence of serious GI ulcer and complications in NSAID users which is four times higher than in nonusers.[20] NSAIDs result in at least 7,000 deaths annually in the United States.[21]

NSAIDs should be prescribed with caution in patients over the age of 65 or with a history of peptic ulcer disease, upper GI bleed, oral glucocorticoid therapy, anticoagulation, and other comorbid conditions such as smoking, alcohol use, and renal disease. A healthy kidney is able to compensate from prostaglandin inhibition, but if baseline renal function is impaired, the kidney will suffer.[22] Expert opinion recommends that NSAIDs, at the lowest effective dose, should be added or substituted for patients who respond inadequately to acetaminophen. There should be careful consideration of risks and benefits before prescribing them for osteoarthritis pain. In patients with increased GI risk, nonselective NSAIDs plus a gastroprotective agent, or a selective COX-2 inhibitor should be used. But, caution should be used in prescribing NSAIDs to patients with increased cardiovascular risk (SOR = C). These strategies are more expensive and only cost effective in patients with greater GI risk.[3]

COX-2 Inhibitors
There is evidence to support a safer GI profile for COX-2 inhibitors as compared to nonselective NSAIDs; however, the combination of a traditional NSAID plus a gastroprotective agent may be equivalent. The relationship of COX-2 inhibitors and cardiovascular adverse effects is a growing concern and studies are currently underway to determine if this is a class effect. COX-2 inhibitors appear to be cost-effective in high risk patients (elderly with multiple concomitant medications and history of GI problems including ulcers or bleeds) that do not respond to acetaminophen.[17] Additional precautions with COX-2 inhibitors include hepatic and renal events similar to nonselective NSAIDs.

Opioids
Opioids are a safe and effective therapeutic option of the treatment of moderate-to-severe osteoarthritis pain that does not respond to acetaminophen or NSAIDs (SOR = A). A systematic review found opioid analgesics, with or without acetaminophen, to be effective for hip osteoarthritis.[3] Opioids have been found to be effective in improving measures of pain, function, and quality of life in patients with chronic, moderate-to-severe osteoarthritis pain.[23]

Extended release forms are preferable to immediate-release formulations at providing consistent stable analgesia. It may be necessary to switch opioid medications, one or more times to achieve an acceptable balance, between adverse events and analgesia as patients have variable responses to different opioids. Side effects with a dose–response relationship include nausea, vomiting, constipation, dizziness, somnolence, and pruritus.

Tramadol

Tramadol is an opioid agonist and centrally acting analgesic not chemically related to opioids. When taken up to 3 months for osteoarthritis, the Cochrane Review gave Tramadol gold level evidence for decreasing pain, improving stiffness, function, and overall well being (SOR = A).[24] A recent RCT in 2006 demonstrated that Tramadol ER was effective for patients with knee or hip osteoarthritis with limited side effects.[25]

Tramadol, in contrast to NSAIDs, does not cause GI bleeding, renal problems or aggravate hypertension and CHF. Compared with narcotics, tramadol does not have significant abuse potential. Common side effects from tramadol include nausea, vomiting, dizziness, sweating, constipation, tiredness, and headache.

Intra-Articular Injectable Therapy

Glucocorticoids and viscosupplementation are the most common intra-articular therapies used for hip osteoarthritis. Due to the location of the hip joint, it is recommended to perform hip injections under direct fluoroscopic visualization or ultrasound guidance (Fig. 14.6). Intra-articular injections of the hip are well tolerated and easy to perform when guided by ultrasound. Overall, the procedure is regarded as innocuous and safe.[26] Contraindications to joint injections include bacteremia, inaccessible joints, joint prosthesis, adjacent osteomyelitis, and overlying infection of the soft tissue.

Corticosteroids

Corticosteroids inhibit the inflammatory and immune cascade at several levels and may be most useful in patients with local inflammation and joint effusion. Intra-articular corticosteroids have an overall anti-inflammatory effect and have been shown to be effective in managing osteoarthritis. However, their long term benefits and safety have not been established definitively.[1] There are no long-term studies examining the risks of multiple injections, but, in general, no more then 3–4 injections per year are recommended.

An RCT of 101 patients with hip osteoarthritis found that patients treated with corticosteroids experienced significant

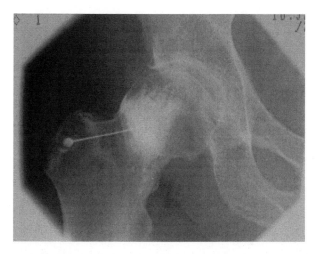

FIGURE 14.6. Fluoroscopic image of intra-articular hip injection (courtesy of Dr. Brian J. McGrory).

improvement during the 3-month intervention period. Although the effect of corticosteroid was short lived, these results support corticosteroid use in the treatment of hip osteoarthritis for acute pain relief. The presence of an effusion in the hip joint was associated with good clinical response to corticosteroid injection.[26]

If total hip arthroplasty (THA) is expected in the near future, caution should be taken in proceeding with intra-articular steroid injection (SOR = C). In a 2006 retrospective review of 224 patients with primary THA implanted within 1 year of intra-articular steroid injection compared with 224 who had not received an injection, there was overall no statistically significant affect on postoperative rates of infection. However, the mean time from injection to THA in patients with deep postoperative infection was 44 days. It is recommended that intra-articular steroids injected into the hip should be avoided for at least 2 months before THA.[27]

Viscosupplementation
Hyaluronan (HA) is a long polysaccharide chain synthesized by type B synoviocytes and fibroblasts in the synovium and secreted into the joint space. Due to its HA content, synovial fluid has both viscous (lubricating) and elastic (shock absorbing) properties.[19] A normal knee contains approximately 2 mL of synovial fluid with a HA concentration of 2.5–4.0 mg/mL. In an osteoarthritic knee, HA

concentration is reduced by a factor of 2–3 due to degradation and dilution, and the molecular weight of HA is reduced as well.[19]

Viscosupplementation is the intra-articular injection of exogenous HA. The dwelling time of exogenous HA in the joint is short lived. However, it exerts its effect over a longer period of time than corticosteroids and may also take longer to achieve this effect. The mechanism is not completely understood, but there are several theories including the restoration of rheologic (viscoelastic) properties of synovial fluid, an anti-inflammatory effect, an antinociceptive effect, normalization of endogenous HA synthesis, and chondroprotection.

In a prospective trial of 56 patients with primary hip osteoarthritis, aged 40 and older, over 50% had a decrease in pain and an increase in function after a single 2 mL dose of hylan G–F under fluoroscopic guidance. The outcomes were better in less severe osteoarthritis and an inverse correlation was seen between the reduction in pain and the joint space narrowing score.[28] One double blind controlled study comparing low molecular weight hyaluronic acid, corticosteroid, and saline (placebo) showed overall no difference at 3 months, but Hyalgan did appear superior to placebo in moderate disease.[26]

In the United States, viscosupplementation is off label use for hip osteoarthritis as it is currently only approved for osteoarthritis use in the knee by the Food and Drug Administration (FDA). Intra-articular viscosupplementation has proven to be safe with ultrasound guidance in the hip.[26] Overall incidence of side effects is 1–4% per injection with the most common being a local reaction which is self limited. Precaution should be taken in patients with avian allergies for many formulations.

In summary, data suggest that viscosupplementation may reduce symptoms in hip osteoarthritis, especially in moderate disease, and is safe and well tolerated. It is indicated for patients who have not responded to non-pharmacologic or oral drug therapy, but due to cost and invasiveness of the procedure, it cannot be recommended as standard therapy. Indications remain highly individualized[26] (SOR = C).

SUPPLEMENTS/ALTERNATIVE THERAPIES

Glucosamine and Chondroitin

Glucosamine sulfate participates in the synthesis of proteoglycans and glycosaminoglycans found in hyaline cartilage. Chondroitin sulfate is a glycosaminoglycan found in cartilage and other connective tissues. They are considered dietary supplements and are, therefore, not regulated by the FDA. Commercial preparations are readily available over the counter, but caution should be used as safety and efficacy may vary from preparation to preparation.[1,29] The recommended dosage of glucosamine is 1,500 mg/day and chondroitin is 800–1,200 mg/day. Onset of effect is variable and results may not be seen for 2 months.

There have been no structure-modifying effects established in osteoarthritis,[3] but results favor glucosamine and chondroitin for pain relief and function compared to placebo as well as glucosamine efficacy in joint space narrowing. However, the majority of the studies have been done in knee osteoarthritis. A systematic review found no direct evidence to support clinical benefit (pain relief, functional improvement) for glucosamine in hip osteoarthritis, but one RCT demonstrated that chondroitin effectively reduces pain and disability from hip osteoarthritis.[3] The Glucosamine/Chondroitin Arthritis Intervention Trial (GAIT) published in 2006 evaluated the efficacy of glucosamine and chondroitin in the treatment of knee arthritis in 1,583 patients. There was a high placebo response in the study and results showed the supplements were not significantly better than placebo at reducing arthritis pain by 20%. Nevertheless, subgroup analysis revealed the combination to be effective in moderate-to-severe knee pain.[30]

Other Supplements

Avocado/soybean unsaponifiables are nutraceuticals shown in vitro to inhibit proinflammatory cytokines and stimulate chondrocyte collagen synthesis. Limited trials suggest improvement in osteoarthritis symptoms; however, long term trials have had negative results.[1]

Rose hips may be beneficial in both early and late stages of osteoarthritis and in a recent RCT of 94 patients, 5 g of a herbal remedy made from the subspecies of rose-hip (*Rosa canina*) taken for 3 months was found to alleviate symptoms of osteoarthritis and reduce consumption of rescue medication.[31]

Acupuncture

Acupuncture, has recently been studied in the treatment of osteoarthritis. A 2006 RCT of acupuncture and osteoarthritis found patients treated with acupuncture in addition to routine care to have significant improvement in symptoms and quality of life compared with patients who received routine care alone.[32] Acupuncture is a safe intervention when administered by physicians, has a small potential for adverse events, and should be considered as adjuvant treatment for hip osteoarthritis[32] (SOR = C).

Diacerein
Diacerein is a symptomatic slow-acting drug in osteoarthritis (SYSADOA) with interleukin-1β (beta) (IL-1β (beta)) inhibitory properties. Not currently FDA approved in the United States, diacerein is available in Europe for the treatment of osteoarthritis. In a meta-analysis of 19 RCTs (2,637 patients), Rintelen et al. found diacerein to be superior to placebo and similar to NSAIDs in active treatment of osteoarthritis. There was no difference in tolerability compared to NSAIDs and diacerein had an additional carryover and prolonged residual effect after the treatment phase.[33] Overall, diacerein shows improvement in symptoms and reduction in cartilage degradation in osteoarthritis with a reasonable safety profile.

Future Directions
Disease-modifying therapies including gene therapy, matrix metalloproteinase inhibitors, and bisphosphonates as well as substances such as green tea and ginger are all potential therapies in need of further study in the treatment of osteoarthritis.

INDICATIONS FOR SURGERY
Before any major reconstruction of the hip is recommended, conservative measures should be exhausted. These should include weight loss, pharmacologic therapy, reasonable restriction of activity, and use of a cane. These measures may delay or obviate the need for surgery. If the patient is experiencing pain at night and pain with motion and weight-bearing activities severe enough to prevent them from working, enjoying a good quality of life, and carrying out the activities of daily living, surgery may be indicated. Pain to this degree with evidence of radiographic degenerative process in the hip is an indication for surgery.

The most important and agreed measures for THR are pain and function[3] (SOR = C). Radiographic change is important to confirm diagnosis, but at this time the importance of the degree of change and indication for THR remains unclear.[3] Vinciguerra et al. found factors associated with the risk of total hip replacement to be of the age older than 54 at diagnosis, BMI greater than 27, and severe radiologic evidence of joint space narrowing at diagnosis.[34]

In young adults with symptomatic hip osteoarthritis, osteotomy and joint preserving surgical procedures should be considered, especially in the presence of dysplasia or varus/valgus deformity.[3]

CASE CONCLUSION
Diagnosed with osteoarthritis, the patient began taking glucosamine and chondroitin and daily acetaminophen. With minimal

results, she attempted a trial of daily NSAIDs without significant results. The pain continued to limit her functional capacity and quality of life. Several cortisone injections under fluoroscopic guidance were done, the effects never lasting more than a month. Given her young age and desire to remain moderately active, she elected to try viscosupplementation. Three weekly injections given under fluoroscopic guidance unfortunately provided very short-term relief. After exhausting all of her non-surgical options, the patient underwent a total hip replacement. She subsequently has been able to return to many activities and overall reports an increased quality of life.

References
1. Fajardo M, Di Cesare PE. Disease-modifying therapies for osteoarthritis current status. Drugs Aging 2005; 22(2):141–161.
2. Roddy E, Zhang W, Doherty M, et al. Evidence-based recommendations for the role of exercise in the management of osteoarthritis of the hip or knee-the MOVE consensus. Rheumatology 2005; 44:67–73.
3. Zhang W, Doherty M, Arden N, et al. EULAR evidence based recommendations for the management of hip osteoarthritis: report of a task force of the EULAR Standing Committee for International Clinical Studies Including Therapeutics (ESCISIT). Ann Rheum Dis 2005; 64:669–681.
4. Jacobsen S, Sonne-Holm S, Soballe K, et al. Radiographic case definitions and prevelance of osteoarthritis of the hip: A survey of 4,151 subjects in the Osteoarthritis Substudy of the Copenhagen City Heart Study. Acta Orthop Scand 2004; 75(6):713–720.
5. Gupta KB, Duryea J, Weissman BN. Radiologic evaluation of osteoarthritis. Radiol Clin North Am 2004; 42:11–41.
6. Tepper S, Hochberg MC. Factors associated with hip osteoarthritis: data from the First National Health and Nutrition Examination Survey (NHANES-I). Am J Epidemiol 1993; 137(10):1081–1088.
7. Lievense AM, Bierma-Zeinstra SM, Verhagen AP, et al. Influence of obesity on the development of osteoarthris of the hip: a systematic review. Rheumatology 2002; 41:1155–1162.
8. Fransen M, McConnell S, Bell M. Exercise for osteoarthritis of the hip or knee. The Cochrane Database of Systematic Reviews 2006; 4.
9. Kellgren JH, Lawrence JS. Radiological assessment of osteo-arthrosis. Ann Rheum Dis 1957; 16:494–502.
10. Croft P, Cooper C, Wickham C, et al. Defining osteoarthritis of the hip in epidemiologic studies. Amer J Epidemiol 1990; 132(3):514–522.
11. Altman R, Alarcon G, Appelrouth D, et al. The American College of Rheumatology criteria for the classification and reporting of osteoarthritis of the hip. Arthritis Rheum 1991; (34)505–514.
12. Tak E, Staats P, Van Hespen A, et al. The effects of an exercise program for older adults with osteoarthritis of the hip. J Rheumatol 2005; 32(6):1106–1113.

13. Brosseau L, MacLeay L, Robinson VA, et al. Intensity of exercise for the treatment of osteoarthritis. The Cochrane Database of Systematic Reviews 2006; 4.
14. Hinman RS, Heywood SE, Day AR. Aquatic physical therapy for hip and knee osteoarthritis: results of a single-blind randomized controlled trial. Phys Ther 2007; 87(1):32–43.
15. Foley A, Halbert J, Hewitt T, Crotty M. Does hydrotherapy improve strength and physical function in patients with osteoarthrits – a randomised controlled trial comparing a gym based and hydrotherapy based strengthening programme. Ann Rheum Dis 2003; 62:1162–1167.
16. Buszewicz M, Rait G, Griffin M, et al. Self management of arthritis in primary care: randomised controlled trial. BMJ 2006; 333:879–882.
17. Kamath CC, Kremers HM, Vanness DJ, et al. The cost-effectiveness of acetaminophen, NSAIDs, and selective COX-2 inhibitors in the treatment of symptomatic knee arthritis. Value in Health 2003; 6(2):144–157.
18. Kuffner EK, Temple AR, Cooper KM, et al. Retrospective analysis of transient elevations in alanine aminotransferase during long-term treatment with acetaminophen in osteoarthritis clinical trials. Curr Med Res Op 2006; 22(11):2137–2148.
19. Brockmeier SF, Shaffer BS. Viscosupplementation therapy for osteoarthritis. Sports Med Arthrosc Rev 2006; 14(3):155–162.
20. Lin J, Zhang W, Jones A, et al. Efficacy of topical non-steroidal anti-inflammatory drugs in the treatment of osteoarthritis: meta-analysis of randomised controlled trials. BMJ, doi: 10.1136/bmj.38159.639028.7C (published 30 July 2004).
21. Schnitzer TJ, Burmester GR, Mysler E. Comparison of lumiracoxib with naprosyn and ibuprofen in the Therapeutic Arthritis Research and Gastrointestinal Event Trial (TARGET), reduction in ulcer complications: randomised controlled trial. Lancet 2004; 364:665–674.
22. Gorsline RT, Kaeding CC. The Use of NSAIDs and nutritional supplements in athletes with osteoarthritis: prevalence, benefits and consequences. Clin Sports Med 2005; 24:71–82.
23. Kivitz A, Ma C, Ahdieh H, et al. A 2-week, multicenter, randomized, double-blind, placebo-controlled, dose-ranging, phase III trial comparing the efficacy of oxymorphone extended release and placebo in adults with pain associated with osteoarthritis of the hip or knee. Clin Therap 2006; 28(3):352–364.
24. Cepeda MS, Camargo F, Zea C, et al. Tramadol for osteoarthritis. The Cochrane Database of Systematic Reviews 2007; 1.
25. Gana TJ, Pascual MLG, Fleming RRB, et al. Extended-release tramadol in the treatment of osteoarthritis: a multicenter, randomized, double-blind, placebo-controlled clinical trial. Curr Med Res Op 2006; 22(7):1391–1401.
26. Qvistgaard E, Christensen R, Torp-Pedersen S, et al. Intra-articular treatment of hip osteoarthritis: a randomized trial of hyaluronic acid, corticosteroid, and isotonic saline. Osteoarthrits Cartilage 2006; 14(2):163–170.

27. McIntosh AL, Hanssen AD, Wenger DE, et al. Recent intraarticular steroid injection may increase infection rates in primary THA. Clin Orthop Rel Res 2006; 451:50–54.
28. Conrozier T, Bertin P, Bailleul F, et al. Clinical response to intra-articular injections of hylan G–F 20 in symptomatic hip osteoarthritis: the OMERACT=OARSI criteria applied to results of a pilot study. Joint Bone Spine 2006; 73:705–709.
29. Adebowale AO, Cox DS, Liang Z, et al. Analysis of glucosamine and chondroitin sulfate content in marketed products and the caco-2 permeability of chondrointin sulfate raw materials. J Am Nutraceutical Assoc 2000; 3:37–44.
30. Clegg DO, Reda DJ, Harris CL, et al. Glucosamine, chondroitin aulfate, and the two in combination for painful knee osteoarthritis. N Engl J Med 2006; 354(8):795–808.
31. Winther K, Apel K, Thamsborg G. A powder made from seeds and shells of a rose-hip subspecies (*Rosa canina*) reduces symptoms of knee and hip osteoarthritis: a randomized, double-blind, placebo-controlled trial. Scand J Rheumatol 2005; 34:302–308.
32. Witt CM, Jena S, Brinkhaus B, et al. Acupuncture in patients with osteoarthritis of the knee or hip. Arthritis Rheum 2006; 54(11):3485–3493.
33. Rintelen B, Neumann K, Burkhard FL. A meta-analysis of controlled clinical studies with diacerein in the treatment of osteoarthritis. Arch Intern Med 2006; 166:1899–1906.
34. Vinciguerra C, Gueguen A, Revel M, et al. Predictors of the need for total hip replacement in patients with osteoarthritis of the hip. Rev Rheum 1995; 62(9):563–570.

Chapter 15
Surgical Interventions in Hip and Pelvis Injuries

Carl Wierks and John H. Wilckens

CLINICAL PEARLS

- Diagnosing the cause of hip pain in the athlete can be difficult, but it almost always can be accomplished with an understanding of local anatomy combined with a thorough history and physical examination.
- For most causes of athletic hip pain, the patient should be given a sustained trial of nonoperative treatment before surgery is considered.
- Femoral neck fractures and hip dislocations in the athlete require emergency treatment.
- Thoughtful imaging of the hip or pelvis is an important diagnostic tool that can distinguish tendon strain from avulsion, help diagnose osteitis pubis, and evaluate for tumor as a cause for pain.
- Adolescents with hip abnormalities commonly present themselves with knee pain. Adolescents with knee pain should have their hips evaluated.

CASE PRESENTATION

Chief Compliant
Right side groin pain

Patient History
A 16-year-old male complains of an insidious onset of right-side groin pain that increases with activity, for the past 2 weeks. He

has recently increased his training regimen to prepare for the upcoming soccer season. He denies any sentinel event, such as a collision or fall, nor has he had similar symptoms in the past. He does have mild night pain.

Physical Examination
As the patient walks into the examination room, a slight antalgic gait is noticed. Hip range of motion, strength, and sensation are normal. There is no snapping as the hip is ranged from full flexion to extension. Focal tenderness is identified in the medial groin. Resisted hip flexion, extension, and internal and external rotation fail to incite pain, but standing on only the affected leg does increase discomfort slightly.

Imaging
An anteroposterior (AP) view of the pelvis and AP and lateral views of the affected hip show a normal pelvis and hip. Magnetic resonance imaging (MRI) shows an increased T2-weighted signal in the superior femoral neck.

INTRODUCTION
Hip and pelvis pain in the athlete can be a difficult diagnosis because of the complexity of the anatomy, multiple potential causes of symptoms (including low back disorders), and the possibility of concurrent disease processes. Pelvic injuries occur most commonly in athletes who participate in sports with frequent cutting, acceleration, and deceleration maneuvers.[1]

Most sports-related conditions resolve with nonoperative treatment, but it is important to identify and treat conditions that could be detrimental to the athlete if not addressed appropriately. A few of these injuries, such as hip dislocation or femoral neck fracture, need to be addressed surgically on an emergent basis, but most injuries require the athlete to undergo extensive nonoperative treatment before surgical intervention is considered.

MUSCLE STRAIN/AVULSION
Muscle strain or avulsion is one of the most common athletics-related injuries to the pelvis. It may occur when a muscle is contracting forcefully, particularly when it is simultaneously lengthening.[2,3] A strain or tear typically occurs at the musculotendinous junction, but it also may occur in the muscle belly.[2] Disability is proportional to the amount of fiber damage.[4]

Patients present themselves with pain or a pulling sensation in the affected muscle group. Provocative testing of the affecting muscle group exacerbates the pain. An AP radiograph of the pelvis may be taken to evaluate for an avulsion fracture, but the fragment may be missed in the skeletally immature athlete whose apophysis may be unossified. MRI can delineate further the extent of injury and potentially can predict recovery.[5]

Muscle strains have been categorized into three grades[6]: grade I, a small disruption of the musculotendinous unit; grade II, a partial tear of the muscle; and grade III, a complete rupture of the muscle. Grades I and II should be treated nonoperatively with a rehabilitation program (SOR = C).[1,2] In grade-III injuries, a palpable defect may be present and can be identified by MRI.[1,7] In addition, loss of function, such as weakness and limited range of motion, may be found. Primary repair of grade-III injuries is difficult and not recommended (SOR = C).[1,2] In chronic cases of muscle belly rupture, scar tissue may replace the native muscle tissue. This scar tissue may contribute to chronic pain and reduced performance.

If a functional deficit is present after a formal therapy program and other potential causes of groin pain have been excluded, then resection of the abnormal tissue at the adductor origin or an adductor tenotomy may provide symptom relief (SOR = C).[7-9] One study that evaluated 16 male athletes 35 months after adductor longus tenotomies for chronic groin pain found that all patients had improved or were free from symptoms; all but one returned to sport, and 10 of 16 performed at preinjury levels.[10]

Avulsions may occur at the origin or insertion sites of the pelvic muscles. They tend to occur with violent muscular contraction (particularly with eccentric contractions), with the hip flexed or extended, and with the knee extended,[11] and in those muscles that cross two joints, such as the rectus femoris (anterior inferior iliac spine) and sartorius (anterior superior iliac spine). When an avulsion occurs at the origin of the hamstring muscles (ischium), it is known as a hurdler's fracture (Fig. 15.1). Since the ischial tuberosity may not fuse completely until the third decade of life (Table 15.1),[12] it is at risk for an apophyseal avulsion injury until that age.[1,2] Surgery may be considered if the avulsed fragment is large enough to be stabilized with hardware and if it is displaced 2 cm or more (SOR = C).[2] Some authors have recommended early surgical fixation of ischial avulsions, quoting improved outcomes compared with those after a rehabilitation program alone (SOR = C).[1,13] Kujala et al.[14] recommended nonoperative treatment as the primary modality for ischial tuberosity apophysitis and avulsion injuries. However, even in that study, 7 of 21 patients with a complete avulsion required surgery to return to sport after initial nonoperative treatment.

A rare complication of an ischial apophyseal avulsion is a late sciatic nerve palsy, which may respond to neurolysis.[15]

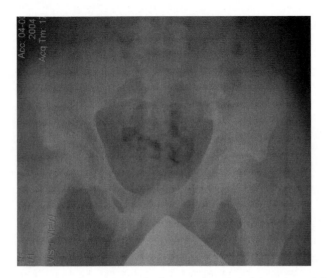

FIGURE 15.1. AP pelvis radiograph of an apophyseal avulsion injury of the ischium.

TABLE 15.1. Appearance and fusion of Pelvic apophyses in adolescents[12]

Location	Approximate age at appearance (years)	Approximate age at fusion (years)
Iliac crest		
Female	13	15
Male	14	16
Anterior inferior iliac spine	13–15	16–18
Ischial tuberosity	13–15	16–18
Lesser trochanter		
Female	11	14–15
Male	12	16–17

From: Metzmaker and Pappas[12]

The differential diagnosis includes tendon strain, hernia, osteitis pubis, internal snapping hip syndrome, and referred low back/discogenic pain.

HIP DISLOCATION

Hip dislocations are rare in sports, but they may occur after high-energy trauma. Hips usually dislocate posteriorly. The hip is at risk when fully flexed or extended, as occurs in head-on collisions.[2]

A posteriorly dislocated hip presents in a flexed, internally rotated, and adducted position. An anteriorly dislocated hip presents in an externally rotated, abducted, and flexed or extended position. Radiographic diagnosis requires an AP view of the pelvis and a lateral view of the hip to confirm the direction of dislocation.

In a controlled setting in which sedation and muscle relaxation can be administered, emergent closed reduction is attempted to decrease risk of avascular necrosis (AVN) and damage to the articular cartilage of the femoral head. A postreduction computed tomography (CT) scan should be obtained to rule out intra-articular fragments and to confirm concentric reduction. Operative intervention may be required if closed reduction fails or if there are concomitant acetabular or femoral head fractures that require surgery. Intraarticular loose osteochondral fragments may be removed arthroscopically.[16]

The most common complication after traumatic hip dislocation is AVN of the femoral head, which, according to Anderson et al.[2] occurs in 10–20% of hip dislocations. For this reason, they have recommended that MRI be performed 3 months after the injury to evaluate for osteonecrosis.

The differential diagnosis includes acetabular fracture.

HIP FRACTURES

Hip fractures, which occur after high-energy trauma such as collisions or falls, present with groin pain. Radiographs should include an AP view of the pelvis, AP and lateral views of the affected hip, and AP and lateral views of the affected femur. These radiographs usually are sufficient for determining the diagnosis.

Fractures of the hip should be managed with anatomic open reduction and internal fixation. Femoral neck fractures require particular urgency because of the risk of AVN. (See the discussion under Stress Fractures for more specific treatment.)

STRESS FRACTURES

Military recruits and athletes with repetitive loading stresses across the hip joint and an increase in training regimen are at risk for stress fractures. Female athletes with amenorrhea and eating disorders also are at risk for developing stress fractures.[2,4] Femoral neck stress fractures present with groin, anterior thigh or knee pain with loading, pain at extremes of range of motion, and, occasionally, night pain.[17] The pain has a gradual onset, is increased with and eventually prevents activity, and is relieved with rest.[4] Physical examination reveals local tenderness, an antalgic gait, and decreased internal rotation of the hip.

Radiographic evidence of fracture may lag 2–4 weeks after the onset of symptoms.[17] Bone scintigraphy or MRI is needed to confirm a clinical diagnosis in the acute setting.[18] Early diagnosis is essential to prevent progression of the fracture to displacement and subsequent risk of AVN and pseudarthrosis.[18,19]

Treatment is based on the fracture pattern. A treatment algorithm has been proposed based on radiographs and MRI of the hip.[20] The algorithm uses the division of compression, tension, and displaced stress fractures as originally described by Fullerton and Snowdy[17] (Fig. 15.2) and then subdivides compression fractures into fractures with a fatigue line less than 50% and greater than or equal to 50% of the femoral neck.[20]

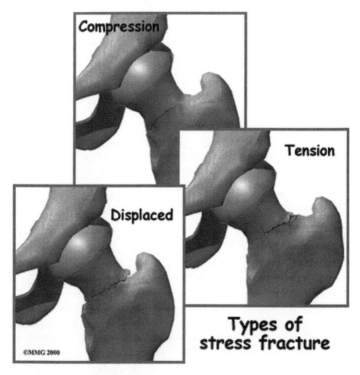

Figure 15.2. Artist's sketch of compression, tension, and displaced types of femoral neck fractures. From eOrthopod. http://www.eOrthopod.com. Image provided as a courtesy of Medical Multimedia Group. http://www.medicalmultimediagroup.com/. Used with permission.

In this algorithm, plain radiography is used initially for diagnosis. If a displaced fracture is present, emergent open reduction and internal fixation is recommended (SOR = B).[17,18,20] If a cortical crack is present on the tension side, then urgent percutaneous pinning is performed (SOR = C).[17,20] If a crack is present on the compression side and is greater than or equal to 50% of the femoral neck width, then percutaneous pinning is done; if the crack is less than 50%, the patient must be nonweightbearing with crutches and is followed closely for progression (SOR = C).[20] If progression occurs, then pinning is done (SOR = B).[17,20]

If plain radiography is negative, MRI of the hip is performed. If the MRI is positive for a tension-side fracture, then urgent percutaneous pinning is recommended (SOR = C).[20] If the compression side is affected, the 50% femoral neck width rule is applied (i.e., pinning of fractures affecting more than 50% and nonweightbearing on crutches for patients with less than 50% affected) (SOR = C).[20] If there is any concern about patient compliance with nonweightbearing, operative intervention is recommended.[19,20]

Percutaneous fixation of compression-side fractures may be performed with three 6.5- or 7.0-mm cannulated screws, and patients may be allowed to bear weight as tolerated postoperatively.[20] Nondisplaced tension-side fractures also may be treated with three percutaneous screws. Displaced fractures may be stabilized internally with a sliding compression hip screw and a side plate or cannulated screws after open reduction. Patients should be nonweightbearing for 8–12 weeks because of the risk of nonunion. Long-term follow up should be done to evaluate for AVN, nonunion, varus malunion, and osteoarthritis.[20] According to one report, approximately two-thirds of patients with displaced fractures develop a clinically significant complication.[21]

ACETABULAR LABRAL TEARS

The acetabular labrum is a fibrocartilaginous rim around the bony acetabulum. The function of the acetabular labrum is to add stability by deepening the hip socket, creating a negative intraarticular pressure, and preserving the fluid-film layer in the joint.[22,23] Inferiorly, the labrum is contiguous with the transverse acetabular ligament and defines the lateral edge of the acetabulum. Free nerve endings have been found in all areas of the labrum, so a tear may cause pain in a way similar to that of a tear of the meniscus.[23]

Labral tears may be caused by trauma, hip dislocation, twisting injuries, or they may have no identifiable cause.[2,23,24] Labral tears also may be a part of a degenerative process.[23,25] Tear have been described as radial flap, degenerative, bucket handle, horizontal cleavage, and peripheral longitudinal types.[26] The most common locations are the anterior[26,27] or anterosuperior[23] labrum.

Labral tears present primarily with groin pain that is exacerbated by pivoting or twisting.[27] Often, "catching" or clicking of the hip and decreased range of motion is present.[2,23,24] Passive range of motion or resisted adduction of the hip reproduces the pain.[23,26]

Diagnostic techniques for labral tears can include a variety of modalities. Radiographs may reveal acetabular dysplasia or degenerative changes such as cysts that often occur in conjunction with labral tears, but alone they usually are insufficient for making the diagnosis.[26] Historically, MRI has not been sensitive or specific enough to make the diagnosis,[22,24,26] except for the presence of a paralabral cyst, which is believed to be diagnostic for a labral tear.[28] Magnetic resonance arthrography is the imaging test of choice because the contrast outlines the capsule and fills the tear.[23] Also, an anesthetic added to the intraarticular contrast injection can be diagnostic. If the pain resolves with this injection, then the source of pain is intraarticular, whether it be a labral tear or a chondral injury. Newer and higher resolution MRI may obviate the need for a contrast study.

Initial treatment for all tear types is protected weightbearing for 4 weeks with nonsteroidal antiinflammatory drugs (NSAIDs) as needed (SOR = C).[2] The natural history of tears, such as whether they will heal spontaneously or become quiescent, is unknown. If nonoperative treatment fails to relieve symptoms substantially, labral resection may be performed. Open resection has been described with some success, but it has a higher risk for complications such as AVN or trochanteric bursitis.[27] For this reason, arthroscopic debridement of the torn aspect of the labrum is the preferred surgical technique (SOR = B).[22–24] It is associated with a decreased risk of surgical complications and allows for visualization of the joint surfaces without dislocation of the hip.[22–24,27]

Postoperatively, patients may be allowed to bear partial weight, with progression to full weightbearing as tolerated.[26] In one retrospective study, 28 patients who underwent arthroscopic labral debridement were divided equally into two groups based on the presence or absence of hip osteoarthritis.[26] The authors reported good results in 71% of patients without arthritis and in 21% of those with arthritis.[26]

Another study that looked exclusively at hip arthroscopy in athletes found that the best surgical outcomes occurred in young patients who had sustained trauma and young patients who had had impinging osteophytes, loose bodies, or ruptured ligamentum teres.[16] Less impressive but marked benefits also were seen in patients with chondral and labral injuries.[16] Complications are rare but those most frequently reported are peroneal, pudendal, and sciatic nerve neuropraxias.[22,29]

The differential diagnosis includes groin sprain, hernia, snapping hip syndrome, and osteitis pubis.

SPORTS/HOCKEY HERNIA

Sports hernia may be a cause of persistent, ongoing pain.[1] It may be secondary to a weakening of posterior abdominal wall, resulting in a direct or indirect hernia. Potential causes are multifactorial but include overuse, congenital weakness of the abdominal wall, and abnormalities in the insertion of the abdominal muscles in athletes who twist or cut forcefully, such as in soccer, ice hockey, and tennis.[1,2]

Typically, presentation is an insidious, progressive, nonspecific deep pain. Bearing down or coughing may increase the pain. Pubic tenderness may be present, but pain with resisted adduction is more common, according to one study.[30] No true hernia is palpated on examination because only the deep fascia is compromised.[31] Although imaging studies may not be helpful in confirming the diagnosis, they are needed to rule out other conditions such as stress fracture and osteitis pubis.

If nonsurgical management for 6–8 weeks fails to alleviate symptoms, then appropriate surgical treatment should be considered.[31] According to one study, 97% of 157 patients with rectus abdominis muscle reattachment returned to their previous levels of activity.[30] In addition, herniorrhaphy via open or laparoscopic approach has had good results.[32]

Inguinal hernias can be an elusive cause of persistent groin pain in the athlete and may represent a later spectrum of a sports hernia. Fortunately, endoscopic preperitoneal herniorrhaphy can be performed to diagnose and to treat effectively athletes with otherwise undiagnosed cause of groin pain.[33] Athletes usually can return to presurgical performance within 3 weeks.[33]

The differential diagnosis includes osteitis pubis, distal rectus abdominis strain, adductor strain, adductor tenoperiosteal lesions, and symphyseal instability.

GILMORE'S GROIN/GROIN DISRUPTION

Gilmore's groin is a severe musculotendinous injury of the groin. It has several reported causes, including torn external oblique aponeurosis, torn or avulsed conjoined tendon, and dehiscence between conjoined tendon and inguinal ligament.[34] Gilmore[34] described his series of soccer players as 98% male; 70% of his patients had unilateral groin pain of insidious onset that increased with increased use. A proposed cause is a muscular imbalance between strong hip flexors, which cause the pelvis to tilt forward and stretch the relatively weaker abdominal muscles, making them susceptible to injury.[34]

The diagnosis is made by palpating the dilated and tender superficial inguinal ring. To rule out pelvic instability, radiographs should be taken while the patient stands on both legs and then on one leg ("flamingo" view). There should be less than a 3 mm shift in the symphysis on the single-leg radiographic view.[34]

All patients should be treated initially with a rehabilitation protocol, with a gradual return to activity over several weeks. If patients do not respond to rehabilitation, surgical restoration of normal anatomy with suture repair has been recommended (SOR = C).[34] In one study, after surgical repair, the average return to sport was within 6 weeks, with a 97% success rate in soccer players.[34]

The differential diagnosis includes hernia, tendon strain, osteitis pubis, and acetabular labral tear.

OSTEITIS PUBIS

Osteitis pubis is a low-grade inflammation associated with mild symphysis pubis instability,[34] sometimes seen in postpartum women returning to athletic activity. It may be caused by repetitive strain on the symphysis pubis from chronic pull of the rectus abdominal or adductor muscles. Presentation typically is increased pain with kicking, jumping, or twisting in runners, soccer players, and hockey players.[2] Diagnosis may be made by an AP radiograph of the pelvis showing sclerosis or resorption of bone adjacent to the symphysis pubis. A step-off across the symphysis also may be seen. Bone scintigraphy shows increased activity at the pubis symphysis but not at the pubic tubercle.[34]

Treatment is with prolonged rest, NSAIDs, and corticosteroid injection is given if symptoms are severe. Symphysis pubis fusion may be required (but rarely) if these modalities fail to provide relief.[34] Additionally, adductor tenotomy has had some benefit in protracted cases.[10]

The differential diagnosis includes hernia, adductor muscle strain or avulsion, Gilmore's groin, and acetabular labral tear.

SNAPPING HIP SYNDROME

Snapping hip syndrome can be divided into internal and external varieties. In the internal variety, a snapping is felt medially in the deep anterior groin when the hip is ranged from flexion through extension.

It is thought that the iliopsoas tendon snaps over structures such as the femoral head, pelvic brim (iliopectineal eminence), or lesser trochanter.[35] In the external variety, snapping is felt laterally as the iliotibial band (ITB) passes over the greater trochanter of the femur with hip adduction and flexion or extension. Both types are seen in distance runners.

Initial treatment of internal and external snapping hip syndromes is relative rest, NSAIDs, and iliopsoas or ITB stretching. Corticosteroid injection to the bursa underlying the ITB also may be attempted.[36] In addition to addressing the tight iliopsoas and ITB, stretching and strengthening and balancing the core musculature is important.

If extensive nonoperative treatment fails, then surgical treatment may be considered (SOR = C).[37] Jacobson and Allen[37] described resolution of snapping symptoms in 14 of 20 patients who underwent a step-cut of the tendinous portion of the iliopsoas muscle. White et al[35] also described using step cuts of the ITB for symptom relief. Glazer and Hosey[36] described surgical release of the ITB with resection of the underlying bursa, and Brignall and Stainsby[38] successfully used a Z-plasty to treat refractory cases.

NERVE COMPRESSION

Nerve compression represents an uncommon cause of pelvic pain in the athlete. Nerves about the pelvis (Table 15.2) may become trapped in scar tissue or fibrous adhesions, or they may be impinged by pelvic masses. Diagnosis and treatment of these problems requires an understanding of a nerve's motor and sensory innervation and its location relative to surrounding structures that may cause impingement. Electromyography and nerve conduction studies may be helpful in localizing the area of compression. Treatment is initially nonsurgical (except for oncologic cases); surgical intervention involves neurolysis around the compressed nerve. Because of the relatively rare occurrence, information about treatment choices comes from case reports.[39–43]

SCIATIC/PIRIFORMIS/HAMSTRING SYNDROMES

Compression of the sciatic nerve may occur from piriformis or hamstring muscle entrapment or adhesions.[2,44,45] Patients may report a history of a fall onto their buttocks or have a history of recurrent hamstring tears, pyomyositis, myositis ossificans, or previous deep muscular injection.[44,45]

Piriformis syndrome presents with pain along the piriformis muscle that may be localized to the sacroiliac joint, may be exacerbated with sitting or internal rotation of the hip, and can radiate

TABLE 15.2. Obturator and femoral nerves

Nerve	Origin	Innervation	Site/type of compression	Presentation
Obturator[39,40]	Ventral rami of the second through fourth lumbar roots	Adductor muscles	Pelvis (tumor or pregnancy) Obturator foramen secondary to inflammation of osteitis pubis Thickened adductor tendons	Deep, acute pain at adduction origin Radiating pain into the medial tibia
Femoral[41]	Ventral rami of L2–L4	Psoas muscle Anterior branch: sartorius muscle, sensation to the anterior thigh Posterior branch: quadriceps muscle, sensation to the anterior medial knee and leg	Inguinal ligament Blunt trauma or stretch injury	Quadriceps weakness Decreased sensation in the anterior thigh and medial knee
Ilioinguinal[42]	First lumbar nerve root	Base of penis or labia, anterior scrotum, and medial thigh	Blunt trauma Abdominal hypertrophy	Groin, genital, or lower abdominal pain
Iliohypogastric[42]	First lumbar nerve root	Sensation to the inferior abdomen and groin/lateral thigh	Blunt trauma Abdominal hypertrophy	Groin, genital, or lower abdominal pain

Genitofemoral[42]	First through the third lumbar nerve roots Ventral rami of the lumbar region, highly variable origin course	Anterior scrotum/labia and medial thigh Sensation to the contralateral thigh and gluteal area	Blunt trauma Abdominal hypertrophy Acute trauma Compression by the inguinal ligament Repetitive squatting	Groin, genital, or lower abdominal pain Pain/paresthesia over the lateral thigh/gluteal area
Lateral femoral cutaneous nerve[43]				

down the leg.[44] Hamstring syndrome is characterized by pain with hamstring stretch, while in a seated position or when running fast.[2,45] Distinguishing the cause of the sciatic symptoms, whether spinal or from the piriformis, can be difficult, but magnetic resonance neurography may help.[46]

Initial treatment is nonoperative, with relative rest, NSAIDs, physical therapy, hip girdle exercises, and trigger point injections.[44] Piriformis syndrome secondary to an inflammatory sacroiliitis is best addressed by initially treating the inciting inflammation rather than by surgical release of the piriformis.[44] Surgery is considered when the above modalities have failed to provide relief (SOR = C).[44,45] If surgery is required, the piriformis may be released or split from its femoral insertion and reattached in a shortened position. In one study of nonathletes, this surgery was performed in seven patients and resulted in 100% return to work, with 70% return to customary work.[44] Similarly, another study found that surgical treatment of hamstring syndrome by division of the tight tendinous structures at the ischial insertion of the hamstring muscles gave complete relief in 52 of 59 patients,[45] but such intervention would be a treatment of last resort in an athlete.

ADOLESCENTS

Slipped Capital Femoral Epiphysis

Slipped capital femoral epiphysis (SCFE) occurs as a result of disruption of the femoral capital physeal plate through a widened zone of hypertrophy. Risk factors include male gender, obesity, and endocrine abnormalities, such as hypothyroidism. Those participating in contact sports also may be at increased risk.[34] Patients with SCFE present with hip, groin, or knee pain and increased pain with ambulation. They have decreased internal rotation of the hip secondary to the relative anterior and externally rotated position of the femoral neck in relationship to the displaced femoral head. Diagnosis is confirmed radiographically with an AP view of the pelvis and AP and lateral views of the affected hip.

Treatment for SFCE consists of ensuring that the patient is nonweightbearing on the affected leg until early single percutaneous screw fixation perpendicular to the displaced epiphysis is performed (SOR = B).[47] Prophylactic pinning of the contralateral hip may be recommended if an endocrine disorder, such as hypothyroidism, is present or the patient has pain but no visible displacement of the femoral head (SOR = C).[48] Although functional and radiographic outcomes worsen with increased severity of the slip, reduction does not appear to be beneficial in long-term results.[47]

The natural history of SCFE is gradual deterioration proportional to the severity of the slip and complications such as AVN and chondrolysis, which are more common with more severe slips.[47]

Apophyseal Avulsions

Apophyseal avulsions occur in skeletally immature athletes, particularly males 14–25 years old[49] after the apophysis appears but before it fuses. The ischium is particularly at risk because of its late age of fusion. One report documents at-risk areas from greatest to least: ischium (53%), anterior inferior iliac spine (22%), and anterior superior iliac spine (19%).[50] Less frequently affected areas were the lesser trochanter and pubic symphysis.[50]

The diagnosis is made by the presence of sudden-onset of severe hip pain after kicking or running.[2,49,51] Patients may hear a "pop" and then may experience severe pain and decrease of function. Frequently, there is no external trauma. Tenderness is found over the avulsion site, along with decreased range of motions and strength of the affected muscle or muscle group. Swelling and ecchymosis may be present.[49] Radiographs may not show an avulsion, particularly if the apophysis has not yet calcified. Ultrasound or MRI are more accurate and can be used to confirm the clinical suspicion of apophyseal injury because ossification may not have yet occurred.

Nonoperative treatment with a progressive rehabilitation program, relative rest, ice, and NSAIDs should be initiated. Surgical fixation may improve results if the displaced fragment is large enough to be stabilized and is displaced at least 2 cm (SOR = C).[52] Others have reported good results even in these conditions with nonsurgical management.[2,4,11]

TUMOR

A tumor may be an uncommon cause of hip pain in the athlete. Among the bone tumors, osteoid osteoma is a relatively common, benign, painful bone lesion (Fig. 15.3.). Typically, the pain is insidious, worse at night, and relieved by NSAIDs. Osteoid osteoma has a characteristic appearance on radiographs and CT scans: each shows a well-defined circular lucency with a sclerotic nidus. Radiofrequency ablation or a limited excisional biopsy may allow for a quicker return to sport.[53]

The differential diagnosis includes osteoma, osteoblastoma, reactive periostitis, osteosarcoma, and bone island (enostosis).

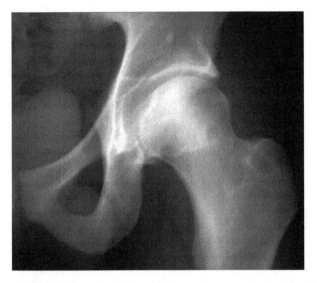

FIGURE 15.3. AP hip radiograph of a patient with an osteoid osteoma of the femoral neck showing the characteristic well-circumscribed lucency with a central sclerotic nidus. Photograph by John C. Hunter, MD. Reprinted by permission from The University of Washington Projects website: http://uwmsk.org/residentprojects.

CONCLUSION OF CASE PRESENTATION

Intervention
Percutaneous screw fixation is performed with three, 6.5-mm cannulated screws.

Follow up
Weekly follow up with radiographs is maintained until the fracture heals and the patient has painless ambulation.

Decision-Making
The decision to obtain an MRI is the key to this situation because if the patient is allowed to ambulate without fracture stabilization, the fracture may progress to a devastating injury. Once the femoral neck stress fracture is diagnosed, the decision is made to stabilize the fracture surgically or maintain a nonweightbearing status until the fracture heals. Even a reliable patient may have difficulty

maintaining strict nonweightbearing, particularly in the case of a slip or fall. Given the low morbidity of percutaneous screw fixation compared with the potentially disastrous consequences of displacement, fixation was performed in this patient.

References
1. Morelli V, Weaver V. Groin injuries and groin pain in athletes: part 1. Prim Care 2005; 32:163–183.
2. Anderson K, Strickland SM, Warren R. Hip and groin injuries in athletes. Am J Sports Med 2001; 29:521–533.
3. Garrett WE Jr, Safran MR, Seaber AV, et al. Biomechanical comparison of stimulated and nonstimulated skeletal muscle pulled to failure. Am J Sports Med 1987; 15:448–454.
4. Lynch SA, Renstrom PAFH. Groin injuries in sport: treatment strategies. Sports Med 1999; 28:137–144.
5. Pomeranz SJ, Heidt RS Jr. MR imaging in the prognostication of hamstring injury. Work in progress. Radiology 1993; 189:897–900.
6. Brown TD, Brunet ME. Thigh. Section A. Adult thigh. In: DeLee JC, Drez D Jr, Miller MD, editors. DeLee & Drez's Orthopaedic Sports Medicine: Principles and Practice, 2nd ed. Philadelphia: WB Saunders; 2003:1481–1505.
7. Hughes C IV, Hasselman CT, Best TM, et al. Incomplete, intrasubstance strain injuries of the rectus femoris muscle. Am J Sports Med 1995; 23:500–506.
8. Martens MA, Hansen L, Mulier JC. Adductor tendinitis and musculus rectus abdominis tendopathy. Am J Sports Med 1987; 15:353–356.
9. Weinstein RN, Kraushaar BS, Fulkerson JP. Adductor tendinosis in a professional hockey player. Orthopedics 1998; 21:809–810.
10. Akermark C, Johansson C. Tenotomy of the adductor longus tendon in the treatment of chronic groin pain in athletes. Am J Sports Med 1992; 20:640–643.
11. Schlonsky J, Olix ML. Functional disability following avulsion fracture of the ischial epiphysis. Report of two cases. J Bone Joint Surg 1972; 54A:641–644.
12. Metzmaker JN, Pappas AM. Avulsion fractures of the pelvis. Am J Sports Med 1985; 13:349–358.
13. Orava S, Kujala UM. Rupture of the ischial origin of the hamstring muscles. Am J Sports Med 1995; 23:702–705.
14. Kujala UM, Orava S, Karpakka J, et al. Ischial tuberosity apophysitis and avulsion among athletes. Int J Sports Med 1997; 18:149–155.
15. Spinner RJ, Atkinson JLD, Wenger DE, Stuart MJ. Tardy sciatic nerve palsy following apophyseal avulsion fracture of the ischial tuberosity. Case report. J Neurosurg 1998; 89:819–821.
16. Byrd JWT, Jones KS. Hip arthroscopy in athletes. Clin Sports Med 2001; 20:749–761.
17. Fullerton LR Jr, Snowdy HA. Femoral neck stress fractures. Am J Sports Med 1988; 16:365–377.

18. Johansson C, Ekenman I, Tornkvist H, Eriksson E. Stress fractures of the femoral neck in athletes. The consequence of a delay in diagnosis. Am J Sports Med 1990; 18:524–528.
19. Devas MB. Stress fractures of the femoral neck. J Bone Joint Surg Br 1965; 47:728–738.
20. Shin AY, Morin WD, Gorman JD, et al. The superiority of magnetic resonance imaging in differentiating the cause of hip pain in endurance athletes. Am J Sports Med 1996; 24:168–176.
21. Visuri T, Vara A, Meurman KOM. Displaced stress fractures of the femoral neck in young male adults: a report of twelve operative cases. J Trauma 1988; 28:1562–1569.
22. Byrd JWT. Labral lesions: an elusive source of hip pain case reports and literature review. Arthroscopy 1996; 12:603–612.
23. Narvani AA, Tsiridis E, Tai CC, Thomas P. Acetabular labrum and its tears. Br J Sports Med 2003; 37:207–211.
24. Hase T, Ueo T. Acetabular labral tear: arthroscopic diagnosis and treatment. Arthroscopy 1999; 15:138–141.
25. Dorrell JH, Catterall A. The torn acetabular labrum. J Bone Joint Surg Br 1986; 68:400–403.
26. Farjo LA, Glick JM, Sampson TG. Hip arthroscopy for acetabular labral tears. Arthroscopy 1999; 15:132–137.
27. Fitzgerald RH Jr. Acetabular labrum tears. Diagnosis and treatment. Clin Orthop Relat Res 1995; 311:60–68.
28. Byrd JWT, Jones KS. Diagnostic accuracy of clinical assessment, magnetic resonance imaging, magnetic resonance arthrography, and intra-articular injection in hip arthroscopy patients. Am J Sports Med 2004; 32:1668–1674.
29. Sampson TG. Complications of hip arthroscopy. Clin Sports Med 2001; 20:831–835.
30. Meyers WC, Foley DP, Garrett WE, et al. Management of severe lower abdominal or inguinal pain in high-performance athletes. PAIN (Performing Athletes with Abdominal or Inguinal Neuromuscular Pain Study Group). Am J Sports Med 2000; 28:2–8.
31. Hackney RG. The sports hernia: a cause of chronic groin pain. Br J Sports Med 1993; 27:58–62.
32. Taylor DC, Meyers WC, Moylan JA, et al. Abdominal musculature abnormalities as a cause of groin pain in athletes. Inguinal hernias and pubalgia. Am J Sports Med 1991; 19:239–242.
33. Azurin DJ, Go LS, Schuricht A, et al. Endoscopic preperitoneal herniorrhaphy in professional athletes with groin pain. J Laparoendosc Adv Surg Tech A 1997; 7:7–12.
34. Gilmore J. Groin pain in the soccer athlete: fact, fiction, and treatment. Clin Sports Med 1998; 17:787–793.
35. White RA, Hughes MS, Burd T, et al. A new operative approach in the correction of external coxa saltans: the snapping hip. Am J Sports Med 2004; 32:1504–1508.
36. Glazer JL, Hosey RG. Soft-tissue injuries of the lower extremity. Prim Care 2004; 31:1005–1024.

37. Jacobson T, Allen WC. Surgical correction of the snapping iliopsoas tendon. Am J Sports Med 1990; 18:470–474.
38. Brignall CG, Stainsby GD. The snapping hip. Treatment by Z-plasty. J Bone Joint Surg Br 1991; 73:253–254.
39. Bradshaw C, McCrory P, Bell S, Brukner P. Obturator nerve entrapment. A cause of groin pain in athletes. Am J Sports Med 1997; 25:402–408.
40. Brukner P, Bradshaw C, McCrory P. Obturator neuropathy: a cause of exercise-related groin pain. Phys Sportsmed 1999; 27:62–73.
41. Miller EH, Benedict FE. Stretch of the femoral nerve in a dancer. A case report. J Bone Joint Surg 1985; 67A:315–317.
42. Harms BA, DeHaas DR Jr, Starling JR. Diagnosis and management of genitofemoral neuralgia. Arch Surg 1984; 119:339–341.
43. Williams PH, Trzil KP. Management of meralgia paresthetica. J Neurosurg 1991; 74:76–80.
44. Foster MR. Piriformis syndrome. Orthopedics 2002; 25:821–825.
45. Puranen J, Orava S. The hamstring syndrome. A new diagnosis of gluteal sciatic pain. Am J Sports Med 1988; 16:517–521.
46. Filler AG, Haynes J, Jordan SE, et al. Sciatica of nondisc origin and piriformis syndrome: diagnosis by magnetic resonance neurography and interventional magnetic resonance imaging with outcome study of resulting treatment. J Neurosurg Spine 2005; 2:99–115.
47. Carney BT, Weinstein SL, Noble J. Long-term follow-up of slipped capital femoral epiphysis. J Bone Joint Surg Am 1991; 73:667–674.
48. Eldridge JC. Slipped capital femoral epiphysis. In: Sponseller PD, editor. Orthopaedic Knowledge Update: Pediatrics 2. Rosemont (IL): American Academy of Orthopaedic Surgeons; 2002:143–152.
49. Waters PM, Millis MB. Hip and pelvic injuries in the young athlete. Clin Sports Med 1988; 7:513–526.
50. Rossi F, Dragoni S. Acute avulsion fractures of the pelvis in adolescent competitive athletes: prevalence, location and sports distribution of 203 cases collected. Skeletal Radiol 2001; 30:127–131.
51. Boyd KT, Peirce NS, Batt ME. Common hip injuries in sport. Sports Med 1997; 24:273–288.
52. Paletta GA Jr, Andrish JT. Injuries about the hip and pelvis in the young athlete. Clin Sports Med 1995; 14:591–628.
53. Ahlfeld SK, Makley JT, Derosa GP, et al. Osteoid osteoma of the femoral neck in the young athlete. Am J Sports Med 1990; 18:271–276.

Appendix 1

EVIDENCE-BASED MEDICINE

Evidence-based medicine is the utilization of the best medical evidence in the clinical decision-making process. Until recently, the majority of the musculoskeletal literature was not based on patient-oriented evidence-based research. Instead, it was formulated via expert opinions, consensus, and case series. While these sources of information are certainly useful, some of these "tried-and-true" dictums of medicine, when tested by controlled trials, have not been found to be as significant as once believed.

The medical community is hungry for evidence-based recommendations that matter to our patients. This is demonstrated by the popularity of reference materials which is Up to Date and the development of various grading scales by organizations such as American Academy of Family Physicians, Center for Evidence Based Medicine,[1] the Cochrane Collaboration,[2] and the U.S. Preventive Services Task Force.[3]

For this handbook, the editors have chosen the system utilized by the American Family Physician journal;[4,5] one with which many primary care providers are already familiar. Within the text, a strength of recommendation (SOR) or level of evidence (LOE) rating is assigned to recommendations and data as appropriate.

STRENGTH OF RECOMMENDATION TAXONOMY

In general, only key recommendations for readers require an SOR grade. Recommendations should be based on the highest-quality evidence available. For example, vitamin E was found in some cohort studies (level 2 study quality) to have a benefit for cardiovascular protection, but good-quality randomized trials (level 1) have not confirmed this effect. Table A1.1 shows the SOR grading scale.

Table A1.1. Sor grades and definitions

Strength of recommendation	Definition
A	Recommendation based on consistent and good-quality patient-oriented evidence.[a]
B	Recommendation based on inconsistent or limited-quality patient-oriented evidence.[a]
C	Recommendation based on consensus, usual practice, opinion, disease-oriented evidence,[a] or case series for studies of diagnosis, treatment, prevention, or screening.

[a]Patient-oriented evidence measures outcomes that matter to patients: morbidity, mortality, symptom improvement, cost reduction, and quality of life. Disease-oriented evidence measures intermediate, physiologic, or surrogate end points that may or may not reflect improvements in patient outcomes (e.g., blood pressure, blood chemistry, physiologic function, pathologic findings

Table A1.2 has guidelines on determining whether a study measuring patient-oriented outcomes is of good or of limited quality. Table A1.3 shows how to determine whether the results are consistent or inconsistent between studies.

LEVEL OF EVIDENCE[4,5]

Level A (randomized controlled trial/meta-analysis): High-quality randomized controlled trial (RCT) that considers all important outcomes. High-quality meta-analysis (quantitative systematic review) using comprehensive search strategies.

Level B (other evidence): A well-designed, nonrandomized clinical trial. A nonquantitative, systematic review with appropriate search strategies and well-substantiated conclusions that includes lower quality RCTs, clinical cohort studies, and case-controlled studies with nonbiased, selection of study participants and consistent findings. Other evidence, such as high-quality, historical, uncontrolled studies, or well-designed epidemiologic studies with compelling findings, is also included.

Level C (consensus/expert opinion): Consensus viewpoint or expert opinion.

It is the editors' hope that the use of these two evidence based grading scales – SOR and LOE – will assist in guiding clinical evaluation through the use of the best evidence available and will enable our patients to receive up-to-date, relevant care.

TABLE A1.2. Determining LOE

Study quality	Diagnosis	Treatment/prevention/screening	Prognosis
Level 1 – good quality patient-oriented evidence	• Validated clinical decision rule • SR/meta-analysis of high-quality studies • High-quality diagnostic cohort study[a][AU1]	• SR/meta-analysis of RCTs with consistent findings • High-quality individual RTCs[b] • All-or-none study[c]	• SR/meta-analysis of good-quality cohort studies • Prospective cohort study with good follow-up
Level 2 – limited-quality patient-oriented evidence	• Unvalidated clinical decision rule • SR/meta-analysis of lower-quality studies or studies with inconsistent findings • Lower-quality diagnostic cohort study or diagnostic case-control study[c]	• SR/meta-analysis of lower-quality clinical trials or of studies with inconsistent findings • lower-quality clinical trial[b] • Cohort study • Case-control study	• SR/meta-analysis of lower-quality cohort studies or with inconsistent results • Retrospective cohort study or prospective cohort study with poor follow-up • Case-control study • Case series
Level 3 – other evidence	• Consensus guidelines, extrapolations from bench research, usual practice, opinion, disease-oriented evidence (intermediate or physiologic outcomes only), or case series for studies of diagnosis, treatment, prevention, or screening		

Table A1.3. Consistency across studies

Consistent	• Most studies found similar or at least coherent conclusions (coherence means that differences are explainable) • If high-quality and up-to-date systematic reviews or meta-analyses exist, they support the recommendation
Inconsistent	• Considerable variation among study findings or lack of coherence • If high-quality and up-to-date systematic reviews or meta-analyses exist, they do not find consistent evidence in favor of the recommendation

References

1. Centre for Evidence-Based Medicine. Levels of evidence and grades of recommendation. At: http://www.cebm.net/levels_of_evidence.asp. Accessed December 13, 2008.
2. Clarke M, Oxman AD. Cochrane reviewers' handbook 4.2.0. The Cochrane Collaboration, 2003. At: http://www.cochrane.org/resources/handbook/handbook.pdf. Accessed November 13, 2008.
3. Harris RP, Helfand M, Woolf SH, et al. Current methods of the U.S. Preventive Services Task Force: a review of the process. Am J Prev Med 2001; 20(3 suppl):21–35.
4. Siwek J, Gourlay ML, Slawson DC, Shaughnessy AF. How to write an evidence-based clinical review article. Am Fam Physician 2002; 65(2):251–258.
5. Ebell MH, Siwek J, Weiss BD, et.al. Strength of Recommendation Taxonomy (sort): A Patient-Centered Approach to Grading Evidence in the Medical Literature. Am Fam Physician 2004; 69(3):548–556.

Appendix 2

PHYSICAL THERAPY MODALITIES

Summary

Category	Modality	Effect
Cryotherapy	Ice packs	Decreased pain
	Ice massage	Minimized secondary hypoxic changes
	Cold water immersion	Increased muscle contractility
	Vapocoolant sprays	
Thermotherapy	Moist heat	Decreased muscle spasm
	Dry heat	Decreased pain perception
	Whirlpool	Increased blood flow
	Contrast baths	Increased metabolic rate
	Laser	Decreased joint stiffness
	Diathermy	Increased collagen extensibility
	Ultrasound	Increased general relaxation
Electrotherapy	TENS	*Based upon mode of application*
	IFC	Increased or decreased muscle tone
	Galvanic stimulation	Decreased pain
	EMS	Decreased spasm
	Iontophoresis	Increased blood flow
	Electroacutherapy	Deliver topical drugs
	Biofeedback	

THERAPEUTIC MODALITIES

Cryotheraphy

Application
- Ice packs
- Ice massage
- Cold water Immersion
- Vapo-coolant sprays such as ethyl chloride
- Principle mode of action (cold transfer) is conduction

Physiological effects
- Decrease in tissue temperature
- Decreased blood flow
- Decrease in muscle spasms
- Decreased pain perception
- Decreased muscle fatigue and maintains muscular contraction
- Decrease in metabolic rate
- Increase in collagen inelasticity increase in joint stiffness
- Increased capillary permeability

Indications
- Acute soft tissue injuries such as sprains, strains, contusions and muscle spasm.
- Chronic inflammatory such as tendinitis, tenosynovitis, and fasciitis.

Contraindications
- Circulatory disturbances
- Hypersensitivity to cold
- Prolonged application over superficial nerves
- Raynaud's phenomenon
- Ice should never be applied longer than 20–30 min at any one time.
- Caution should be used in applying cryotherapy to individuals on blood thinners

THERMOTHERAPY

Superficial effect

Application
- Moist heat
- Dry heat
- Whirlpool
- Contrast baths
- Laser – both superficial and deep based upon the type of laser utilized
- Mode of action is conduction, convection, radiation, conversion

Physiologic effects
- Depends on the type, intensity, duration and unique tissue response to heat
- Decreased muscle spasm

APPENDIX 2

   Decreased pain perception
   Increased blood flow
   Increased metabolic rate
   Decreased joint stiffness
   Increased collagen extensibility – when used before stretching may increase ROM
   Increased general relaxation
Indications
   Typically subacute injuries used to increase blood flow and promote healing
Contraindications
   Application to decreased or insensate areas
   Application of heat immediately after an injury
   Never apply heat when there is decreased arterial circulation
   Never apply heat directly to the eyes or genitals
   Never heat the abdomen during pregnancy
   Never apply heat to a malignancy
Caution should be used when applying heat to the elderly or infants who cannot report their reactions
   Research shows that prolonged application of heat (heat wrap) is beneficial in reduction of muscle spasm
Modality
   Laser – Is applied to trigger points, acupuncture points, or nerve roots within the focal area.
   Helium-neon, or HeNe – shallow penetration of 2–5 mm
   Gallium arsenide, or GaAs – deep penetration 1–2 cm beneath the skin

Mode of action is radiation

Physiologic effects
   Pain reduction
Indications
   Acute, subacute, and chronic conditions
Contraindications
   Active or suspected carcinoma
   Direct irradiation of the eyes
   Irradiation over the pregnant uterus
   Irradiation of the gonads
   Irradiation of patients with a history of epilepsy
   Irradiation of areas of altered skin sensitivity
   Active epiphyseal regions in children
   Cognitive difficulties or unreliable patients
   Increased sensitivity to light

Deep effect

Modality
Ultrasound
Application
Generation of high frequency sound waves causing molecules in the tissue to vibrate producing heat and mechanical energy

Mode of action is conversion

Physiologic effects
Thermal, nonthermal, or both
Thermal effects
Deep heating 7–8° up to 5 cm below the skin's surface
Nonthermal effects
Stimulates chemical activities in tissue
Alters cell membrane permeability
Two modes – pulsed and continuous
(a) Cavitation – the physical force of the sound waves on dissolved gases within the fluid
Acoustical streaming – the unidirectional movement of fluids along cell membranes
(b) Continuous modes produces both thermal and nonthermal effects
Pulsed modes produces primarily nonthermal effects due to interrupted flow and less total energy
Indications
Post acute soft tissue trauma
Bursitis
Tendonitis
Fasciitis
Contraindications
Acute inflammatory conditions with the continuous mode
Areas with limited vascularity or sensation
Treatment over the ears, eyes, heart, reproductive organs, endocrine glands, central nervous system, or open epiphyses
Treatment must be given with a coupling medium, typically gel or under water which allows treatment on contoured surfaces
Modality
Phonophoresis
Application
Ultrasound with medications
Mode of action is conversion
Physiologic effects
Nonthermal – as with ultrasound
Effects and actions of the applied medication
Typical mode of application is pulsed
Indications
Used as a medication delivery system to sub dural areas
Contraindications
Same as with ultrasound
Sensitivity or allergy to dosing medication
Phonophoresis is generally of lower intensity but longer duration than standard ultrasound therapy
Modality
Diathermy
Short wave (SWD) – high frequency electrical currents converted to heat
Microwave (MWD) – electromagnetic radiation converted to heat

Mode of action is conversion
Physiologic effects
  SWD
    Deep-penetration up to 2 in.
    Increase in temperature to between 109.4°F and 113°F (43 C–45 C)
  MWD
    Superficial-localized heat
    More concentrated than SWD but less penetration than SWD
    Increase temp to 106°F
Indications
Post acute soft tissue trauma
Bursitis
Tendonitis
Fasciitis
Arthritis exacerbation
Contraindications
Use in the presence of metal – implants, surgical fracture fixation hardware, etc
Use over joints with effusion or cavities within fluids
Active malignancy
Patients with pacemakers
Deep X-ray treatment or other ionizing radiation (in the last 6 months) in the area to be treated
Advanced cardiovascular conditions
Active tuberculosis
Avoid irradiation to the abdomen or pelvis during menstruation
Patients should remove contact lenses and jewelry during therapy

Electrotherapy

Application
<u>Electrical Stimulation</u> – using electrodes or probes in contact with the body.
Mode of action is electrical energy that displays magnetic, chemical, mechanical, and thermal effects on tissue
General contraindications
Pacemakers
Pregnancy
Application over:
Eyes or testes
The stellate ganglion
The cardiac area in advanced heart disease
The cranium
Active epiphyseal regions in children – due to premature closure
When muscular contractions are not desired
Nonunited fractures
Areas of active bleeding
Near malignancies

Modality
Transcutaneous electrical nerve stimulation (TENS)
Physiologic effects
Stimulate peripheral nervous system via electrodes attached to the skin producing pain relief via gate theory
Indications
Acute pain control
Neuropathic pain – complex regional pain syndrome, RSD, causalgia
Phantom pain
Post-therapeutic neuralgia
Post surgical pain
Peripheral neuropathy
Musculoskeletal pain
Contraindications
Pacemakers are a relative contraindication- based upon location of TENS application
Modality
Interferential electrical stimulation (IFC)
Physiologic effects
Alternating medium frequency electrical currents with the amplitude modulated at low frequency to produce therapeutic effects
Relief of pain
Reduction of swelling
Indications
Subacute relief of pain
Chronic pain with or without swelling
Spasm
*IFC is not effective in post traumatic pain in the acute phase
Contraindications
Arterial disease – theoretically could produce emboli due to stimulatory effect of IFC
Deep vein thrombosis – in the acute phase could increase inflammation of the phlebitis or dislodge the thrombi
Skin infections due to the risk of spreading
Pregnant uterus
Danger of hemorrhage
Direct stimulation of malignant tumors
Pacemaker
Stimulation over the carotid sinuses – may lead to a decrease in blood pressure
Large open wounds in the area of stimulation due to distortion of the IF field
Modality
Galvanic stimulation – high volt pulsed galvanic stimulation
Physiologic effects
Reduction of swelling
Indications
Acute/subacute edema
Contraindications
DVT – in the acute phase could increase inflammation of the phlebitis or dislodge the thrombi

Skin infections due to the risk of spreading
Pregnant uterus
Danger of hemorrhage
Direct stimulation of malignant tumors
Pacemaker
Modality
Electrical muscle stimulation (EMS) – low voltage current to stimulate motor nerves causing muscular contraction
Physiologic effects
Muscle reeducation
Retarding atrophy
Muscle spasm reduction/elimination
Improvement in localized blood circulation
Increased range of motion.
Indications
Acute/subacute Injury
Post surgery
Contraindications
Same as general E-stim contraindications
Modality
Iontophoresis – the use of an electrical current to deliver medications to a localized area of the body
Physiologic effects
Localized erythema – temporary
Localized itching – temporary
Effect of the medication delivered
Indications
Delivery of medications/substances that need local penetration in order to avoid systemic effects
Areas where oral absorption is variable or contraindicated.
Contraindications
Same as general E-stim contraindications
Modality
Electroacutherapy – use of an electrical current and probes to stimulate acupuncture points
Physiologic effects
Localized erythema – temporary
Local or regional pain relief
Specific to the point stimulated and the resultant effect
Indications
Acute, subacute, and chronic conditions of the musculoskeletal and nervous system
Contraindications
Relative contraindication is pregnancy – must avoid stimulation of points that effect uterine contractility
Relative contraindication during menses – may not be effective during this period.
Assess on a case by case basis

Allergy to metal
Patients on anticoagulant drugs
Patients with a bleeding disorder

Modality
Biofeedback – use of an electrode(s) to register and display muscular activity – used in muscle reeducation/relaxation

Physiologic effects
None through the biofeedback device
Effects are the result of volitional training and reinforcement of repeatable actions.

Indications
Skeletal muscle reeducation, including pelvic floor
Can be used to increase tone or decrease tone depending on instructions and protocol used

Contraindications
Dermatological conditions such as eczema and dermatitis
Allergy to electrode or contact material
Patients who are unable to understand and follow commands
Diminished skin sensation may reduce the full benefit of therapy

Index

A

Acetabular fractures. *See* Legg–Calvé–Perthes disease (LCPD)
Acetabular labral tears
  cause, 323–324
  description, 323
  diagnostic techniques, 324
  plain radiographs, 129
  symptoms, 129
  treatment, 324–325
Acetaminophen, 306
Acute fracture
  description, 96
  diagnosis, 97, 98
  SCFE, 97–98
Adductor strain
  cause, 118
  treatment, 119
Adult hip and pelvis disorders
  anterior pain
    acetabular labral tear, 129
    adductor strain, 118–119
    athletic pubalgia, 131–132
    AVN, femoral head, 128
    femoral neck stress fracture, 125–127
    femoroacetabular impingement, 130
    hip dislocation, 127–128
    iliopsoas/iliopectineal bursitis, 130–131
    iliopsoas strain/hip flexor strain, 121–122
    internal snapping, 132–134
    osteitis pubis, 123–124
    osteoarthritis, 129
    pubic ramus stress fracture, 124–125
    pubic symphysis dysfunction, 122–123
    quadriceps contusion, 120–121
    rectus abdominis strain, 122
    rectus femoris, 119–120
  differential diagnosis, 117
  intermittent hip pain, 115–116
  lateral pain
    external snapping hip, 134–135
    greater trochanteric bursitis, 136
    hip pointer, 135
    Meralgia paresthetica, 137
    TFL syndrome, 135–136
  leg length discrepancy
    measurement, 143
    types, 142–143
  pain causes, 117–118
  posterior pain
    coccygeal injury, 142
    gluteus maximus and medius strain, 139
    hamstring, 137–138
    ischial bursitis, 139
    piriformis syndrome, 141–142

SI joint dysfunction, 140–141
Amputee athlete. *See also* Special populations, hip and pelvis injuries
cycling, 199
running
involved and uninvolved extremity, 195
phases, 196
transtibial and transfemoral amputations, 196–197
skiing
alpine skiers, 198
three-track system, 197–198
water sports, 198–199
Anterior superior iliac spine (ASIS)
anterior inferior iliac spine, 98, 164
patellas position, 30
posterior innominate dysfunction, 141
PSIS, 279
superior pubic shear, 243–244
Apophyseal avulsions
occurence, diagnosis and treatment, 331
radiograph, 320
Apophyseal injuries
avulsion fractures, pelvis, 163–164
diagnosis
five-step rehabilitation program, 166–167
sonography, 166
surgical excision, 167
incidence, 162
ischial tuberosity, 162, 163
pelvic epiphyses, characteristics, 165
physis, 162

Articulatory technique, 252–254, 255
Athletic pubalgia, 131–132
Avascular necrosis (AVN)
femoral head, 128
femoral neck stress fracture, 125
idiopathic, 100
mimicking, 96
risk factors, 160
SCFE child, 159

B

"Big 3" exercises
bird–dog, 227
curl-ups, 224, 227, 228
Bone
description, 172–173
FRACTURE index, 173–175
gradual loss, 173
mass and drugs, 173, 174
Bracing
compression shorts, 266–268
molded thermoplastic protection, 269
vs. taping, 266

C

Childhood and adolescence
apophyseal injuries
avulsion fractures, pelvis, 163–164
diagnosis, 166–167
incidence, 162
ischial tuberosity, 162, 163
pelvic epiphyses, characteristics, 165
physis, 162
DDH (*See* Developmental dysplasia of the hip)
LCPD (*See* Legg–Calvé–Perthes disease)
rightsided knee pain, 149–150

SCFE (*See* Slipped capital femoral epiphysis)
transient synovitis, 156–158
Core muscles
  anatomy
    anterior, 209, 210
    components, 209
    diaphragm and pelvic floor, 214
    erector spinea, 212
    external and internal oblique, 210
    thoracolumbar fascia, 212–213
    tissue arrangement, 209–210
  assessment exercises, 223
  groups
    athletes, 230–231
    gluteus maximus, 229
    hip abductors function, 229–230
    low back pain, 230
  kinetic chain
    anchoring, 215
    coupling, 216
    inherent connection, 214
    instability, 217
    link theory, 215–216
    multifidi and transverse abdominis, 218
    transverse abdominis muscle, 217–218
  musculature
    balance, 218
    endurance, 222–223
    flexors and extensors, torso, 223–224
    hamstrings test, 220
    lumbar spine, 218–219
    narrow lunge and deep squat test, 222
    neutral spine, 219
    prone and lateral bridge, 223, 224
    rotational and hurdle step test, 221
    screening examinations, 219
    torso extension test, 225
  strengthening and endurance, 225–229
Core strengthening. *See also* Core muscles
  exercise programs
    "Big 3" exercises, 228
    diaphragm breathing, 228
    goal, 225
    plyometrics, 229
    stages, 227
    training levels, 226
  low-back, left buttock and lateral thigh pain, 207–208
  muscle groups, 229–231
Corticosteroid
  exogenous, 279
  hip osteoarthritis, 308–309
  injection
    contraindications, 278
    hyperglycemia, 279
    sports injuries, 273
  intra-articular, 308
  oral, 124
  preparation, 275–276
Craig's test, 32–33

D

Developmental dysplasia of the hip (DDH)
  changes, radiographic, 100–101
  diagnosis
    maneuvers, 151–152
    Pavlik harness, 152
    ultrasound, 151
  genetic and mechanical risk factors, 150
  radiographs, 151
  right hip pain, 101

E

Ely's test, 27, 28, 116
External snapping hip
  iliotibial band, 134
  physical therapy, 135

F

FABER test, 21–22, 24
FAI. *See* Femoroacetabular impingement
Femoral neck stress fracture
  compression and displaced, 126
  management, 127
  physical exam, 125–126
  risk factors, 125
Femoroacetabular impingement (FAI)
  cause and recognition, 130
  chronic impaction, 103–104
  hip pain and synovial herniationpit, 106
  left hip pain and cam-type, 102, 103
  mechanical impaction, 101–102
  osacetabulum and left hip pain, 105
  pincer type, 102–105
  sign, 102
FRACTURE index
  bone mineral density (BMD), 175
  osteoporosis, 175
  questions and scoring, 174–175
Fulcrum test, 33
Functional and kinetic chain evaluation
  anatomic concepts and neuromuscular control
    gamma loop mechanism, 42
    MAPs, 42
    neuromuscular imbalance, 42–43
  assess posture, 59
  athletes, 41–42
  biomechanics, hip joint
    abdominal musculature *vs.* spine erector muscles, 45–46
    atraumatic instability, 44
    EMG, 47
    flexion and extension, 43
    force closure, 45, 46
    gait cycle, 47–49
    HLR movement impairment, 43–44
    joint dysfunction model, 45
    lumbopelvic-coupled movement, 44
    muscle imbalance patterns, 51
    sacroiliac joint motion, 46
    static stabilizers, 44
    stressors, muscle imbalance, 50
    suboptimal posture model, 49
    thoracolumbar fascia, 46–47
    tonic muscles, 49–51
  description, 39
  diagnostic imaging, 60
  dysfunctions
    acetabulum, 56
    adductor group strains, 51
    femoroacetabular impingement and tears, 56–57
    hamstring strains, 53–54
    iliopsoas muscle, 52, 53
    labrum, 56
    MR arthrography (MRA), 58
    osteitis pubis, 54

pain, 52–54
plain radiographs and computed tomography (CT), 57
snapping hip syndrome, 57–58
soccer players, 51–52
symptoms and stress fractures, 55
osteoarthritis
  knee, 40–41
  risk, 41
physical examination, 38–39, 59
right hip and low back pain
  physical examination, 38–39
  spasm, 38
  waxing and waning discomfort, 37–38
sports injuries, 40
standing flexion test, 38
treatment
  exercise prescription, 61
  initial, 60

G

Gaenslen sign, 31–32
Gait assessment
  age and differences
    adults, 81–82
    ankle power output, 82
  case assessment and treatment, 82–84
  cycle, 76
  determinants, 80–81
  elements
    kinematics, 75–78
    kinetics, 79–80
    muscles, 79
    walking and running, 74–75
  male and female, 82
  presentation, case
    anatomic plane classification, 73
    illness, 71–72
    physical examination, 72
    testing, 74
Geriatric athletes
  balance, 179
  bone, physiological changes
    description, 172–173
    FRACTURE index, 174–175
    gradual loss, 173
    mass and drugs, 174
  cartilage, ligaments and tendons, 178–179
  exercise after surgery
    consensus recommendations, 183–184
    hip fractures, 181–182
    revision, 183
    THA, 182
  exercises, injury prevention
    flexibility and balance, 181
    weight-bearing, 179–181
  intertrochanteric hip fracture, 171–172
  low-trauma hip fracture, 184–185
  muscle
    sarcopenia, 178
    strength, 177
  osteoporosis evaluation, 175–177
Gillet test, 31, 141
Gilmore's groin
  description, 325–326
  diagnosis and treatment, 326
Greater trochanteric bursitis, 136
Groin pull. *See* Adductor strain

H

Hamstring strain
  biceps femoris, 137–138
  diagnoses and treatment, 138
  occurence, 53
Heterotopic ossification (HO)
  description, 109
  right hip, 189
  SCI population, 202
  surgical resection, 203
High velocity low amplitude techniques
  right posterior innominate, 250–251
  sacral base posterior, 251–252
  unilateral sacral shear, superior inominate shear, 248–250
Hip abductors
  function, 229
  gluteus medius, 136
  left hip pain and calcific tendinopathy, 108
  muscle testing, 208
  Trendelenburg's sign, 20–21
Hip and pelvis injury
  bony joint, 11–12
  case report presentation
    analysis, 1–2
    assessment, 5–6, 34
    complaint, 1, 9–10
    follow-up, 34
    plan, 5–6, 34
    results, 10–11
  causes, 2, 13
  description, 2, 11
  diagnosis, 2, 12
  gender, 6
  muscular anatomy, 12
  patients age
    Legg–Calvé–Perthes disease, 3
    school-aged *vs.* adolescent, 3–4
  skeletal development, 2–3
  physical examinations
    Craig's test, 32–33
    Ely's test, 27, 28
    FABER test, 21–22, 24
    fulcrum test, 33
    Gaenslen sign, 31–32
    Gillet test, 31
    lateral pelvic compression test, 33
    leg length assessment, 28–29
    log roll test, 25–26
    neurologic testing, 19–20
    Ober's test, 22–23, 25
    palpation, 17–18
    passive abduction and resisted adduction, 33
    piriformis/FAIR test, 24
    prone knee flexion test, 31
    range of motion, 14–17
    scour test/quadrant test, 33
    standing flexion test, 31
    Stinchfield test, 26–27
    straight leg raise test, 27–28
    supine to sit test/long sitting test, 31, 32
    Thomas test, 23–24, 26
    Trendelenburg's sign, 20–23
    Weber–Barstow maneuver, 29–30
  radiating symptoms, 13–14
  sport activity
    ballet dancers, 4
    hip osteoarthritis, 5
    runners and soccer players *vs.* athletes, 4
Hip dislocations
  AVN, 321
  posterior, 127, 320–321
  prompt reduction, 127–128
Hip fractures, 321

Hip pointer, 135
Hip spica technique, 267–268
HO. *See* Heterotopic ossification
Hydroxyapatite deposition disease (HADD), 107–108

I

Iliopsoas
  mechanisms, 130
  pain and symptoms, 130–131
Imaging
  arthrography, magnetic resonance, 91
  magnetic resonance, 90–91
  pelvis normal AP view, 89
  radiography, 88–90
  radiologic diagnosis, athletes
    articular pathology, 98–108
    muscle, 109–111
    osseous, 92–98
    snapping tendons, 108–109
  ultrasound (US) and computed tomography (CT), 90
Inferior lateral angles (ILAs)
  PSISs and, 252
  sacral sulci, 246
  treatment, 248–249
Internal snapping hip
  extra and intra-articular, 132–133
  plain radiographs, 133
  treatment, 133–134
Intra-articular injectable therapy, 308, 309
Ischial bursitis, 139

J

Jansen's test/Patrick's test. *See* FABER test
Joint injections
  hip, 288–289
  pubic symphysis, 289–290
  sacrococcygeal, 290–291
  sacroiliac, 287–288

K

Kinesiotape
  action mechanism theory, 265
  application, 265
  functions, 266
  muscle injuries, 265
Kinetic chain theory. *See* Link theory

L

Labral tears, 104–106
Lateral femoral cutaneous nerve, 291–292
Lateral pelvic compression test, 33
Legg–Calvé–Perthes disease (LCPD)
  children and adolescents, 3
  description, 152–153
  diagnosis
    Catterall and Herring classification, 154
    hip abduction and internal rotation, 153–154
    home-based physiotherapy program, 156
    left hip radiograph, 155
    limp, 153
    radiographs, 154
    surgical intervention, 154, 156
    unilateral hip involvement, 153
Leg length assessment, 28–29
Link theory
  core strength, 208–209
  definition, 216
  musculoskeletal motion, 215
Log roll test, 25–26

M

Manual medicine
  activating forces, 240
  differential diagnosis, 237–238
  functional anatomy, 236–238
  manipulations, 239
  right hip pain, 233–234
  techniques
    articulatory, 252–254
    counterstrain, 241–242
    high velocity low amplitude, 248–252
    muscle energy, 242–248
    stretching, 254–259
    table assisted, 252
  treatment goal, 240
Meralgia paresthetica, 137
Muscle activation patterns (MAPs), 42–43
Muscle energy techniques
  abduction, restricted, 243–244
  adduction, restricted, 244
  anteriorly rotated inominate/inferior pubic shear, 242–243
  extension and flexion, restricted, 245
  external rotation, restriction, 245
  internal rotation, restricted, 246
  posterior rotated inominate/superior pubic shear, 243
  sacral base anterior, 246–248
  sacral torsion, same axis, 248
  SI joint dysfunction/pubic shear, 243

N

Nerve compression, 327–329
Neurologic testing, 19–20
Non-pharmacologic therapy
  assistive devices, 305
  exercise
    adherence and risk, 304–305
    benefits, 303
    type, 303–304
  hydrotherapy, 304
  patient education and self management programs, 305
  weight loss, 305–306
Nonsteroidal anti-inflammatory drugs (NSAIDs)
  acetaminophen, 306
  acute muscle injury, 120
  pain control, 123
  pelvis radiograph, 155
  prescription, 307
  vs. tramadol, 308
  use, 306–307
Nonsurgical interventions
  anatomy, 279–280
  anesthetic/corticosteroid injection, 292–293
  contraindications, 278
  diagnostic injections
    blocks, 274–275
    image guidance and fluoroscopy, 274
  documentation, 280
  fundamentals, injection technique, 280–282
  injection therapies, 273
  joint injections
    hip, 288–289
    pubic symphysis, 289–290
    sacrococcygeal, 290–291
    sacroiliac, 287–288
  nerve blocks, 291–292
  pharmacological agents

anesthetics, 276–277
corticosteroid, 275–276
hyaluronic acid, 276
proliferants, 277
potential complications
  exogenous corticosteroids, 279
  injection site preparation, 278
  soft tissue atrophy and skin depigmentation, 278–279
  systemic effects, 279
right hip and groin pain
  differential diagnosis and imaging, 272–273
  mild relief, 271–272
  physical examination, 272
safety considerations, 277–278
soft tissue injections
  greater trochanteric bursa, 282–283
  hamstring origin, 284–285
  hip adductor origin, 286–287
  iliopsoas bursa, 285–286
  ischial bursa, 284
therapeutic injections, 275

O

Ober's test, 22–23, 25
Obturator and femoral nerves, 328–329
Osteitis pubis
  cause, treatment and diagnosis, 326
  etiologic factors, 122
  physical examination, 122–123
  therapy program, 124
Osteoarthritis
  acupuncture, 311
  avocado/soybean unsaponifiables (ASU), 311
  bilateral hip, 100
  depression and fibromyalgia, 297–298
  diacerein, 312
  diagnosis
    joint space width (JSW), 300–302
    physical symptoms, 299–300
  epidemiology, 298–299
  glucosamine and chondroitin, 310–311
  joint space narrowing, 99
  morphology, 100
  nonoperative management
    non-pharmacologic therapy, 303–306
    pharmacologic therapy, 306–310
  right hip, 298
  risk factors, 299
  surgery, 312
Osteoporosis
  bone mineral density (BMD) testing, 177
  definition, 176
  falling, risk factors, 175
  nonpharmacologic interventions, 176
  pharmacological treatments, 177

P

Palpation, 17–18
Passive abduction and resisted adduction, 33
Perthes disease.
  See Legg–Calvé–Perthes disease (LCPD)

Pharmacologic therapy
  acetaminophen, 306
  corticosteroids
    intra-articular, 308–309
    total hip arthroplasty (THA), 309
  COX-2 inhibitors, 307
  intra-articular injectable, 308
  NSAIDs
    prescription, 307
    use, 306–307
  opioids, 307–308
  tramadol, 308
  viscosupplementation
    hip osteoarthritis, 310
    hyaluronan (HA), 309–310
Piriformis/FAIR test, 24
Piriformis syndrome
  muscle, 141, 327, 330
  surgery, 330
  tender points treatment, 242
  treatment, 141–142
Plyometrics, 229
Posterior superior iliac spine (PSIS)
  ILAs, 251–252
  piriformis muscle, 237
  sacral compression medial, 140
Prone knee flexion test, 31
PSIS. *See* Posterior superior iliac spine
Psoas, 241–242
Pubic ramus stress fractures
  periosteal reaction, 124
  treatment, 125
Pubic symphysis dysfunction
  pain control, 123
  pregnancy, 122

Q

Quadriceps contusion
  active knee flexion, 121
  myositis ossificans, 120–121

R

Radiologic diagnosis, athletes
  articular pathology
    developmental dysplasia, 100–101
    FAI, 101–104
    hip ligaments, 106–107
    labral tears, 104–106
    osteoarthritis, 99–100
    tendons, 107–108
  muscle, 109–111
  osseous, fracture
    acute, 96–98
    stress, 92–96
  snapping tendons, 108–109
Range of motion testing, 14–17
Rectus femoris strain/quadriceps strain
  hematoma, 120
  origins, 119
  pain, 119–120
Right posterior innominate, 252, 254

S

Sacroiliac (SI) joint dysfunction
  articulation, 140
  multiple dysfunctions, 141
  treatment, 140–141
Sarcopenia, 178
SCFE. *See* Slipped capital femoral epiphysis
Scour test/quadrant test, 33
Slipped capital femoral epiphysis (SCFE)
  classification, 159
  diagnosis
    anteroposterior (AP) radiography, 160
    pain, 159–160
    prophylactic fixation, 161

surgical treatment, 160–161
weight-bearing, 162
pre-adolescent/adolescent athlete, 97
risk factors, 330
site, 158
treatment, 320–321
Snapping hip syndrome
division, 325–326
external, 134–135
internal, 132–134
treatment, 327
Snapping tendon, 108
Soft tissue injections
greater trochanteric bursa, 282–283
hamstring origin, 284–285
hip adductor origin, 286–287
iliopsoas bursa, 285–286
ischial bursa, 284
Special populations, hip and pelvis injuries
amputee athlete
adaptive devices, 194
computerized knee, 197
cycling, 199
hyperextension, 195
lower-extremity, 195
running, 195–197
skiing, 197–198
water sports, 198–199
athletes, categorization, 190–193
cerebral palsy (CP)
ambulatory to non-ambulatory athletes ratio, 200
patellofemoral dysfunction, 200–201
spasticity, 200, 201
disabled athletics, 193–194
exercise benefits, 188
heterotopic ossification, 189
SCI, 187–188
unique body region, soft tissue injury, 191
wheelchair athlete
basketball athletes, 202
HO, 202–203
paraplegia, 201
surgical resection, 203
Spinal cord injury (SCI)
heterotopic ossification, 188, 202
wheelchair athletics, 201
Sports/hockey hernia, 325
Sportsman's hernia, 108–109
Standing flexion test, 31, 38
Stinchfield test, 26–27
Straight leg raise test, 27–28
Stress fractures
military recruits and athletes, 321–322
presentations, 94–96
radiographs, 93–94
subchondral bone, 96
treatment
algorithm, 322–323
magnetic resonance imaging and percutaneous fixation, 323
Stretching techniques
doctor-assisted resisted piriformis, 259, 260
gluteal, 256, 259
groin, 259, 260
hamstrings, 254
iliopsoas, 254–255, 257
iliotibial band, 255–256, 258
piriformis, 257, 260
quadriceps femoris, 258
Supine to sit test/long sitting test, 31, 32

Surgical interventions
  acetabular labral tears, 323–325
  adolescents
    apophyseal avulsions, 331
    SCFE, 330–331
  dislocations, hip, 320–321
  Gilmore's groin, 325–326
  hip fractures, 321
  muscle strain/avulsion
    description, 318
    grades, 319
    occurence, 319–320
    provocative testing, 318–319
  nerve compression, 327
  osteitis pubis, 326
  right-side groin pain, 317–318
  sciatic/piriformis/hamstring syndromes, 327, 330
  snapping hip syndrome, 326–327
  sports/hockey hernia, 325
  stress fractures, 321–323
  tumor, 331–332

T

Table assisted technique, 252
Taping
  vs. bracing, 266
  drawbacks, 264
  indications and efficacy, 264
  right lateral hip pain, 263
  tape types
    kinesiotex (See Kinesiotape)
    zonus, 264
  techniques, 266
Tendon
  calcific tendonitis, 107–108
  cartilage, ligaments and, 178–179
  degeneration/tear, 108
  iliopsoas, 132–133
  rupture risk, 279
  snapping, 108–111
Tensor fascia lata (TFL), 135–136
THA. See Total hip arthroplasties
Thomas test, 23–24, 26
Total hip arthroplasties (THA)
  consensus recommendations, 183
  end-stage osteoarthritis, 181, 182
  hip fractures, 182
Tramadol, 308
Transient synovitis
  diagnosis
    clinical prediction algorithm, 157–158
    laboratory and radiographic studies, 157
  pain, 156–157
  recurrence, 158
  septic arthritis, 157, 158
  synovium, histological examination, 156
Trendelenburg's sign
  compensated, 22
  defined, 20
  diagnoses, 21
  positive, 23
Tumor, 331–332

W

Weber–Barstow maneuver, 29–30
Wheelchair athlete
  basketball, 202
  HO, 202–203
  paraplegia, 201
  surgical resection, 203